The

Mother's Guide to Sex

The Mother's Guide to Sex

ENJOYING YOUR SEXUALITY THROUGH

ALL STAGES OF MOTHERHOOD

ANNE SEMANS *and* **CATHY WINKS**

THREE RIVERS PRESS • NEW YORK

Published by Three Rivers Press, New York, New York.
Member of the Crown Publishing Group.

Random House, Inc. New York, Toronto, London, Sydney, Auckland
www.randomhouse.com

THREE RIVERS PRESS is a registered trademark and the
Three Rivers Press colophon is a trademark of Random House, Inc.

Printed in the United States of America

Design by Jo Anne Metsch

Library of Congress Cataloging-in-Publication Data
Semans, Anne.
The mother's guide to sex: enjoying your sexuality through all stages of motherhood/
Anne Semans and Cathy Winks. — 1st ed.
1. Sex instruction for women.   2. Mothers — Sexual behavior.   3. Pregnant
women — Sexual behavior.   4. Parenting.   I. Winks, Cathy.   II. Title.
HQ46 .S46 2001
306.874'3 — dc21
00-060735

ISBN 0-8129-3274-9

10 9 8 7 6 5 4 3 2 1

First Edition

For our mothers,

Diane Semans and Pat Winks—

if you hadn't had sex,

we never could have written this book.

ACKNOWLEDGMENTS

Heartfelt thanks to the hundreds of women who filled out our survey about mother-hood and sex—you were our inspiration—and to our on-line pals who posted the survey: Krissy Cababa of GoodVibes.com, Heather Corinna of ScarletLetters.com, Jane Duvall of JanesGuide.com, Christopher Filkins of SaferSex.org, Wyyrd of HootIsland.com, and most especially, Bee Lavender of HipMama.com. Our appreci-ation and admiration go to the courageous, outspoken women who participated in the Sex and Parenting panel featured in SexTV's "Sexy Mamas" documentary: Helen Behar, Susie Bright, Ariel Gore, and Rachel Pepper—and to Michelle Melles for pro-ducing the show.

We are very grateful to our interview subjects, who were so generous with their time and expertise: Helen Behar, Joani Blank, Stephanie Brill, Colette Choate, Meg Hickley, Lisa Keller, M.D., Ann Langely, Harriet Lerner, Pat Love, Andrea O'Reilly, and Maryl Walling-Millard. Thanks to Robin Brooks and Staci Haines for their refer-rals. We're greatly indebted to Erica Breneman, M.D., for reviewing the pregnancy chapter, and to Cheri Van Hoover, C.N.M., for her prompt and thoughtful answers to a wide variety of medical questions. Needless to say, any factual errors that remain are our own.

Much love and thanks to Becky Abbott, who first suggested we write a sex book for mothers. We appreciate the work of our agent, Amy Rennert; our editor, Betsy Rapoport; and Betsy's assistant, Stephanie Higgs. Special thanks to two of the most sex-positive parents we know: Michael Castleman, for his unfailing kindness and encouragement, and Susie Bright for being an inspiration and mentor for many years. Anne is eternally grateful to all Roxanne's wonderful baby-sitters: Trish, Caroline, Christine, Cathy, Becky, Diane, Bill, Doug, and Sandie, but especially to her sister and unofficial coparent, Sheila Semans, for selflessly logging in hours of adventures, meals, and bathtimes. Most of all, Anne thanks Roxanne for being the sun that for-ever shines. Cathy thanks her coworkers at The Sperm Bank of California, Jeffrey Abbott, and Becky, for providing an abundance of practical and moral support dur-ing the writing of this book.

CONTENTS

INTRODUCTION

MOMS HAVE SEX? WHO KNEW!

As soon as we started spreading the word about our idea for this book, we knew we were on to something. Parents instantly responded with curiosity, enthusiasm, and almost desperate nods of approval, while folks without kids looked politely puzzled. And who could blame them? Although volumes have been written about motherhood and sex, the two subjects lie on parallel tracks that rarely intersect. Parenting books never explore how a mother can expect her sex life to be transformed by the demands of child rearing. Sex and relationship books for parents suggest tips for "keeping the flame alive" that depend on creating the illusion that you don't *have* kids. And neither ever addresses how honoring your own sexuality through all the phases of your life sets a powerful example that enables your children to grow into responsible, sexually fulfilled adults.

The Mother's Guide to Sex reaches out to women who want to integrate the joys of a satisfying sex life with the joys of motherhood. We offer tips, anecdotes, and practical information about sex and parenting, supported by advice from medical experts, sex experts, and the most valuable experts of all—other mothers.

MOTHERS FIRST

While we like to think that all parents can glean useful information and perspective from this book, it is written first and foremost for mothers. We are unabashed in asserting that mothers need and deserve a book of their own—their sex lives have been invisible for far too long. Women simply aren't raised with a sense of entitlement to sexual expression, and mothers face the double bind of social attitudes that deem maternity and sexuality mutually exclusive. Most mothers can testify that the desire for a fulfilling sex life didn't disappear when they had children; it simply got buried under an avalanche of conflicting demands on their time and attention. A woman's sex life undergoes significant changes from the moment she decides to have a child, and she has to navigate these changes with no more than the occasional tidbit of information from a kindly nurse or relevant anecdote from a straight-shooting friend. The legions of mothers who visit sex-related discussion boards on parenting Web sites— swapping tips on everything from waning desire to remaining kinky—reveal a profound hunger for an explicit discussion of sexual issues.

Ask a mom about her sex life and you'll get responses ranging from "Sex? What's that?" to "It's better than ever, but it took a lot of work." If you're partnered, you're probably not surprised by the statistic that parents living with children spend only about twenty minutes each week being intimate with each other. If you're single, perhaps you wonder how to be fully present for your kids without neglecting your own desires. You may have picked up this book because a sexual drought is making you long for "the good old days," or you may be curious to explore how your newfound maternal power and passion can enhance your sex life. Either way, we hope you'll find much in these pages that challenges your assumptions and fuels your desires.

THE MOMS SPEAK

We wanted our discussion of mothers' sexuality to reflect the concerns and experiences of a full spectrum of moms—married, single, heterosexual, lesbian, adoptive, and biological—so we posted a survey in several places on-line, including *Hip Mama*'s Web site. Imagine our delight when over seven hundred impassioned responses poured in. We heard from women whose experiences ran the gamut of maternal sexuality, from sexually confident fertility goddesses who were reveling in a sexual rebirth to mothers stymied by the practical and cultural restrictions on their sexuality. Their poignant and often humorous quotes appear throughout this book, and their comments guided our writing.

We owe a debt of gratitude to the moms who shared their thoughts—not just because they sacrificed some of their precious free time to contribute to our book—but because their stories reveal how every aspect of becoming and being a mother has sexual repercussions: from the stresses of trying to conceive to the hormonal shifts of pregnancy and postpartum to the challenges of prioritizing personal pleasure with children on the scene. It's our goal to take as comprehensive an approach as possible in affirming a mother's identity as a sexual being. Throughout this book, we refer to your sexual "partners": a neutral term we use deliberately, since we believe that exploring your sexuality with a long-term spouse or a short-term fling is equally valid.

USING THIS BOOK

Whether you're pregnant and wondering which sexual activities are safe, the mother of a toddler curious about why your sex drive flew the coop, or the mother of a teenager in need of sex education, you'll find help here. We understand if you'll want to make a beeline for the chapters specific to your own stage of motherhood, but we hope you'll also peruse the entire book, as it encompasses a philosophy and range of material that can't be contained in a single discussion of postpartum sex or the physical changes of puberty. We've organized the material into the following four areas:

Part One: Building Blocks of Sexuality

Core components define a woman's relationship to her own sexuality, whether she is young or old, single or partnered, a mother or childless. In this section, we discuss the basic building blocks of a satisfying sex life—sexual self-image, self-esteem, masturbation, desire, and communication—and suggest ways to integrate each into your changing life.

Part Two: The ABCs of Becoming a Mom

Certain sexual concerns are specific to the time period during which a mother is planning to have a child, is pregnant, or has just given birth. Few times in a woman's sex life are as hemmed in by proscriptions, some medically justified and others not. In this section, we cover the basics of conception, pregnancy, and postpartum.

Part Three: Reinventing Sex as a Parent

Every mother is faced with a staggering array of obstacles to her love and sex life. This section offers practical advice on how to make sex a priority, how to share the responsibility for a fulfilling sex life with a partner, how to manage a sex life when you're single, and how to expand your definition—and experience—of sex.

Part Four: Raising Sexually Healthy Children

If we want to create a world in which a woman's right to be both a maternal figure and a sexual figure is assumed and celebrated, we need to raise a generation of sexually literate, responsible adults. We discuss the steps that parents can take to model good attitudes and to provide appropriate sex information to their children.

In order to provide accurate medical information, we interviewed a host of professionals—from midwives to doctors to psychologists—and their advice appears throughout the text. However, we are not licensed medical practitioners, and we strongly advise you to consult your health-care provider if you have a pressing medical concern or need a second opinion. We know how difficult it can be to articulate your sex questions to a medical expert, so we've included a chapter on doing just that.

WHO WE ARE

We're lifelong friends and colleagues motivated by the philosophy that everyone is entitled to a happy, healthy sex life. Together we've written two nonfiction sex guides that offer up-to-date information and practical advice on how to enjoy safe and satisfying sexual explorations. Our first book, *The New Good Vibrations Guide to Sex*, was born out of our decade-long careers as vibrator saleswomen at San Francisco's women-owned erotic emporium, Good Vibrations. Our second book, *The Woman's Guide to Sex on the Web*, was inspired by our appreciation of the Internet's contribution to women's sexual empowerment and self-expression. Both endeavors have given us a provocative glimpse into the bedrooms of ordinary women and men of all ages and backgrounds.

In our lives and in our work, we're dedicated to furthering women's sexual emancipation. Anne writes the "Sex and Parenting" column for the popular on-line magazine *Hip Mama* and enjoys firsthand experience as the currently single mother of a four-year-old. Having been raised in a large Catholic family where any sexual expression was as forbidden as Eve's juicy apple, Anne longs for a day when parents can experience, model, and teach healthy sexuality to their children without inviting criticism or shame. Cathy, who's not a mother, currently works at The Sperm Bank of California, providing information and support to women who are building alternative families. After years of writing and talking about sex to strangers, as well as years in a long-term relationship, she's learned that it's a lot easier to communicate about sex from a soapbox than up close and personal — but that both are well worth the effort.

AS *YOU* PLEASE

We realize that advice books, particularly parenting books, can make you feel like you're back in school, struggling to keep up with homework assignments — after you've finished absorbing details relevant to one developmental stage, you take a breather, and then it's on to the next stage. If you, or your child, lag behind, you can start to feel like a screwup, or that you're missing out on some grand opportunities. The last thing we want is for readers of *The Mother's Guide to Sex* to feel inadequate as a result of our advice or other mothers' experiences. We offer tools, information, and a lot of encouragement to explore your maternal sexuality, but please honor your own experience and explore at your own pace.

Most of all, we want to send you on your way with our thanks and praise. It takes courage and determination to challenge the cultural conditioning that mothers should practice self-sacrifice rather than pursue their true sexual desires. We hope this book gives you the inspiration and the means to pursue a lifetime filled with sexual pleasure.

ANNE SEMANS
CATHY WINKS
April 2001

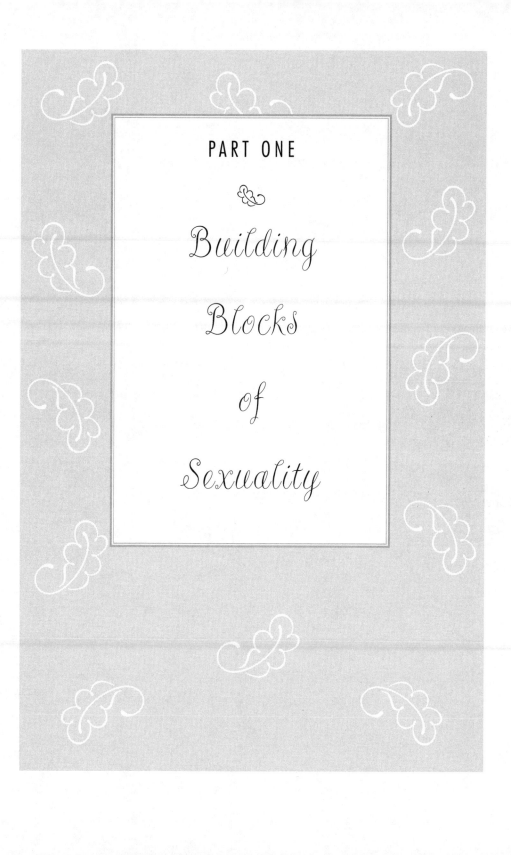

PART ONE

Building

Blocks

of

Sexuality

SEXUAL SELF-IMAGE

EXY moms." Let's admit it, these two words don't exactly conjure up the same wealth of images as, say, "voluptuous vixens" or "smokin' hotties." Sure, you may have qualified as one of the latter before becoming a parent, but your new identity as "somebody's mom" trumps every identity you've had before. Why are moms desexualized? The reasons are complex—a cultural view of sex as dirty, a religious tradition that celebrates chaste motherhood, and a socioeconomic system that demands maternal self-sacrifice. The irony that sex is what makes many women mothers in the first place probably isn't lost on you.

> The looks I get if I walk into a store like Victoria's Secret are hysterical! I feel like asking people if they know how my son got here in the first place. I'm no less a sexual being now then I was before my child. In fact, I feel like more of a sexual being now that I'm a mom. I mean, I created a whole other person in my body with the help of the person that I love! How much more sexual can you get?

This mother speaks for countless others—both biological and nonbiological—who have found that becoming parents inspires them with a new sexual confidence and vitality. A renewed respect for their bodies, an increased capacity for love, a powerful connection to humanity: These are the reasons women cite most often for the improved self-image that unites the best of their maternal and sexual selves.

Yet few mothers arrive at sexual independence without a bumpy ride en route. You, like many others, may have lost sight of your sexual self as a result of physical changes, logistical challenges, hormonal fluctuations, or negative messages from partners, friends, and strangers. We don't intend to suggest that if motherhood prompts a sabbatical from sex, you've somehow failed to "be all you can be." Everyone goes through natural cycles of sexual activity. But we are arguing that our *identity* as sexual beings is nonnegotiable, and that no one is ever justified in making you feel that motherhood and sexuality are mutually exclusive. Sexuality is an important source of your creativity; it infuses you with love, energy, and a sense of well-being; it improves all your relationships; and it makes you more human to your own children. Whether you're carving a new notch in the bedpost every night or you can't remember the last time you got a little action, your erotic nature is your undeniable birthright.

Much "expert" advice has been proffered on good mothering — from nutrition to schooling to family bonding — but experts tend to remain silent on the subject of sexuality, serving only to confirm our suspicions that good moms don't have sex. Knowledge is power, and the more you know about the cultural forces conspiring to drive a wedge between maternity and sexuality, the better equipped you'll be to kick them to the curb. In this chapter, we provide a context for today's challenges by looking back at cultures where mothers' sexuality was revered and at those where it was reviled. And we hear from contemporary moms who struggle and succeed in integrating their maternal and sexual identities.

SEXY MOMS OF OLD

Goddess Worship

Any mother embarrassed by or afraid of her sexual nature need only look to the myths of ancient cultures for reassurance that her sexuality is not just natural, it is positively divine. Before humankind had any idea of men's role in procreation, women's ability to reproduce was viewed as magical, and the world itself was envisioned as the creation of a Great Mother. Early agrarian civilizations linked female reproduction to the earth's fertility. Even after the connection between semen and pregnancy became clear, goddess worship continued to flourish. The Great Mother was joined by a male consort, often a young god whose life cycle paralleled the annual seasonal cycle; he died when the crops died and was resurrected through sexual reunion with the goddess, thereby making the land fertile again.

The Venus figurines

Among the oldest examples of ancient civilizations' reverence for female fertility are the Venus figurines (circa 20,000 B.C.), statuettes of women with exaggerated stomachs, butts, breasts, thighs, and clearly delineated vulvas. Historians debate whether they are fertility symbols, representations of the Great Mother, or Paleolithic porn, but our favorite theory posits them as self-portraits carved by pregnant women, which would explain the enlarged breasts and belly and relative insignificance of the feet or limbs.[1] In other words, maybe these figurines are the Stone Age equivalent of a proud mom-to-be's snapshot!

Inanna

The Sumerian civilization of Mesopotamia was the first to produce written texts (circa 2300 B.C.), many of which hymn the praises of a supreme sexy mama. Inanna, the Queen of Heaven (also known by the name Ishtar), was goddess of love, procreation, and fertility. Ancient hymns describe how the young Inanna revels in her sexuality: "rejoicing at her wondrous vulva, the young woman applauded herself." The sacred marriage between Inanna and her lover and consort, the shepherd Dumuzi, is celebrated in explicit, erotic verse.

> He shaped my loins with his fair hands,
> The shepherd Dumuzi filled my lap with cream and milk,
> He stroked my pubic hair,
> He watered my womb,
> He laid his hand on my holy vulva.
> He caressed me on the bed.[2]

Inanna's priestesses re-created this sacred marriage bed with the reigning king every new year, thereby revesting the king's power and ensuring fertility in the land and its people. Children born of these couplings were considered semidivine. Would that Sumerian sexual attitudes had survived into the modern day: Sexual intercourse and prostitution were considered sacred acts, masturbation was believed to enhance potency, and anal intercourse was practiced by high priestesses as a means of contraception.

Isis

Isis, the most beloved of Egyptian goddesses, was worshiped in ancient Egypt and throughout the Hellenistic world. Although pharaohs themselves were considered divine, their power ultimately issued from Isis, a powerful Mother Goddess, who is often depicted with a pharaoh suckling at her breast. One of the best-known stories of Isis tells of her marriage to her beloved consort and twin brother, Osiris. The two engage in divine incest while still in their mother's womb (pharaonic succession was based on marriage between brothers and sisters). They fall hopelessly in love, marry, and rule over a great civilization until their jealous brother Seth murders Osiris. Isis seeks far and wide for her husband. In some versions of the story, his body has been torn into many pieces, and she is able to find every piece except his penis. Undeterred, she fashions a penis from clay and impregnates herself before restoring Osiris to life. The son she conceives is Horus, whose wife, Hathor, the cow-goddess, is known as "mistress of the vulva," ruling fertility, conception, and childbirth.

HELLO MADONNA, GOODBYE GODDESS

While it's a joy to excavate images and stories of powerful and sexy goddess-moms whose fertility and sexual assertiveness were essential to the survival of their people, we all know that's not the tradition we inherited! The two dominant influences on Western culture are patriarchal Greek civilization and patriarchal biblical civilization. That's a lot of patriarchy . . . which means we haven't heard much about sexy matriarchs for the past two thousand years.

The Old Testament

The first woman in the Bible doesn't even make an appearance — that would be Lilith, Adam's uppity first wife. According to Jewish folklore, Lilith was banished from Eden when she refused to lie beneath her husband in the missionary position. Instead, she preferred sex with demons (who must have let her get on top) and went on to give birth to hundreds of demon children. These demon spawn — the succubi — were feared by pious Christians up through the Middle Ages and were blamed for infertility, miscarriage, and wet dreams.

Although the sexuality of untamed female outlaws such as Lilith is depicted as dangerous and manipulative, the Old Testament contains plenty of positive portrayals of powerful mothers who do have sex. The Hebrew Bible may present procreative sex as the only acceptable form of sexual expression, but it is also seen as a pleasurable and blessed duty. Under Jewish law, marital sex is a *mitzvah*, a good deed, in and of itself.

Greeks

Early Christianity was as much influenced by Greek philosophy as by Judaism. Greek philosophy was one source of the Church's dualistic view of soul and body and, by extension, of men and women. In the Greek worldview, men, culture, and the soul line up on one side; women, nature, and the body on the other. Classical Greeks believed that it was natural to struggle with bodily desires and to succumb on occasion, but that it was the goal of civilized men (by definition, civilized people were men!) to strive for moderation. Sex (of any kind) wasn't any more or less shameful an appetite than a taste for certain foods and wines — it was overindulgence that was shameful. The aspects of this philosophy passed down to us through the Church, however, are that the soul is superior to the body, and women are more susceptible to irrational, natural urges than men.

Certain ideas about reproductive biology first expressed by Classical Greek writers persisted in medical thinking until well into the eighteenth century. Both Hippocrates, the fifth-century B.C. father of medicine, and Galen, a second-century physician who influenced medical thought until the Renaissance, wrote that successful conception depends on the mingled sexual fluids and sexual enjoyment of both men and women. Aristotle, writing in the fourth century B.C., was a dissenting voice; he held that semen alone contained the vital life spirit necessary for conception, and that women were just the receptive vessel — like earth for the seed. All these writers shared the belief that men are born with a finite supply of semen; ejaculation, therefore, was considered wasteful of a vital substance and physically debilitating. This almost mystical view of semen bolstered later Christian arguments that sex for other than reproductive purposes was sinful.

Christians

While a variety of early Christian sects were body-positive and sex-positive and allowed women positions of authority, several centuries' worth of social and political power struggles resulted in an orthodox Christianity that blended sex-negative, misogynist strands from both Jewish and Greek traditions.[3] To achieve the life of the spirit, Christians were urged to give up the life of the flesh; sex was cast as the ultimate sin, and women were cast as the ultimate sinners — let's not forget Eve, who caused humanity's fall from grace through her weak and greedy ways. Procreation was the only possible justification for sex. In her riveting book *The Mythology of Sex*, Sarah Dening describes this devolution.

> In earlier times, above all the Goddess had represented the sacredness of natural life, and this included sexuality. Once the spirit alone came to be considered sacred, all that she stood for was necessarily devalued. The feminine now became identified with nature, the serpent, the temptations of the flesh. Sexuality had been transformed into something evil, to be feared

and at all costs kept under control lest it lead man astray and make him a sinner.[4]

Mother Mary

Yet no religion could have survived as long as Christianity without incorporating feminine imagery. In the process of converting "heathen" all across Europe, the Church appropriated many of the myths, customs, and rituals from the preexisting traditions. For example, ancient Celtic carvings known as Sheila-na-Gigs—which depict squatting, naked female figures parting the lips of their prominent vulvas with both hands—are found over the doorways in churches throughout Ireland and Britain. Some interpret the overtly sexual symbolism as a warning of the sins of the flesh, with the vulva as the gaping gates of hell (one theory holds that the Sheilas are the children of Lilith).[5] The carvings were frequently touched by churchgoers, especially brides on their wedding days, so it seems more likely that they are vestiges from a previous fertility-goddess culture.

Mother Mary herself is simply another version of the Great Mother; in fact, the earliest depictions of the Madonna and Child were clearly inspired by images of Isis and Horus. During the Hellenistic era, myths abounded of heroes who were born under unique circumstances, suffered, died, and were reborn. The concept of virgin birth, which also appeared in these stories, didn't refer to sexual virginity. *Parthenos*, the Greek word that early biblical translators have handed down to us as "virgin," literally translates as "she who is unto herself," meaning a woman who is unmarried or not dependent on any man. The goddess Ishtar's temple prostitutes were considered holy virgins, and their semidivine children were referred to as virgin-born. As Christianity evolved, Mary's virginity was likely reinterpreted to emphasize a sexual purity that ordinary sinful women should aspire to.

Puritans and Victorians

In the United States, we trace much of our discomfort with sex to the Puritans, who fled England's religious repression only to found their own sexually repressive New England community. We're all familiar with the idea of Puritans as sex-negative, hysterical hypocrites—reinforced by the tale of Hester Prynne's infidelity with a priest in Nathaniel Hawthorne's *The Scarlet Letter*, and in the infamous Salem witch trials. It's certainly true that the Puritan community punished all nonmarital forms of sexual expression (adulterers were publicly flogged) and that the Puritan clergy urged sexual repression, railing against all manner of sexual vice, immodesty, and wantonness. In colonial homes, however, attitudes toward sexuality were probably more nuanced. Believing that sex should be only for procreation doesn't preclude a belief that procreative sex should be pleasurable. Marital guides of the day promoted sexual pleasure for both men and women as necessary for conception and gave the clitoris its due as an organ of pure pleasure. While the Christian idea that women were prone to excessive licentiousness still held sway, mothers were expected to enjoy sex.[6]

The tides turned in the mid–nineteenth century as the social and political changes of the Victorian era brought a new emphasis on sexual self-control for the sake of social productivity. The classical Greek theories that ejaculation saps a man's strength were revived, and middle-class men were encouraged to practice sexual moderation even within marriage so they would have more energy for business endeavors. (The late nineteenth century was the high-water point of a flood of anti-masturbation literature aimed at both men and women.) Middle-class women were expected to serve as both inspiration and support for upholding sexual moderation, and the myth of the innately chaste woman was born. Eve the temptress gave way to the Angel in the House, who was her husband's moral (if not intellectual) equal by virtue of her utter lack of sexual desire. Women's lust, which had been feared and demonized for millennia, was thoroughly and convincingly denied—to this day, we can't quite shake the Victorian notion that women are by nature less sexual than men.

Presumably many of these Victorian women were willing to embrace their new passionless identity, since it not only freed them from conjugal duties but allowed them to enter the public arena as social reformers. (Many contemporary women still see sexuality and political activism as an either/or choice.) Yet Victorian medical and marital advice books didn't deny the positive aspects of sexual expression. Elizabeth Blackwell, the first woman to earn a medical degree in the United States, wrote:

> Women have been taught to regard sexual passion as lust and as sin—a sin which it would be a shame for a pure woman to feel, and which she would die rather than confess. She has not been taught that sexual passion is love, even more than lust, and that its ennobling work in humanity is to educate and transfigure the lower by the higher element. The growth and indications of her own nature she is taught to condemn, instead of to respect them as foreshadowing that mighty impulse towards maternity which will place her nearest to the Creator.[7]

Dr. Blackwell's words hint at a new attitude in which intimacy and eroticism are as important to sexual expression as procreation, which sets the stage for a major cultural shift. In the twentieth century, sexuality is reframed—not as original sin, nor as a necessary evil—but as an instinctual life force, evident through every stage of life, which should not be repressed or denied. The ideas of Sigmund Freud and sexologists such as Havelock Ellis paved the way for our modern notion of sexual expression as *self-expression*. In our day, sexuality and reproduction are clearly separated, and sexuality is viewed as a crucial aspect of how we discover and define ourselves. Yet our attitudes remain shaped by outmoded cultural beliefs: Heterosexual sex is still considered the defining norm (because it's potentially procreative); intercourse is still considered the defining sexual activity (because it's potentially procreative); and women's sexuality is still defined by the either/or equations—Madonna *or* whore, frigid ice princess *or* irrepressible slut—that make it so difficult to honor our whole selves.

MODERN MOMS: COMING UP SHORT

If it was easy to shake off our cultural heritage and seamlessly integrate our sexual and maternal selves, you probably wouldn't be reading this book right now. Every woman's self-image gets an overhaul in the transition to motherhood, and sexuality is just one of the aspects of identity that is temporarily dismantled. It takes a while to complete a transformation that allows you to feel true to yourself; in fact, the process is ongoing. We review some of the common challenges to your postbaby sexual identity below, and address them in greater detail throughout the book.

Unattainable Ideals

All moms experience a period when they're too tired to care how they look, and stained clothes dominate the wardrobe. Biological moms have the double whammy of major physical changes, and some experience a certain disconnect from their dual-purpose bodies. When genitals or breasts are serving a utilitarian purpose, seeing them as sexual isn't always easy.

> Breast-feeding and taking care of a small infant who lived IN MY BODY for nine months changed my perception of my sexual self. I thought of my body as more of a tool for a while, and so many things hurt physically for so long. I feel that just now, two years after the birth of my daughter, I have come full circle. I am able to separate my sexual self from my parent self, and it feels like a great personal change, so healthy.

> Now being the somewhat dumpy stay-at-home mom that I am, it's difficult to reconcile that with the sexy sweet young thang I once was. I'm learning to love myself as a GODDESS with the broad hips, low breasts, and the incredible life experience that implies.

It doesn't help that media images of motherhood tend to swing between one extreme—down-and-out welfare moms—to the other—high-powered professional or celebrity moms who are leading lives completely unattainable for the rest of us. The former are blamed for having a sex life, and the latter are praised for having a sex life. When *People* magazine ran a cover story on "Sexy Moms" several years ago, this quote was typical of the dozens of readers who complained.

How come being sexy means you must look like you never gave birth at all?
Why can't round, curvy, real women and moms be considered sexy too?

Since most moms don't see themselves in these images, they find the notion of sexy motherhood almost depressing. If motherhood means not only keeping a clean house and raising well-adjusted kids but looking like a million bucks too, who wouldn't feel like a failure? And we're right to be suspicious of this version of sexy motherhood. With her glamorous, never-a-hair-out-of-place veneer, the twenty-first-century celebrity mom bears a certain suspicious resemblance to the perfect 1950s housewife—she just gets a personal trainer and private nutritionist instead of a vacuum and blender.

Marriage manuals from the 1930s through the 1950s emphasized that husbands and wives needed to prioritize their sex lives for the health and stability of the family. A wife's way of contributing to this otherwise laudable goal was to stay sexy and feminine and not to "let herself go" for fear that her neglected husband might be driven to stray. Freudian theories were widespread during this time period, and most middle-class American women knew they were supposed to sever their immature attachment to clitoral stimulation and adopt a "mature" sexuality focused on vaginal intercourse. Gynecologists of the day advised wives of "the advantage of innocent simulation of sex responsiveness"; in other words, the advantage of faking orgasm![8]

Your parents may not have read these marriage manuals, but chances are good they absorbed the philosophy that a good wife takes responsibility for her husband's sexual satisfaction—and that you inherited some version of this idea. Numerous retro parenting guides are still printed every year, urging wives to sustain some kind of sex life with their partners, come hell or high water. But who wants to sustain a sex life if her own sexual pleasure is secondary? Many mothers find that it takes some time after becoming a parent to get back in touch with their sex drive, and you'll be a lot more motivated to do so if the goal is exploring how your sexual responses may have changed—not "slimming down" and greeting your hubby at the front door wearing nothing but Saran Wrap! Sure, we all want to retain our sexual attractiveness—for ourselves as well as our partners—but setting the bar unreasonably high can lead to a vicious cycle of self-loathing: We end up feeling undesirable, which inhibits our ability to project a sexual confidence that others might find attractive. The experience ends up confirming our suspicions that we've lost our sex appeal.

I feel so gross and emotionally drained. I no longer appeal to men on the street, nobody takes a second look anymore. I feel old and haggard, like I am no fun anymore.

The challenges to your self-image won't all revolve around physical appearance. If your initial experience of motherhood isn't one of instinctive, effortless love and bonding, you may feel like a terrible fraud—but you should know that you're not alone. Communicating with other mothers—particularly in the anonymous, candid environment of on-line forums—can be hugely reassuring.

I felt as though I had lost myself, and it was such an awful and scary feeling. I've only recently begun to locate me again. I remember feeling as though the light that I had, which was so bright, was losing its strength. I felt like I was the only woman who wasn't absolutely ecstatic and in love with her baby. Oh yes, I love him dearly, but these feelings were real and weighed very heavy on my conscience.

Everyone Wants a Piece of Mom

It's easy to be so overwhelmed by the very real demands of motherhood that your sexuality is the last thing on your mind. For some, the sheer increase in responsibility saps their sexual energy.

I have a lot more insecurities now than I did before I was a mother—body issues, single-mother issues, time and privacy issues, potential stepfather issues. It's hard to even view myself as a sexual being sometimes.

My sense of self changed the day he was born. I was given tons more responsibility. I took on this "role" right from the beginning. I saw myself as a mother and a housekeeper. Sexual being was not on my list.

Other feel demoralized by the pressure to become the ultimate self-sacrificing mom, an unrealistic and unhealthy ideal that society tends to shove down our throats.

I had to struggle to hang on to the me who was me—as opposed to the MOM me. It is always a struggle for women, I think. So many demands, expectations, etc. So many perfectly coifed PTA moms wearing holiday theme sweaters and bright smiles.

Unless you actually *are* a celebrity mom (in which case we apologize for our snotty comments) with a bevy of personal trainers, chefs, drivers, nannies, and assistants who can manage the mundane details of your life, you're bound to run into what we've dubbed "scarcity" issues. If you don't have enough time or energy to make sexual expression a possibility, let alone a priority, in your life, check out the Surviving Scarcity chapter (page 175).

Not You Two Again! Madonna and the Whore

We all inherit the same double standard of female sexuality. You and your partner may contend with a fear that sex has the power to transform a sainted mother like you into a selfish, slutty whore. Even if your fears don't take such extreme forms, you've probably experienced at least a fleeting anxiety that the sexual activities you enjoyed before becoming a mother just aren't quite "appropriate" anymore.

> I felt that mothers couldn't be sexual—that the roles were pretty specific: Mothers took care of the kids, mistresses took care of the fathers.

> Mothering is not traditionally seen as a sexual role and I felt castrated! My hormones changed and I just didn't feel like a sexual person anymore. Moms are not sexy. They lactate. They make lunches. They clean the house and then they are supposed to transform at evening into this sexy thing for the husband's pleasure. I didn't transform at all. I just mothered.

> My husband wants me to be more conservative now. He feels some of the things I wear are not suitable. I want to feel sexy again—it was always such a big part of me.

Then again, violating a taboo does have some erotic potential.

> A lot of men find me more desirable—it's that whole "perfect mommy" by day, slut by night syndrome.

Many moms internalize the Madonna/whore double bind so thoroughly that they begin to censor not only their sexual activities but their sexual fantasies too, according to some unwritten rules regarding how to be a good mom.

> I no longer enjoy reading porn as I did occasionally before we became parents, and wish he wouldn't even bring it into the house, ditto with X-rated videos, they actually make me sick now.

I have heard many girlfriends say that they felt sex was too "dirty" after their children were born.

I sometimes feel guilty for thinking sexual thoughts, like as a mom I shouldn't feel that way.

By repressing your sexuality—and all its colorful kinkiness—you lose access to an important part of yourself. While you can't very well avoid experiencing anxieties that have been drummed into our collective consciousness, you can cultivate awareness of your self-censoring moments and thereby open yourself up to a world of sexual self-discovery.

Sometimes I catch myself thinking that I shouldn't be having the thoughts I have sometimes because I'm a mom! Then I remind myself what BS that is.

Andrea O'Reilly, the president of the Association for Research on Mothering, theorizes that our cultural uneasiness over sexually expressive mothers stems from their being too powerful for men: "Women have power two ways, sexually and as mothers. Under the old tradition, women's sexuality could lead men astray—women, as with Helen of Troy, could cause the ruin of civilization because of beauty and sex appeal. Women also have power as mothers, in their ability to create life. I think there's an unconscious fear of women's power as sexual beings and mothers, and if you put both of them together it's too much for men to handle."

We like to hope that men are evolving toward an ever increasing comfort level with powerful women, but this can't happen unless women become comfortable with their own power first. Perhaps envisioning yourself as an extraordinarily potent being is just the inspiration to assert your maternal sexuality.

The Naysayers

When it comes to self-image, a mother has enough internal demons to deal with. Morphing bodies, shifting priorities, unprecedented demands—our ability to weather these tumultuous changes directly affects our sexual self-confidence. But even if we successfully navigate our way through a maze of self-doubt, there's no predicting what obstacles those around us have stored up to throw in our paths. Approach the subjects of sex and motherhood separately, and there are plenty of people on their soapboxes, ready to pass judgment. But blend them together into one real-life human called a "sexual mom" and you've opened a Pandora's box of criticisms.

If the history of attitudes toward women's sexuality has taught us nothing else, it should have taught us not to believe everything we read or hear. Society, science, religion, and your nosy neighbors may seek to define what's appropriate, but only you know what sex is and should be in your own life. If you can identify the illogic, inconsistency, or misinformation fueling every attack on your sexual expression, you can reveal the attack for what it is: not a personal indictment of your motherhood, but a mask for someone else's hang-ups. Each time you deflect a poison arrow aimed at your sex life, your self-esteem gets stronger and your self-image more clearly defined.

Our survey respondents were not at a loss to identify the myths they encountered when they became mothers:

Myth #1: Sex is for procreation

Despite the sexual revolution, the invention of birth control, and a self-help movement which trumpets that sex can be enjoyed solely for the sheer, body-arching pleasure of it, some people continue to assume that parents are only having sex to reproduce — or alternately, that once you become parents, you forget how to have sex for any other reason.

> Some of my partners seemed really surprised that I was interested in sex at all — one girlfriend told me, "You'd think you'd have learned your lesson after three kids, wouldn't you?"

> Some people that I knew just assumed that I would never have that "normal" young-people sex life again, like "Too bad you're parents now — no more sex for you guys."

Myth #2: Moms aren't sex objects

One of the biggest shocks to our self-image comes from the realization that many people can't conceive of a mother as a sex object. We become objects of pity, reverence, or dismissal in the eyes of those we used to count on for a little simple sexual validation.

> I was more grounded and sexually confident than ever before, but other people saw me as a "mom." Men quit looking at me in the grocery store when I had the baby with me. They looked at me like they look at my mother. I felt a little disappointed.

> I felt like I was invisible while I was pregnant, and this is true even now

when I'm in public with my son. Oddly enough, I still find men flirting with me when my son is NOT with me.

I was in college while raising my son. A lot of the boys there were intimidated by my mom status and I think they found it hard to view me as anything other than someone's mother. I guess it's just the age that college boys are, they can't separate their own mothers from someone who is a mother.

There are many reasons for this sexual invisibility—people assume you're unavailable, they treat you by extension as they would treat their own mothers, they don't want to interfere with your family—but the important thing to remember is, it's no reflection on your actual sex appeal. You may find, as some moms do, that it's a relief to experience a little less unsolicited sexual attention.

I have a lot of male friends and now that I am a mom we are all closer in a new way. They don't seem threatened by me the way they would be by other girls. My friend is always trying out his lines on me and that sort of thing, because I am a woman, but I am also a mother. I think this makes him feel safe around me.

Myth #3: Dads are sexy, but not moms

While many people can't quite wrap their head around the idea of a sexy mom, nobody has too much trouble conceiving of dads as sexy.

I notice that when I walk around with our daughter, I become invisible. When my husband is alone with her, he gets all kinds of attention. Why are men who look like single dads perceived as such chick magnets, yet women who look like they might be single moms cease to exist?

In another example of the double standard, a father's sex life is a given—the biggest cause for concern is whether he's getting enough—but a mother's sex life is not. Mothers who make their sexual needs a priority are deemed oversexed, promiscuous, or even neglectful; fathers who do so are simply exerting their conjugal rights.

When I left my kids' dad, I was considered a "slut" because it was obvious I left for a sexual relationship. Moms who prioritize a sexual life are perceived as irresponsible, selfish, even abusive.

Myth #4: All parents are Ozzie and Harriet

If your family doesn't fit the white-picket-fence ideal, no matter how rock-solid your self-esteem is, dealing with all the inaccurate assumptions you encounter on a daily basis is a challenge.

> I get so sick of people asking about the baby's dad — I just want to whip out my girlfriend's picture and say, "Here's papa!"

> Being an adoptive mom, I did come across some rude statements by other moms that implied I wasn't a "real" mom.

> Sometimes I feel like wearing a sign when I'm out with my daughter that says "Hey, I am an available, desirable, sex-loving single mom. Date me!" It seems like people just assume I'm taken.

And not every woman who conceives through intercourse with a man appreciates the assumptions that ensue about her sexual orientation.

> I think that people's image of me changed because my hubby was the first man I'd had a long-term relationship with in a while. I'm one of the few in my circle who is openly bi. That gave me a certain sexual cachet. Now, people seem to think that just because I married a man, I'm not bi anymore. That's hardly true. I'm just in a straight marriage.

> Lesbians thought I "had to be" hetero! It was a scream since I had been with women nine of the ten previous years before my son was born.

MATERNAL SEXUALITY REDEFINED

But enough about challenges! Motherhood is also an amazing opportunity to create a richer and more fully integrated self-image. Many women discover that they now feel more whole and have a greater appreciation for the spirituality inherent in sexuality.

> Being a mom made me feel more complete as a woman. Like two halves coming together. The maternal side and the sexual side combining to form this one magnificent being: Woman. My desire for sex is greater than ever

because I feel that sex is integral to being a complete person, which in turn makes me a much better mom.

I feel even more comfortable with my sexuality because I feel more connected with the whole circle of life. It sounds corny, but it's true.

I feel more sensual. I feel very connected to the earth, I feel very spiritual. This has affected my sexuality immensely.

Others identify motherhood as the wellspring for a newfound power, which translates into more sexual confidence and assertiveness.

I became a sexual goddess in that my beliefs about my body and the power of woman are so much clearer. I became cougar mama! You know, that "don't fuck with me or my kids or I'll kill you" mentality. For some reason, this made my sexual being more powerful for me and for those around me, male and female.

You may have found that motherhood has inspired a renewed respect for your body. Many biological mothers find that a changed body—weight gain, stretch marks, expanded hips, pendulous breasts, and all—is an unexpected boon to their sexual self-image. Discovering your body's creative capabilities, your strength, and your resilience can yield surprisingly erotic results.

I think I am way more beautiful and powerful and sexy than I used to be. I feel freer sexually. Because we were able to make these amazing creatures through pure fucking! It's great! I appreciate my body so much more, because it has done some wondrous shit, I am just so in awe of it!

The heightened state of awareness from labor hasn't really ended. I'm also really comfortable with my body now, I'm rounder but I feel delicious. I feel sexier than I used to. I stepped beyond a lot of early-twenties hang-ups.

And, as this survey respondent discovered, sex can also bring you back to your creative capabilities if you've lost touch with them after motherhood.

I had a special experience with sex after the death of our first child. After the premature birth, hospitalization, and eventual death of our firstborn, my body was completely numb. I couldn't feel a thing. It was through sex that I started to regain feeling and the awareness of the physical sensations of my body. Sex reconnected me with my body. Our second baby was born unassisted on the side of the road on the way to the midwife. It was one of the most empowering experiences of my life.

Moms Make Better Lovers

This may sound like bumper-sticker hype, but plenty of mothers confirm the slogan, because the qualities that make us good mothers—being caring, nurturing, and generous—are precisely the qualities that make us better lovers.

> My children taught me how to truly love someone with total surrender. I learned how to express my love with my partner better than before, which led to better sex.

> I didn't know how to love anyone seriously till I had a child. It expanded my humanity, which in turn enhanced my sexuality.

As author Susie Bright points out in her book *Full Exposure,* distinctions between mother love and sexual love are arbitrary: "Maternal love is just one facet of erotic love—because it is the erotic imagination and generosity in our spirit that makes such 'maternal' sacrifice and unconditional appreciation possible."[9]

Many women find that motherhood brings them greater sexual maturity. Competitiveness, vanity, and status-seeking are replaced by authenticity and self-expression.

> I feel sexier in a different way than I used to. I feel more experienced and whole and less like a seductive teenybopper.

> I feel more sexually charged, I can tell other people can feel it, too, but it is more mellow and confident than before. I am not as much of a flirt.

> Becoming a mom at the age of twenty was an awakening. I had thought of myself as sexual only in the sense of being desirable, or manipulating my sexuality for my physical, monetary, or psychological benefit. Becoming a mother acquainted me with the elemental, sacred aspects of sex that are now a permanent part of my sexual identity. I find my maternal sexu-

ality to be much more appealing to myself and others. I feel that I am in control.

Becoming a mother teaches you true intimacy. A child demands intense closeness and offers utter trust; once you discover your own capacity for maternal intimacy, you may find it translates into the realm of sexual intimacy, resulting in a sexuality that is radiantly attractive to your partners.

I soon realized that my new assertiveness (the protective-mom factor) made me even more attractive to partners. I have improved with age, and being a mother has only made me softer, harder, more well rounded, and generally more interesting.

Time to Upset the Apple Cart, Eve

Nothing will improve your self-image quite like bucking the system, asserting your individuality, and reclaiming your right to sex as a woman and a mother. In the process, you challenge others to see you in a different light, and you participate in a cycle of change and growth that we hope will restore mothers' sexuality to the place of reverence it held long ago. Here's some parting advice from your fellow moms:

I was told by my family to tone down the Commie Red lipstick and penchant for not wearing slips with see-through dresses. I didn't listen. I see myself as sexier now, like the eternal Earth Mama!

The thing that turned our sex life around was simply my attitude. At some point, I just decided that both I and my husband needed and deserved a good sex life. I started wearing stuff I found sexy. I made exercise a bigger priority because doing it not only actually makes me look better, but it makes me more confident and unapologetic about my body. I started pushing my body in my husband's way and talking sex up to him even on nights when we couldn't do it. At first, he thought it was weird, but I refused to be embarrassed, and he eventually stopped thinking of me as a tired, dried-up "soccer mom" and started seeing me as some kind of a sexpot, which is a huge turn-on to him.

Your sexuality has the capacity to fill your life with the same vitality and joy your children do. When you unite the two powerful forces of motherhood and sexuality, you vastly improve your self-image and make a gift to your children. Canadian hip-hop artist Michie Mee says it best:

> You have to open up as a woman in society. You're not just a hot girl, you're a hot mama, and you have to coordinate the two. You cannot put one down; it's a package that doesn't go away, it's an outfit that you do not return. I want to show my son his mom is kooky and sexy. It's more than makeup, hair and clothes—strong sexuality comes from within.[10]

SEXUAL SELF-ESTEEM

ELF-ESTEEM is a big business in our culture. Countless books, magazine articles, and inspirational tapes encourage one and all to banish any nagging sense of inadequacy by standing before the mirror and proclaiming, "I'm swell just the way I am." Let us confess up front that we approach this topic with some trepidation; we're not equipped to compete with the best hucksters of our generation. We're all too conscious of the fact that affirmations are only skin-deep, that our grip on personal self-esteem is tenuous at best, and that we can't bully you, esteemed reader, into self-confidence. But we are also genuinely angry at how many unjust and unnecessary obstacles block women's access to sexual self-esteem. All those pocket-size affirmation books are products of the same popular culture that fuels our sexual anxiety with misinformation and mystification. You can't shrug off a sexual inferiority complex by clicking your heels together three times and repeating, "There's no one as sexy as me." But you can *distract* yourself from your insecurities — pay no attention to the man behind the curtain! Curiosity can be the key to a whole new realm of sexual empowerment. When you stop scrutinizing how you measure up and start exploring your own unique sexuality, you've taken the first step toward a flourishing self-esteem.

CULTIVATING A POSITIVE BODY IMAGE

For most women, sexual self-esteem is inextricably entwined with body image — if you feel unattractive, you feel undesirable and tend to limit your sexual interactions.

Your Sexual History

We're often too busy worrying about sex, obsessing about sex, or wishing it would just plain go away to take the long view. But reviewing the patterns in your personal sexual history can shed a lot of light on where you'd like to go from here. You'll probably get the most out of this exercise if you write out your answers (and they'll be of great interest to read later on), but even just pondering these questions as you sit in traffic or lie in the tub can be enlightening.

- What were the early messages you received from relatives, teachers, and peers about sex, reproduction, bodies, masturbation, and gender roles?
- What are your earliest memories of sexual feelings? Of sexual experimentation?
- What was your experience of puberty? Of adolescence?
- What was your first sexual experience with another person?
- What have been the most positive and most negative sexual experiences of your life?
- What are your most and least favorite things about your body? About your sexual responses?
- If relevant, how has your history of birth control, pregnancy, and childbirth affected your sexuality? If relevant, how has your history of sexual or medical problems affected your sexuality?
- What are your current sexual practices?
- What are your current fantasies?
- What would you like to change about your sex life?
- What do you imagine your sexuality will be like in ten years? Twenty years? etc.

Conversely, if you feel comfortable in your body, you're more likely to feel deserving of sexual satisfaction and therefore even more likely to get it. Nothing is quite as sexually appealing as simple self-assurance.

What Stands in Your Way

For most of us, women in particular, learning to accept our bodies is a lifelong battle. We all know that media depictions of "beautiful" or "sexy" are ludicrously limited, yet it's hard to shake the sense that we'd be a whole lot happier if we could just bridge the gap between our own appearance and the fantasy ideal. The media is only part of the problem—our inability to stay in the here and now is another; we tend to postpone appreciating our body until that unspecified future point when we'll have attained sufficient perfection to allow ourselves to stop and smell the roses. Even if we move in circles where a wider range of body types is appreciated, nearly every one of us sees something to envy in somebody else's appearance, or something that needs improvement in our own.

To a certain extent, our obsession with improvement reflects a yearning for some manageable sphere of influence; if we can't exert our will over the body politic, we can at least bring our body into line. After all, despite expanded professional opportunities, fundamental social inequities haven't budged—women still have less earning power than men, and mothers still juggle more than their fair share of responsibility for child care, housework, and child support. No wonder some of us turn to gyms, plastic surgeons, and diet docs to experience a sense of control.

The problem is that when your body is a work in progress, it's hard to find the time amid all that shaving, exfoliating, toning, and slimming simply to enjoy being in it. A 1998 *Glamour* magazine poll of twenty-seven thousand women found that over half the respondents were dissatisfied with their bodies, and that 40 percent spent more than one third of their time dieting. As a result, more respondents said they would rather lose weight than spend a romantic evening with someone they really liked.[1]

We all fight the tendency to scapegoat our bodies, and some of us face greater challenges than others. Survivors of sexual abuse or assault often struggle with negative body image, either feeling detached from, betrayed by, or ashamed of their bodies. Eating disorders are more common in abuse survivors. Even those of us without the devastating disempowerment of sexual assault in our history contend with a lesser, low-grade disempowerment: the ongoing commodification of women's bodies.

Why do women fret more about how they look than how they feel? Because we are *judged* more on how we look than how we feel. Standards of beauty may come and go, but the bottom line never wavers: Looks are a woman's ticket to validation and power. Although women tend to be one another's (and our own) harshest critics, our point of reference is always the male gaze. Even the staunchest feminist man inherits the entitlement to judge a woman's appearance, and even the staunchest feminist woman inherits the justifiable anxiety that any man could flex his birthright at a moment's notice. If you don't believe this is so, have a lesbian affair, and watch how your body image blooms and your belly relaxes, how an extra five pounds here or there recedes in importance. We're not suggesting that lesbians don't care about physical attractiveness, just that aesthetic standards become a lot more inclusive once you detour away from mainstream consumer culture.

And we're not blaming men; both sexes suffer equally when woman's bodies are treated as status symbols. Sadly, the latest development in popular culture is equal-opportunity objectification; instead of expanding our standards of beauty, we're beginning to enforce equally narrow and unattainable standards for men. Now young boys are mainlining steroids and pumping iron in a quest to cultivate the rippled chest and washboard abs that are fixtures of contemporary advertising. "Body anxiety for all" seems to be the rallying cry of the twenty-first century, which we hope will inspire you to cry, "Enough is enough!" and step off the treadmill.

Why Take Action?

We're encouraging you to develop a more positive body image for three reasons: You owe it to yourself, you owe it to your partners, and you owe it to all the young women in your life.

For yourself

Let's start with you. You're probably already well aware that nothing dampens libido more thoroughly than a negative body image. One third of the *Glamour* survey respondents reported that "feeling fat" sometimes prevented them from having sex (and an even higher percentage reported that a compliment was more likely to make them feel good than having sex).[2] The paradox is that nothing can boost your body image and take your mind off feeling fat as effectively as enjoyable sex.

Did you ever stop to consider how many of the people you see out in the world — of all sizes, ages, and abilities — are enjoying active sex lives? The chances are good that if you tried to guess which one of your fellow bus passengers was enjoying the most satisfying sex life, you'd be wrong. Sexual chemistry transcends standards of beauty and subverts expectations, but we remain locked into the assumption that sex is for the young and jiggle-free largely because we don't receive much evidence to the contrary. As psychologist Lenore Tiefer puts it:

> Cultural messages, whether they are coming from religion or commercialism, are influential in part because they're not counteracted by your own observation. . . . If you stopped to think, you might say to yourself, "I've never seen ordinary people make love. What do they do with a big stomach? How do they undress each other?" The lack of a bridge between people's own experience and the culture serves to depress us about sexuality.[3]

But when you set aside cultural messages, sex can be a holiday from the cult of perfection. In their excellent sex-enhancement guide, *Let Me Count the Ways*, therapists Marty Klein and Riki Robbins advise:

> Experience your body's perfection during sex. Notice how good kissing doesn't require you to lose weight; notice how having more hair or whiter

teeth wouldn't make your orgasms any better. In this sense, sex can be a mental vacation from all the self-criticism your body endures.[4]

You can create your own bridge to authentic sexuality by looking around you for role models of women who exude sensual assurance. Surely you've noticed that plenty of women who don't fit into a size-six dress have vigorous self-esteem (and plenty of cover models don't). Despite the cultural fetish for sexy youth, you'll probably find your best role models among women who aren't spring chicks. This book is filled with quotes from women who testify that maturity and motherhood have brought them a deeper self-acceptance and sexual fulfillment than they had known before.

I was a very thin, nubile woman before having children. After two children, I'm a little Rubenesque, but much more comfortable with it. I'm turning forty in a week or so and am relishing myself these days. I still feel very much the sexual woman. And I try to convey this sense to my daughters in a way that makes sense: "Mommies are loving, caring, *and* sexual beings."

Too many girls grow up feeling inadequate because they don't match up to the bodies they see on television or movies. It's taken me forty years to realize that I'm beautiful and desirable at my size (currently 315 lbs.), and that I've wasted too many of those years trying to alter the way I look, while feeling that I was unappealing to the opposite sex. It's all an illusion. Confidence and attitude are the most attractive qualities any person can possess.

For your partners

All too often, low self-esteem becomes a way not only to punish yourself but to punish your partner as well. Women who are feeling dissatisfied with their appearance are liable to either tune out their partner's expressions of affection and appreciation or deflect advances. But if your partner wants to make love to you, he or she really doesn't need to hear about how fat you feel, or that you have to get to the gym first thing in the morning. If you were to pause in that headlong rush to turn off the lights, and take a moment just to focus on what it feels like to touch your lover's body, the unself-conscious joys of sexual satisfaction could be closer than you think.

Negative body image makes us unnecessarily threatened by a lover's appreciation for other people or fantasy materials; we automatically see any desirable other as a reflection of our own inadequacy. Just because your husband drools over a porn star's long legs doesn't mean yours don't feel pretty darn great wrapped around his back, and just because your girlfriend religiously watches each and every *Xena: Warrior Princess* episode doesn't mean she's going to leave you for a kickboxing vixen. Let go of that pinched, scarcity-based fear that you're not good enough, and switch your focus to an examination of all the different people and situations that arouse *your* sexual desires. Sexual curiosity is the first step on the road to sexual generosity.

For girls everywhere

Finally, modeling a positive body image is the single best gift you could bequeath the girls and young women in your life. They are growing up in a world where casual female self-deprecation, if not self-denigration, is the name of the game. We ourselves used to work in a women-owned, feminist sex business, where sexual diversity was sincerely honored and celebrated. You might think that this environment would have been an oasis from negative body image, but we still heard regular variations on those age-old junior high refrains: "You look great, did you lose weight?" or "You're so skinny—I hate you!"

Every time your daughter, younger sister, or niece sees you stand in front of the mirror with a furrowed brow or disgusted expression, she's getting the message that a woman's physical appearance is anxiety-inducing. The *Glamour* survey found that 62 percent of the women who described their own mothers as having had a negative body image inherited this sense of dissatisfaction. And girls who are unhappy with their bodies are girls at risk. As historian Joan Jacobs Brumberg puts it:

> As long as they feel so unhappy with their bodies, it is unlikely that they can achieve the sexual agency that they need for complete and successful lives in the contemporary world. Girls who do not feel good about themselves need the affirmation of others, and that need, unfortunately, almost always empowers male desire. In other words, girls who hate their bodies do not make good decisions about partners, or about the kind of sexual activity that is in their best interest. Because they want to be wanted so much, they are susceptible to manipulation, to flattery, even to abuse.[5]

Sure it's hard to silence the negative tapes in your own head, or to break the habit of companionable fretting with other women, but if you can't do it for yourself, try doing it for the next generation of women, who deserve to blossom into Warrior Princesses one and all. Be vigilant, cultivate perspective, and hold on to your sense of humor. Who knows, maybe the next time somebody asks, "You look great, did you lose weight?" you'll be inspired to answer, "Actually, I've gained a couple of pounds, but I just had a terrific orgasm, which always makes me look good!" And then take a young girl out to lunch and tell her how beautiful, strong, and smart she is.

Positive Steps

We've offered plenty of reasons to cultivate self-esteem. Here, in no particular order, are some practical tools for exploring your relationship to your body and your sexuality:

- *Review your assets.* Make a list of the qualities you've always admired in yourself (you don't need to limit yourself to the physical). Describe why you appreciate these qualities and whether you think they're sexy.

- *Compare and contrast.* Make a list of people you find attractive, friends and strangers alike. Can you pinpoint what it is about them that's so appealing? Which of their appealing characteristics conform to the norm, and which don't?

- *Define your terms.* What does being a sexy woman mean to you? When you feel sexy, what do you look and feel like, and how are you expressing yourself? If you're not sure you've ever felt sexy, what's your fantasy of what this would be like?

- *Take your own sex history.* Your background (family, religious, and cultural) and relationship history are all formative influences on your sexual identity. Write your own sex history (see the sidebar for details) to get a sense of where you've been and where you might like to go.

- *Talk about it.* Talk to friends and lovers about what comments or situations hinder or help your self-esteem. Swap tips on coping mechanisms. Talk about what's depicted as sexy in movies, TV, ads, and music videos compared to what's been sexy in your own experience.

- *Don't talk about it.* Declare a moratorium on conversations about body fat, dieting, cellulite, and skin care. Every time you feel yourself on the verge of a self-critical comment, imagine the snappy retort you'd make if anyone criticized someone you love in those terms (it's so much easier to be generous and gallant to our loved ones than to ourselves).

- *Develop friendships on-line.* People rave about the faceless environment of the Internet, which allows them to get to know one another for who they are, not what they look like. You might get to know and appreciate aspects of yourself that you rarely express face-to-face.

- *Go to a nude beach.* You'll benefit from the healing sensation of sun and air kissing every inch of your skin — along with a powerful reality check about just how many body types are out there.

- *Flaunt it.* Give yourself permission to invest in your favorite physical attributes. Try a new hairstyle that draws attention to your lovely eyes, clothes that accentuate your shapely derriere, or a manicure that says, "Kiss my hands, please!"

- *Indulge yourself.* Give your partner a fifteen-minute body massage. Touch in ways that delight or feel good to you (your partner should give you feedback only if he or she is uncomfortable or in pain). What's it like to touch someone purely for your own pleasure?

- *Move it.* Walk, dance, bicycle, swim, stretch, masturbate. Move your body in whatever ways feel good.

APPRECIATING YOUR SEXUAL ANATOMY

Even if you have a good attitude about your figure, your sexual self-esteem can suffer if you don't have an equally good attitude about what's between your legs. An astonishingly large number of women lack the basic physiological information to put them in control of their own sexual satisfaction. As children, too few of us receive accurate information about our genital anatomy; if anything, we're usually taught that girls have a vagina "down there," and that babies come out of this place. It can be highly disorienting for a girl who's heard not a peep about pleasure, and has been given no language to describe the clitoris and vulva, to discover that it feels good to rub her clitoris. The adult embarrassment or disapproval that ensues if she's "caught" engaging in self-exploration only reinforces the message that genitals are unmentionable at best and shameful at worst.

The willful ignorance that many women pick up during childhood often extends to our sexual responses. All too many of us take a hands-off, romantic attitude toward sexual pleasure; Prince or Princess Charming is supposed to gallop in on a white steed and take care of the mysterious mechanics of sex without our ever needing to say, "A little to the left, please."

As two women who came of age right along with the women's sexual self-help movement, we're convinced that every woman alive would benefit from sitting down with a hand mirror and taking a long, loving look at her own genitals. For one thing, they are utterly, miraculously beautiful. For another, every woman's labia, vagina, and clitoris are different, and you deserve to know how you're unique and to experiment with the unique stimulation styles that will please you. Finally, every mother owes it to her children to cultivate a healthy comfort with and appreciation of her genitals, as she's bound to communicate her own attitudes.

A Valentine for Your Vulva

You may be the most self-assured, body-loving, bold-faced nudist in town, but if you don't have a genuine appreciation for your own genitals, your sex life will suffer. Have you ever felt a flicker of anxiety as a lover's mouth headed between your legs? Have you ever worried "Does he think I look/smell/taste okay?" or "Isn't she getting bored down there?" Then it's time for a crash course in vulva love.

- Draw a picture of your labia. Get out the hand mirror and sketch what you see. Your efforts to capture the artful nature of every fold could arouse a new appreciation for your intimate architecture.
- Tour your genitals. Take a manual tour, touching and caressing every inch of your vulva, labia, and clitoris. Consider this an information-gathering expedition rather than an effort to arouse. Just let yourself experience the different types of skin and sensation.
- Have a taste. Forget about those fish jokes—a healthy vagina smells and tastes just dandy, but you're going to have a hard time believing this unless you test it for yourself. Check how your natural secretions change in texture and taste throughout your menstrual cycle. (If your vagina does veer too far from its sweet, tangy norm, there's probably a bacterial imbalance you'll need to address.)
- Rock around the clock. Explore your vagina to discover your own personal pleasure spots. Envision your vagina as a clock face, and your fingers as the hands of the clock; travel round the clock, pressing your fingers firmly into the vaginal walls and noting where you're extra sensitive. Time will fly.

With that lecture out of the way, let us take you on a whirlwind tour from top to bottom of your genital anatomy.

A Genital Tour

The external female genitals are referred to as the vulva and consist of the labia, the clitoral glans, the vaginal opening, and the urethral opening. The two long fleshy folds of the outer lips, the labia majora, are composed of fat and erectile tissue and are covered with pubic hair. The most distinctive portion of the vulva tends to be the labia minora, the smooth, hairless inner lips that enclose the urethral and vaginal openings. Labia come in a range of sizes, colors, and shapes, and they are not likely to come as a matched pair. Many women have suffered shame thinking that their labia were deformed or unsightly because one lip hung lower than the other, or because they weren't tucked discreetly inside the vulva. Women simply aren't exposed to much vulva imagery and don't necessarily have any frame of reference (no, Georgia O'Keeffe paintings do *not* count!). If you've ever thought your own or any woman's genitals were ugly or abnormal, we encourage you to check out the art-work in Betty Dodson's *Sex for One* for glorious depictions of women's genitalia in all their variety.

The labia minora meet in small folds at the top of the vulva, right above the clitoral glans. If you pull back this hood of skin to take a closer look, you may be intrigued to see how much the clitoral glans resembles a miniaturized version of the glans of a penis (sans urethral opening). Small as it is, it's power-packed; the clitoris is made up of some eight thousand nerve fibers, a higher concentration than in any other part of the body (and twice as many as in the penis). The exquisitely sensitive glans sits on top of the short clitoral shaft that runs beneath the skin in the direc-tion of the pubic bone—if you press down on the skin above your clitoris, you can feel the shaft rolling beneath your fingers. The shaft is attached to the two clitoral legs (also called *crura*), which are about three inches long and extend beneath the labia, arcing like two halves of a wishbone on either side of the vaginal and urethral openings.

The clitoral shaft and legs have far fewer nerve endings than the glans but are made of spongy erectile tissue that is rich in blood vessels. During sexual arousal, increased blood flow to the vulva engorges the labia as well as the entire clitoral body, which swells and becomes firmer—it's not exactly like a man's erection, but darn close. There's really no such thing as a clitoral versus a vaginal orgasm, because a woman can't stimulate any part of her genitals without indirectly stimulating the clit-oral body. The labia and vagina are sensitive erogenous zones, but while some women can orgasm with general genital stimulation, the majority of women require direct stimulation of the clitoral glans to get over the top. In fact, although Freud's decree that clitoral pleasure was "immature" cast a long shadow over our understanding of women's sexuality during the twentieth century, for thousands of years before that, the clitoris was well known as the main site of female sexual pleasure. A typical passage from a nineteenth-century marital guide describes the clitoris as an organ that can "stir up lust and give delight in copulation, for without this the fair sex neither desire nuptial embraces nor have pleasure in them."[6]

The urethral opening lies between the clitoris and the vaginal opening. The skin around the opening is rich in nerve endings, and some women find stimulation of this area highly pleasurable. The urethra itself is a slender, short tube that conducts urine out of the bladder. It runs above and parallel to the vagina and is surrounded by spongy erectile tissue, containing paraurethral glands and ducts ("para" means "beside" or "near"). This urethral sponge is what's come to be hyped as the "G-spot." Why a spot? Well, the urethra itself is only one and a half to two inches long, so the urethral sponge isn't very large. The erectile tissue of the urethral sponge swells during sexual arousal, at which point you can feel the G-spot by pressing hard against the front wall of the vagina. Some women find G-spot stimulation highly arousing; it can also lead to ejaculation of a clear, odorless fluid. Although this fluid is ejaculated through the urethra, it's chemically distinct from urine. All women have a urethral sponge, but not every woman ejaculates.

The vaginal opening lies just below the urethral opening. If you have witnessed or experienced vaginal delivery firsthand, you have doubtless developed great respect for the muscular expansiveness of the vagina. Made of muscle and tissue, lined with mucous membrane, the vagina is about four inches long and curves at roughly a 45-degree angle up toward the cervix—the neck of that other amazingly muscular organ, the uterus. While the vagina is often compared to a tunnel or hole, the vaginal walls rest companionably against each other most of the time and expand outward only upon sexual arousal (or during childbirth).

Reach just inside your vaginal opening and you'll feel a slightly ridged surface, especially along the front wall just behind the pubic bone, where the urethral sponge protrudes. The outer third of the vagina, which contains more nerve endings than the inner two thirds, can be quite responsive to touch. The inner two thirds of the vaginal walls are smoother and more responsive to pressure than touch.

The perineum is the small stretch of skin between the vaginal opening and the anus and is an erogenous zone in its own right. Another body of erectile tissue, referred to as the perineal sponge, lies between the back wall of the vagina and the rectum and probably contributes to pleasurable sensation during both vaginal and anal penetration. During vaginal labor, the perineum may tear, or the laboring woman may be given an episiotomy, a surgical cut through the skin of the perineum designed to reduce the risk of further tearing during delivery. Since the perineum is the site of many nerves and crisscrossing pelvic floor muscles, an episiotomy can result in some loss of sexual sensation, though most women find that a tear or episiotomy has no long-term effects on their genital sensitivity.

The anus is also loaded with nerve endings, which is why anal stimulation can be just as arousing as genital stimulation. While anal play carries a taboo as being somehow dirty or dangerous, it's a natural, safe form of eroticism. Many folks of all sexualities enjoy the pleasurable pressure of anal penetration. If you're going to explore this form of eroticism, you should practice relaxing your anal sphincter muscles; the external sphincter muscle is under voluntary control, but the internal sphincter is involuntary and will tighten if you rush or force penetration, with painful results.

Any anal penetration, whether with a pinkie or a penis, should always be accompanied by a generous application of lubricant, since the rectum doesn't self-lubricate, and rectal tissue is much more delicate than vaginal tissue.

Pelvic Muscles

Pelvic muscles play a major role in a woman's experience of sexual pleasure—and in her overall health. The pelvic muscles lie about an inch beneath your pelvic floor and are attached like a sling to your pubic bone at one end and your tailbone or coccyx at the other; that's why they're also referred to as the pubococcygeus, or "PC," muscle. The singular term, PC muscle, actually refers to a group of interconnected, multilayered muscles that support the entire pelvic floor and form a figure eight encircling the vagina, urethra, and rectum in women and the base of the penis and rectum in men.

Pelvic muscles play a key role in sexual sensation—they're loaded with nerve endings and contract involuntarily during orgasm. Learning to control these muscles not only has numerous health benefits, it heightens sexual responsiveness. If your pelvic muscles are well toned, you'll have increased genital sensation, greater vaginal lubrication, and more powerful orgasms.

The importance of pelvic muscle control is known and taught around the world; belly dancing, hula, and much African dance depend on it. But true to form, in America we trace our information on pelvic muscle exercises back to a medical authority. Gynecologist Arnold Kegel devised a simple series of exercises in the 1940s to treat urinary incontinence, and these exercises have since become known as "Kegels." If you're a biological mother, these are all too familiar to you, as you'll have been encouraged to do Kegels both in preparation for labor and to speed recovery postpartum. Kegels entail repetitive tightening and relaxing of the pelvic muscles— either in a sequence of quick squeezes, or in a slower pulling up and bearing down. The easiest way to identify the pelvic muscles is to stop and start the flow of urine; the muscles you use to do so are the pelvic muscles.

You can do Kegels any time, but these exercises beg to be incorporated with sexual activities. A penis or dildo inside your vagina is particularly helpful as a resistive device while doing Kegels. Since Kegels increase sensation in and blood flow to the genitals, they can enhance any sexual encounter. You can heighten your arousal by coordinating Kegels with breathing—inhaling as you contract and exhaling as you relax—or with pelvic rocking.

What About Sexual Response?

We're not going to give you a song and dance about the sexual response cycle, largely because, throughout this book, we'll encourage you to get to know your own body and to identify your unique sexual responses and preferences. Sure, certain constants of physiological response are common to all individuals: the increased blood flow, genital swelling, and muscular tension of arousal, and the discharging of this tension through the muscular contractions of orgasm. But there's a wide range of subjective experience that the monolithic model of one sexual response cycle is woefully inadequate to express. If you are someone who has never reached, or doesn't reliably reach, orgasm, we refer you to the Resources section for some recommended reading. If you are someone who does reliably orgasm, we doubt the experience would be enhanced for you by learning that sex researchers Masters and Johnson clocked orgasmic contractions as occurring every eight tenths of a second.

Sexual self-knowledge is not a onetime journey of discovery in which you map out your personal terrain once and for all. In fact, our experience of sexual response is ever evolving over the course of a lifetime, and why should it be otherwise? Our bodies change over time, and our relationship to our bodies changes over time—the pattern of sexual response we develop in adolescence is no more likely to remain relevant through adulthood than our adolescent relationship style. If you're able to put aside societal messages about what's sexually "normal" and simply listen to your own body's responses, you'll be able to reap the greatest sexual pleasure out of your evolving experience.

ATTITUDES ABOUT SEXUAL PLEASURE

Wouldn't it be great if, instead of talking with other moms at the playground about our kids' latest accomplishments, we could swap stories about our own latest erotic adventures? You gasp. But think about it: We share intimate details about our children's biological functions with near strangers; what prevents us from talking about our own urges and desires? Unfortunately, we live in a society where such sexual frankness is discouraged—a profound loss for mothers, considering how much we could learn from one another about loving our bodies, keeping the flame alive, and exploring our fantasies.

Instead, we're left to decipher the mixed messages we receive about sexuality. Our society places great value on the family and on sex for procreation, yet we receive no reality-based sex education or relationship training, so we muddle through our first sexual and emotional experiences, risking embarrassment and failure. We slowly gain confidence and expertise but may be hounded throughout our lives by the questions "Am I good enough?" or "Is what I'm doing normal?" As we grow more adventurous, we confront one label after another: If we enjoy having sex often, we're promiscuous. If we enjoy alternatives to vaginal intercourse, we're kinky. If we are taking a break from partner sex, we're frigid. We receive so many conflicting messages from parents, friends, religious institutions, medical professionals, magazine articles, and lovers about what, when, where, how, and why (or why not) to have sex that it's easy to forget why we have it in the first place: because it feels good and because it's good for us.

After all, we share a Victorian heritage that values self-control over self-expression and considers abstinence a virtue. Women in particular have internalized the message that it's possible to have too much pleasure, and that the pursuit of pleasure is necessarily a selfish act. As mothers, we're subjected to specific scripts that play right into this philosophy, inhibiting intimacy and curbing sexual expression. Somehow, children come first, our needs come second, and sex winds up last on our agenda. The desire to be good parental role models can lead us to limit or closet our own sexual behavior for fear that we'll set some sort of bad example.

You need confidence and self-awareness to reject these messages and proudly embrace your sexuality. You also need self-acceptance. Nurturing sexual self-esteem is an ongoing process, and you're bound to hit some bumps in the road. When you're feeling negative about yourself, your body, or your sexuality, just look at what's fueling these feelings and keep in mind that they'll pass. After all, every time you assert your right to be sexual—whether you're buying a tight new dress that highlights your womanly figure or hiring a baby-sitter so you can enjoy a sensuous afternoon masturbating—you'll reap the undeniable rewards.

SELF-LOVE

E'D be happy to put our cards on the table and tell you just what we think about masturbation . . . but then we'd have to take our hands out from under the sheets! Few topics inspire our personal gratitude or stimulate our inner cheerleaders as much as as masturbation. What's to celebrate? So many things: Masturbation is fun, easy, relaxing, pleasurable, and available to individuals of all ages, sex styles, and abilities—it's even free! Masturbation is a crucial component of any satisfying sex life, and an unparalleled way to honor and express your sexuality from cradle to grave.

My satisfaction comes from my willingness to take good care of my own sexual needs rather than let my desires fall by the wayside.

WHY DO IT

If you've never masturbated, you may not be sure how to go about it. Take heart—there are some excellent guidebooks written especially for women which offer detailed instructions and encouragement (look in the Resources section, page 340, for information on Lonnie Barbach's *For Yourself* and Betty Dodson's *Sex for One*). Even if you

The Many Ways to Masturbate

With water: bathtub faucets, shower massagers, hot-tub jets

With vibrators: clitoral, insertable, hands-free, waterproof

With dildos: anal plugs, vaginal dildos, produce, strap-ons

With oil: anoint your erogenous zones and be a sacred priestess of love

On the sly: pressed up against the washing machine, riding a motorcycle, climbing a pole, rubbing against the seam of your tightest jeans

Quietly: get under the covers and breathe softly

Loudly: breathe deeply, moan, don't hold back

With Kegels: contracting and releasing your pelvic muscles will enhance arousal

With a lover: I'll do you if you do me

Any way you want!

already enjoy masturbation, you may not have thought much about why it's such a delightful form of sexual expression. Read our list of just a few of masturbation's many benefits and you may develop new insights and ideas.

It Boosts Your Sexual Energy

When your time, energy, and personal space are limited, your libido usually disappears. It's not that you wouldn't *like* to feel the pulsing, tingling thrill of good old-fashioned arousal, you just can't exactly be bothered to pursue it. But with sex, nothing succeeds like excess. The more sexual pleasure you experience, the more you're motivated to have. Masturbation can be a great way to jump-start your stalled sex drive because it's unconstrained. You don't have to coordinate desire with a partner or contend with performance anxiety; simply go at your own pace and focus on what feels good.

It Teaches You About Your Own Responses

We aren't born knowing what pleases us sexually, and chances are you've gotten to a relatively ripe age without knowing every possible quirk of your sexual responses. Masturbation is a brilliant way to explore your genital anatomy and sensual preferences. Many girls and women have their first orgasms, multiple orgasms, or G-spot orgasms from masturbation. Unrestricted by the "rules" and expectations that dog partner sex, you can intensify your own arousal through techniques such as deep breathing, flexing and releasing your pelvic muscles, moving your hips, stopping and starting stimulation, and building tension. Think of all the time you've probably put into activities like perfecting your cheesecake recipe or coming up with a thoughtful handmade holiday craft—don't you deserve at least that much time to discover just how much sexual pleasure you're capable of having?

> I used to masturbate in the same way, always getting very rigid, taking short breaths, and cramping up. A friend told me to try taking deep breaths while approaching orgasm, and I was shocked at a) how hard it was to give up my tried-and-true method and b) how strongly I felt that orgasm to the tips of my toes when I did breathe into it!

It Allows You to Fantasize Freely

Exploring your fantasies during partner sex may seem awkward if you believe that your attention should be focused on the matter at hand. Masturbation is a powerful tool for mental, as well as physical, self-exploration. On your own, with nobody else present to inhibit or censor you, you can let your fancy wander. Determining what thoughts, feelings, or images stimulate your desire is just as crucial to a fulfilling sex life as determining what kind of touch stimulates your clitoris. Masturbation allows you to explore both in tandem.

It Feels Good

If masturbation *doesn't* feel good to you, we suggest you review the information on the masturbation taboo below. Many of us have been raised to believe that masturbation is an immature, self-polluting, inappropriate form of behavior, and it can be difficult to shove these negative messages aside long enough to access the pure and simple pleasure of touching yourself. Trust us, you did it as a tiny baby, and you can do it again.

It's Good for You

We bet you don't exercise as much as you feel you should. And even though you clip all those nutritious recipes, we doubt you're adhering to the healthy diet you resolve to follow every January first. Well, take heart, masturbation is an activity that doesn't force you to choose between looking good and feeling good. Masturbation is a form of exercise: It increases blood and oxygen flow to your genitals, strengthens your pelvic muscles, and serves as a mild cardiovascular workout (ankle weights are optional). Like all exercise, it relieves stress, releases endorphins, and promotes a general sense of health and well-being.

It's Creative

Masturbation has the power to renew, refresh, invigorate, and heal largely because it's a creative act. As parents, we get so little private time in which to gather our thoughts and marshal our resources that we tend to compensate by seeking refreshment through consumption; we take our breaks by having a cigarette, drinking a latte, eating some chocolate, or shopping for treats. But masturbation isn't about consumption; it's about creation. It blends the soul-satisfying joys of privacy and erotic self-expression, leaving you more energized and exhilarated after the fact than when you started.

> Since I'm not partnered, I masturbate whenever it doesn't interfere with child raising—like when my son is watching TV. It gives me some crucial time all to myself.

You Can Share It with a Loved One

If the above reasons sound just a wee bit too self-serving, keep in mind that all the information you glean about your sexual preferences, responses, and stamina will be of great interest to your partners. One of the all-time best ways to learn how you and a partner can please each other is to masturbate together.

> We masturbate, alone and together, more often than we have intercourse. Sometimes we just want to come. Enjoying my own body has really helped me to enjoy my partner's body also.

HISTORY OF A TABOO

By now you may be thinking, Gosh, if masturbation's so swell, why does everybody treat it like one great big sniggering joke? We've inherited a grab bag of religious and cultural beliefs about masturbation that are relentlessly negative. In the Western world, our attitudes about sexuality are rooted in Judeo-Christian and Greek philosophy and grafted onto the medical "wisdom" of the day. Here's a brief survey of masturbation's checkered career:

It Ain't Necessarily So

The Old Testament writers emphasized procreative sex as the only acceptable form of sexual expression for the ancient Israelites, both because population growth was their only means of expanding social and political power and because the Israelites used dietary and sexual prohibitions to symbolically distinguish themselves from surrounding cultures (in which cult prostitution and homosexuality were common). Many modern-day assumptions about sexual morality derive from biblical stories taken out of context or, in some cases, completely misinterpreted: The story of Onan, who "spilled his seed upon the ground" and was struck dead for this sin, is popularly believed to be a story about masturbation (which explains the derivation of the word "onanism"). In fact, it's a story about how he chose the withdrawal method of birth control when tradition dictated that he should impregnate his dead brother's widow. Although religious teachings may leave you with the vague sense that the Bible says masturbation is wrong, the Bible actually has nothing to say on the subject.

Woodsman, Spare That Seed!

So where does Greek philosophy come in? As far back as the fifth century B.C., Hippocrates was writing that semen is a precious, finite fluid, and that depleting this valuable substance would sap a man's strength. The idea that semen is an almost magically potent fluid that shouldn't be squandered is found around the world. Chinese Taoist philosophy holds that women's yin energy is inexhaustible, but men's yang energy is a river that can all too easily run dry (hence, male Taoist sexual techniques focus on achieving orgasm without ejaculation).

This economic metaphor was taken to new extremes in the mid–nineteenth century, when the Swiss doctor Samuel Tissot's 1758 tract, *Onanism: Treatise on the Diseases Produced by Masturbation*, was first published in English. Tissot railed against the debilitating effects of masturbation, which he felt leeched women and men alike of vital life force. Although women clearly didn't have to worry about wasting a limited allotment of semen, masturbation nonetheless rendered them vulnerable to losing their minds and being driven to a uterine fury "which deprives them at once of modesty and reason and puts them on the level of the lewdest brutes, until a despairing death snatches them away from pain and infamy."[1]

"The Most Degrading Act That a Human Being Can Commit"[2]

Throughout the nineteenth century, masturbation was viewed as a dangerous activity that resulted in all manner of ill health, from acne to dementia. Basically, any disease of unknown origin was blamed on "the solitary vice," and all the scare stories you've ever heard about masturbation's terrible side effects (hairy palms, blindness, etc.) probably date back to this era. An entire industry grew up around preventing young boys and girls from playing with themselves. Bondage belts, mittens, and dire injunctions to keep hands outside the covers were the milder forms of treatment. Spiked penile rings (designed to inhibit erections) and clitoridectomy were among the more horrifying treatments; the last clitoridectomy in the U.S. intended to "cure" masturbation was perpetrated on a five-year-old in 1948.[3]

Damned with Faint Praise

By the twentieth century, masturbation lost its notoriety as a life-threatening hobby. Americans gleaned the message from Sigmund Freud and sexologist Havelock Ellis that to suppress sexual desires was potentially more dangerous than to express them. Freud's theory that all humans pass through a variety of stages on the road to sexual maturity (oral, anal, narcissistic) simultaneously removed masturbation from the category of *unnatural* activities and deposited it neatly in the category of *immature* activities. Despite the fact that every sex researcher from Alfred Kinsey on has hammered home the fact that the vast majority of people masturbate, and despite the fact that sex educators practically get down on their knees and plead with one and all to explore its many benefits, to this day countless people still consider masturbation to be at best a childish activity.

THE LOVE OF A LIFETIME

Even if you've studied up on the history of the taboo, you may remain somewhat guilt-ridden about masturbating. Most folks who are embarrassed, touchy, or sheepish about masturbating are under the thrall of the most tenacious stereotype of all: that masturbation isn't really sex.

Maybe you think sex doesn't count unless two people are present. Maybe you think masturbation is acceptable only if you're doing field work to report your findings to your lover. Maybe you think it's somewhat shameful to touch your very own genitals just for the fun of it, to stroke your very own skin and admire how smooth and silky it feels beneath your fingers. Please make every effort to address these feelings head on, and in the immortal words of one of Cathy's favorite soap-opera characters, "feel it, deal with it, get over it!"[4]

If you're feeling sexual excitement, stimulating your genitals, arousing your senses, and striving for the delicious release of orgasm, you *are* having sex. It doesn't matter if there's nobody, one lover, two lovers, or a crowd of spectators in the room with you (the crowd of spectators *is* an excellent fantasy enhancer). Take a tip from your young children and let yourself marvel and delight in how interesting, amazing, and stimulating your body truly is. Masturbation is a lifelong pleasure, and you shouldn't deny yourself this pleasure at any age. You'll masturbate as a baby, as a teenager, as an adult, as a gorgeous old woman. Your partner sex life will have its ups and downs, and lovers will come and go. Through it all, masturbation keeps you in touch with your own innate eroticism. Enjoy.

THE EBB AND FLOW OF DESIRE

DEFINING OUR TERMS

YOU can be intimately acquainted with your sexual anatomy and responses, utterly comfortable with your body, and an exquisitely skilled communicator, but if you don't have desire, you won't want to have sex. Desire is the alchemist's stone that transforms the raw matter of reproductive biology into the glittering gold of sexual expression (and inspires lyrical language in even the most pragmatic sex writers!). Throughout this book, we use terms such as "sex drive" or "libido" to describe a basic physiological ready-willing-and-ableness, but we use the term "desire" to point to the ineffable spark of eroticism that makes sex so—well—desirable. Desire is the essential component to a satisfying sexuality, yet it can be so unpredictable and complicated. And well it should be! Desire brings into play your anatomy and biochemistry, certainly, but also your memories, fantasies, life experience, and cultural beliefs—everything that makes you the unpredictable and complicated woman you are. In this chapter, we'll look at the various forces influencing desire and suggest ways to identify and appreciate your own unique patterns.

DESIRE AND CULTURE

Your expectations and understanding of sexual desire are inevitably shaped by the world around you. Sure, sexual impulses are perfectly natural, but the way we think and feel about them is profoundly influenced by culture.

The More Things Change . . .

Don't be surprised if you experience a certain amount of ambivalence about exploring your own sexual yearnings. After all, you are challenging millennia of cultural conditioning simply by asserting your entitlement to sexual desire. You're familiar with the expression "The more things change, the more they stay the same"? For thousands of years, cultural attitudes around female desire have seesawed between "Women are insatiable, lusty devils whose sexual appetites must be controlled" and "Women are innocent, chaste angels who must be protected from men's sexual appetites." In trying to control the means of reproduction, male-dominated societies through the ages have established restrictions on women's bodies—including the highly effective restriction of telling women what is appropriate for them to think or feel about sex. So, twenty-first-century women still grow up believing that men want sex, women want romance, or that women have lower sex drives than men. Just because you might be able to find examples in your own life that seem to support these assertions doesn't mean they reflect biological truths. The last thing a fish is likely to notice is water, and we all—women and men alike—are swimming in the same sea of cultural expectations. Furthermore, sex is a much riskier proposition for women than for men. As one primatologist points out:

> It seems premature to attribute the relative lack of female interest in sexual variety to women's biological nature alone in the face of overwhelming evidence that women are consistently beaten for promiscuity and adultery. If female sexuality is muted compared to that of men, then why must men the world over go to extreme lengths to control and contain it?[1]

Consider what a woman risks by expressing herself sexually: Heterosexual women risk pregnancy and disease. Women of all sexualities risk being dismissed or attacked as sluts, nymphomaniacs, or bad mothers if they so much as display interest in, let alone pursue, sexual pleasure. Women make up the overwhelming majority of sexual assault victims. Given this social backdrop, it's a testament to the power and tenacity of women's desire that so many of us find a way to embrace, enact, and celebrate our eroticism.

Medical Models

The first generation of modern sex therapists and educators in the 1960s, heirs to the work of Alfred Kinsey and Masters and Johnson, generally believed that inhibition and ignorance were the only impediments to a satisfying sex life. Kinsey's documentation of the varieties of sexual behavior expanded the definitions of sexual normalcy, while Masters and Johnson's research on the physiology of sexual response gave a clinical stamp of approval to orgasms for both women and men. In the first flush of the new dawn of sexology, many therapists were understandably confident that, given accurate information about sexual anatomy and response, a few sensate focus exercises, and encouragement that sex is normal and healthy, any individual could walk into the sunset of orgasmic fulfillment. Indeed, many could and still do—as former vibrator saleswomen, we can vouch for the power of simple information (most women need clitoral stimulation to reach orgasm) and encouragement (there's nothing *wrong* with needing clitoral stimulation to reach orgasm) to transform an individual's experience of sex.

However, man can't live by bread alone, and woman can't experience sexual pleasure from clitoral stimulation alone. If sexual satisfaction were simply a matter of locating the right buttons to twiddle, sex wouldn't capture our imagination, tug at our heartstrings, and stimulate our mind the way it does. Basic anatomical information is not enough to guarantee sexual pleasure. People need to desire sex to enjoy having sex. By the late 1970s, sex therapists had to expand their nuts-and-bolts approach to include issues of desire. Sex therapist Helen Singer Kaplan amended the sexual response cycle proposed by Masters and Johnson (excitement, plateau, orgasm, and resolution) to include desire as a necessary prerequisite to excitement and orgasm, and her model (desire, excitement, orgasm) has been widely followed ever since.

Twenty years ago, sex professionals broke away from the notion that sex is solely a matter of biological responses and acknowledged the power and primacy of desire. Yet in recent years, the pendulum has swung back toward physiology as the be-all and end-all of sexual satisfaction, taking desire right along with it. The concept of desire has been medicalized to such an extent that a list of so-called desire disorders are now clinically categorized as sexual dysfunctions in the DSM IV (the *Diagnostic and Statistical Manual of Mental Disorders*). If you, dear reader, are experiencing difficulty with arousal or orgasm, or have sexual urges less often than is decreed "normal," you have a medically treatable condition. And you better believe that drug companies are lining up to treat you with Viagra-style products that work to increase blood flow to the genitals or to increase vaginal lubrication. In 1999, *The Journal of the American Medical Association* published a study reporting that 43 percent of American women experience sexual dysfunction (lack of interest in sex being most commonly reported). Both the authors of this study just happened to be paid consultants to Pfizer, the company raking in big bucks on Viagra.[2]

So how did desire become a medically treated condition? Probably because of our culture's deep-seated discomfort with sex. Sure, popular magazines, advice columns, and TV shows are filled with tips on how to make your sex life bigger, harder, hotter, and simultaneously better than but as normal as that of the folks next door. But the all-American preference is always for quick-fix solutions at the expense of any thoughtful, potentially discomfiting examination of what actually turns us on and why. Ultimately, designing ways to keep penises erect and vaginas supple and well lubed takes less time than reevaluating the social forces that conspire against authentic expressions of eroticism. Instead, we conflate sexual desire and sexual function as engineering problems that can be resolved with mechanical solutions. This approach is a gold mine for modern-day snake-oil salesmen, such as the doctor who promotes a vaginal cream that "basically eliminates the need for foreplay" and enhances "sexual response in three to four minutes."[3] Somewhere along the line, the sexual reflexes of a fourteen-year-old boy became our society's normative model for human sexual response.

The fact is, desire involves so much more than physical responsiveness. Your genitals can be displaying every sign of physical arousal, but that doesn't mean you're any more interested in sex than is a man who gets an erection during a rectal exam. Throughout this book, we discuss ways to enhance your physical responses — blood flow to the genitals is indeed conducive to arousal, and ample lubrication is indeed essential to pleasurable penetration. But, and this is a big but, you can't separate your genitals from the rest of your body and mind — and why would you want to?

A 1994 study by University of Amsterdam psychologist Ellen T. M. Laan is revealing on the distinction between physiological and subjective experiences of arousal. She showed the forty-seven women in her study group two different explicit videos — one a generic mainstream porn video, and the other a video by feminist filmmaker Candida Royalle, which depicted a sexual encounter that the actress clearly enjoyed. The women's physiological responses to both videos were the same — increased genital blood flow and lubrication — but they reported finding the Candida Royalle video highly arousing and the mainstream video an annoying turnoff. In other words, the enjoyable video boosted their desire, and the other video did not, despite the knee-jerk physiological responses. Context is everything. Of course, the study didn't look at the ways in which women might be culturally conditioned to enjoy — or be willing to admit enjoying — only certain kinds of erotic imagery. There are plenty of women who might report as much arousal from hard-core "wall-to-wall" porn as men — but that's a separate issue. The issue for this researcher boils down to one practical point: Just because a woman is wet doesn't mean she's ready.[4] We're willing to bet you've had experience with this phenomenon yourself.

The trouble with the medical model of desire and arousal is that it establishes penis/vagina intercourse as the only acceptable game in town and folks with firm, youthful, well-oiled genitals as the only acceptable players. Many sex educators and therapists are tearing out their hair over Viagra. Sex educators used to be able to counsel people that growing older meant growing wiser, that slower responses or less reliable erections could open up a whole new world of erotic experimentation in which the goal shifted from pure performance to pure pleasure. It's difficult to hear the voices challenging the cult of intercourse over the din of all that erection construction.

Don't get us wrong: Penetration is nifty. And truth be told, as women who came of age in the 1970s, we have friendly feelings toward recreational drugs and would even be curious to try Viagra once or twice. Certainly, if age and disease cause vascular problems that impede genital arousal, we'd never argue with a person's right to explore medical treatment. But an adult's experience of sex is supposed to *evolve* over the years. That's the beauty of it. As you age, your physical abilities change—maybe even deteriorate in some ways—but your emotional life gains depth, your imagination becomes bolder, your sense of self becomes stronger, and you have the capacity to access and enact sexual desires that the three-minute-orgasm contingent would, at the very least, never have time for. How's a grown woman supposed to sustain her sexual appetite over a lifetime if dreary, wham-bam adolescent sexual intercourse is the only item on the menu for decades? The "intercourse or bust" model of sexual desire doesn't exclude only same-sex couples, it excludes everyone who enjoys a richer, more varied palette of sensual pleasures.

As you make your way through a sexual lifetime, cultural attitudes about what it means to be a woman and a mother are bound to influence or even inhibit how you express yourself sexually. Let your experience be your teacher, let your desires be your guide, and keep in mind that both of these will be in constant flux throughout your life. Sometimes you'll crave a three-minute orgasm, sometimes you'll orchestrate a three-hour sensual symphony, and sometimes you'll want no genital activity at all. What you yearn for today won't necessarily be what you yearn for tomorrow, but each and every one of your desires has something to teach you about who you are and who you're becoming.

DESIRE AND YOUR BODY

The current emphasis on the physiology of desire also reflects a recent surge of research into the role hormones play on human behavior. Hormones are substances produced in the tissues of one part of the body which travel to other parts of the body and stimulate activity there. (For instance, estrogen produced by the ovaries during the first half of your menstrual cycle prompts your cervix to produce mucus and your uterine lining to plump up.) The hormones that play a big role in a woman's reproductive life—estrogen, testosterone, progesterone, oxytocin, prolactin—also have an impact on her sexual experiences. All these hormones are present in both men and women; however, women have up to ten times more estrogen than men during their reproductive years, and men have over ten times more testosterone than women. Therefore, when research is done on the links between estrogen, testosterone, and libido, these studies are often interpreted to explain desire differences between women and men.

Even if you've read very little on the subject, you've almost certainly picked up the idea that testosterone is the hormone of lust and aggression. Some researchers believe that testosterone levels are the primary determinant of how libidinous you will be and distinguish between "low T" and "high T" individuals. According to this model, your biochemistry—specifically, your body's testosterone levels—predisposes you for either a low or high sex drive. Since men, by definition, have higher levels of testosterone than women, presto: There's your explanation for the "fact" that "women have lower sex drives than men."

But perhaps you've also picked up the idea that estrogen plays a role in women's libido. Or maybe you've noticed a fairly regular rise and fall in your own interest in sex over the course of your menstrual cycle. There are studies that suggest that, all other factors being equal, women tend to experience an increase in libido right before ovulation, when their estrogen levels are highest. There's some evidence that, to the extent that testosterone boosts libido in women, this phenomenon occurs only because proteins that would normally bind to and interfere with estrogen bind to testosterone instead, thereby freeing estrogen to go about its inspirational business.[5] Bear in mind that hormone research is in its infancy; hormones were isolated less than a hundred years ago, and scientific understanding of how they operate is still evolving, theories overturning on a regular basis.

Throughout this book, we'll pay all due respect to the powerful influence hormonal fluctuations can have on your state of mind, emotions, body, and sex life. Pay attention to the ways in which your own levels of energy and desire may rise and fall cyclically. Hormones fluctuate in daily, monthly, seasonal, and situational cycles which researchers are only beginning to identify—for instance, studies of testosterone levels in men show that they peak in the morning and dip in the late afternoon; increase in the autumn; and decrease during times of stress. Women are familiar with the impact of hormones during physiological life changes such as puberty, pregnancy, breast-feeding, and menopause. If you are a biological mother, your sex life may well have been affected by the well-being that often results from increased estrogen levels during pregnancy, and the fatigue that results from the dramatic decrease in estrogen postpartum.

> The biggest challenge is definitely lack of desire due to physical tiredness and the hormonal changes resulting from on-demand breast-feeding. Before I was pregnant, my desire was directly affected by my fertility cycle, and now that I am not ovulating, things are different.

> GIVE ME ESTROGEN! I would like to WANT sex again, not just want to make my husband happy.

Hormones will affect you sexually whether they're manufactured in your body or prescribed. If you are postmenopausal or combating long-term depression, you may find that taking testosterone reinvigorates a waning sexual appetite.

Chronic depression over the last year and changing medications twice (I had been stabilized before on Prozac, which didn't work anymore after two years) completely destroyed any vestige of a sex drive. I'm now taking two grains of testosterone daily to see if I can get it back!

If you use contraceptives containing progesterone (birth-control pills, Depo-Provera, Norplant), you may experience a sexually depressing effect.

The first few weeks postpartum were a sexual awakening of sorts because it was the first time in my menstruating life that I wasn't on some sort of birth control or hormone, and wow did I feel great. I would have had sex five times a day if my husband had wanted to. But then, sadly, came the inevitable, and after the Depo shot I haven't felt like having sex more than once a week.

While we encourage you to investigate the impact of hormones on your sexual well-being, we'd also urge you not to assign an exaggerated power to these biochemical messengers. Physiology is only one of the many factors that affect how sexually desirous — and desirable — you feel. Stress, self-esteem, depression, body image, fatigue, being single, being partnered, and access to time, space, and privacy all impact your libido. Again, context is everything.

My sex drive increased after the birth of my first child. I felt empowered by the birth process and proud of the great job I was doing raising my boy. I was also less tolerant of nonsense in my life. All these things led to greater self-esteem, therefore greater sex drive.

DESIRE ESSENTIALS

I do not have the desire to have sex. I really wish that I could. I really miss that feeling.

I have a newfound zest for sex. I have no idea why, or how it came about. I just hope that it stays!

Like the women quoted above, you may think of desire as a mysterious force outside your control. Weeks or even months can pass without your thinking much about sex, then one sunny afternoon you catch sight of a cute butt on the bus and it all comes rushing back to you. Desire may feel like a random gift from fickle gods, but it's actually more like the lottery ticket in this old joke: A man gets on his knees day after day, always with the same prayer, "God, please let me win the lottery, just let me win the lottery." Finally, after months of this routine, he's answered one day by a voice from the clouds saying, "Abe, meet me halfway—buy a lottery ticket!"

Desire Motivators

As any aspiring actor could tell you, you've got to know your motivation. When you're yearning for sex, what is it that you're yearning for? If you understand what you get out of sex, you'll be in a better position to figure out what inspires your desire. And since we aren't all motivated by the same reasons, each individual in a relationship should understand what sex means to the other. For most folks, motivation tends to fall into the following categories, none of which are mutually exclusive, and most of which are equally applicable to solo or partner sex.

Pleasure: Because it feels good. Good sex grounds us in our bodies, places us in the moment, and suffuses us with a sense of well-being. The physical release of orgasm is nothing to sneeze at, either.

Sensuality: Because it involves physical touch. When we're aroused, our entire body is exquisitely sensitive to tactile stimulation. For many people, a sexual encounter is one of their only opportunities to enjoy flesh-to-flesh contact with another adult.

Validation: Because it's an ego boost—who doesn't enjoy reveling in her body's potential for pleasure during masturbation, or feeling desired, appreciated, and catered to during partner sex? The flip side is that it's a great way to express desire and appreciation for someone else.

Relationship: Because it creates an emotional connection. When you're engaged in a mutually pleasurable sexual encounter, you can enjoy a deeply satisfying sense of harmony.

Transcendence: Because it takes you out of yourself. You can simultaneously experience total self-awareness and a total lack of self-consciousness.

Self-expression: Because it integrates your body, mind, emotions, fantasies, past, present, and future in a way that is utterly unique.

Our point is, you're not going to feel desire unless you *allow* yourself to feel it. We like to conceive of desire as an instinctual passion that wells up and sweeps away all obstacles in its path. Sometimes—particularly in the first flush of a new romance—desire does feel like a force of nature. However, most of the time we aren't able to access our oh-so-primal urges unless our hearts and minds are in it, and our hearts and minds are designed to generate inhibitors. Motherhood is a mother lode of situational inhibitors in and of itself. But don't despair—becoming conscious of common obstacles to desire is the first step toward making an end run around them. If you can satisfy all of the following prerequisites, you'll be well on your way to hitting your own erotic jackpot.

You Have to Feel That Sex Is Worthwhile

To want to be sexual, you have to believe that sex is a worthwhile activity. We get conflicting messages in our society: On one hand, sex is treated like an important status symbol ("My sex life is bigger and better than the Joneses'."), and on the other, it's treated like a waste of time ("Those shiftless Joneses are never going to get ahead if they spend all their time in the sack."). Either way, sex is rarely presented as a valuable means of self-expression. When you're a busy mother, it's easy to view sex as a luxury that demands time, energy, and resources you don't have to spare. But feeling temporarily unable to get motivated about sex is different from feeling that sex is fundamentally frivolous. *Eroticism is a necessity.* Whenever you feel the surge of sexual desire, you're experiencing connection: a connection of body and mind; a connection to your own emotions, drives, and fantasies; a connection to other people; and a connection to something outside yourself. If you acknowledge sex as intrinsically meaningful, you'll always be receptive to the tug of desire.

You Have to Feel That You Deserve Sexual Pleasure

Many of us struggle with internalized scripts that say we're not entitled to sexual pleasure. It's difficult to muster up much desire if you feel fundamentally unworthy. Some women feel ashamed of their sexual inexperience, while others feel equally ashamed of their experience.

> I need to hold on to the idea that I deserve to be held, loved, appreciated, kissed, hugged, and all that. Here in the South, the pervasive attitude toward single moms is "You made your bed, now lie in it." On bad days, it is easy to adopt that attitude myself. I remind myself that I am twenty-three and beautiful, and just as worthy of love as before my "moral downfall."

Mothers face particular pressure to sublimate all personal urges and focus on developing a purely selfless persona.

> There is a certain amount of self-involved vanity which goes hand in hand with feeling sexual. Now that I've got children, I've become so fucking Mother Teresa that getting off is damn near impossible.

Yes, sex is deeply selfish. Sexual self-expression is selfish just as creative self-expression is selfish. Do you really want to go through life without either? Feeling that you're not entitled to be sexual is like feeling you're not entitled to be fully human. Why not choose to explore and express every aspect of yourself?

You Have to Feel Desirable

Concerns about physical appearance often derail women's desire. It's common for women to tell themselves that they *will* feel perfectly entitled to sexual pleasure as soon as they make themselves presentable—the "If I just lose five pounds, I'll feel more like having sex" syndrome.

> Body image makes all the difference between whether I want sex or not. I know it sounds weak, but if I don't feel sexy then I don't wanna have sex.

Needless to say, attitude is everything. If you're dealing with a deep sense of dissatisfaction with yourself, you won't feel desirable for long, even if you're showered with constant praise. Plenty of beautiful women are too insecure to be relaxed about sex, and plenty of ordinary-looking women are secure in their appeal. Feeling desirable is a matter of confidence and perspective. Most of us find it easiest to access desire when we're feeling healthy, strong, and in harmony with our bodies.

> My biggest turn-on is nothing external but rather when I've been treating myself right and feel good in my body.

When you're partnered, you often need to feel desired by your partner. It's usually more important to feel that the person who's most intimate with you finds you desirable than to get hit on at a party (not that *that* isn't nice too). Of course, sometimes feeling desirable is inextricable from feeling desire. If your erotic appetites and imagination aren't being stimulated by your environment, they may decline.

> I recently moved to a more repressed town, and I don't think of anyone here in a very sexual manner (except my partner). I find that there just seem to be fewer people I find attractive, which somehow reduces my own interest in sex.

You Have to Have Your Own Space

Many of us think of sex as a subcategory of relationships, as something we do with or for a partner. But you're a sexual being even if you never have sex with another person in your life. You're much more likely to access your truest desires if you have private time and space to explore what makes you tick erotically.

> I need enough time to myself to let my sexuality flourish, rather than clear-cutting it to make room for other people's needs and demands.

> What would satisfy me? A quiet room ALONE. Two words: SHOWER MASSAGER.

You Have to Feel That Your Desires Deserve Respect

Feeling motivated sexually is difficult if you don't expect to get what you want out of the encounter. Too often, we go through our lives as sexual adults in reactive mode: soliciting, responding to, or accommodating our partners' desires. Mothers—who are expected to thrive in the role of solicitous, responsive, accommodating caretaker—have to make an extra effort to assert their own erotic needs. You may have a hard time naming your own desires because they seem so unmaternal.

> When I do feel like changing our routine sex, the role of sex initiator still feels incompatible with the role of mummy. I think my biggest challenge is to try and make the two roles exist together. Can mums be sexy?

Or you may find that becoming a mother has both boosted your self-esteem and reduced your tolerance for pussyfooting around!

> I have a much easier time with my sexuality now that I am a mom. I feel stronger and am more able to see that my needs are met. I am also more honest about when I do or do not want to have sex.

You may have no trouble accepting your theoretical right to be sexual but a harder time accepting your right to do the things you want to do. If you feel that your sexual desires are somehow ridiculous, kinky, or otherwise "abnormal," you're likely to do what you can to suppress them, which means your interest in any kind of sex will fade. Throughout this book, we emphasize the utter futility of distinguishing between "normal" and "abnormal" sexual desires. After all, the only norm you can count on is that any sexual activity you could come up with has been considered normal at some time and place in history, and equally abnormal at some other time and place. However, if you're interested in exploring certain fantasies or activities and your partner is not, you'll need to come up with an explicit mutual compromise to avoid short-circuiting your desire. See the Communication chapter (page 56) and the Desire Revisited chapter (page 197) for more on this subject.

You Have to Accept Contradictions

By now you may be thinking, Hey, wait a minute. I've actually been in relationships where my self-esteem was low, I had no personal space, and my desires weren't particularly catered to . . . but I couldn't get enough of the insensitive jerk who was my lover. Well, we did warn you that desire is complicated. If you appraise your sexual history honestly, you'll doubtless discover what psychotherapist Jack Morin has termed "the paradoxical perspective . . . that anything that inhibits arousal—including anxiety or guilt—can, under different circumstances, amplify it."[6] For sex to be desirable, there has to be something in it for you, so even if you've been in the classic "woman who loves too much" relationship, you probably were accessing important aspects of your sexual self. If you can tease out the individual components of every highly arousing situation and identify what Morin calls your "Core Erotic Theme," you have information you can use to channel your desires into new and healthier avenues of pleasure (his book, *The Erotic Mind*, is a particularly useful tool). Perhaps you repeatedly find yourself in situations of unrequited love because you get an erotic charge from sensations of longing and uncertainty, in which case you can work toward incorporating elements of anticipation and unpredictability into a relationship with a more reliable partner.

While we don't argue that sexual desires can make total losers ineffably desirable and total winners unaccountably unappealing, we are by no means implying that you should strive to repress your desires. For one thing, you simply can't do it, and for another, you have much more to gain if you take the risk of erotic self-exploration. Nor are we implying that some desires are automatically "inappropriate" for mothers, as the survey respondent below seems to feel.

> I'm not sure I like the fact that I don't really dig nice, sensual lovemaking and instead want the dirty "who's your daddy" sex. Maybe having a daughter and hoping to give her a healthy attitude about sex has made me wonder about my own. I'm sure this has a lot more to do with my pre-baby history.

If you bring consciousness to bear on what fuels your flame, you'll increase both your sexual pleasure and your self-knowledge. These are powerful examples to set for your children.

I'm able to separate my mother role from my lover role and let go of the hang-ups that one might think go along with parenting. By that I mean if my partner and I want to role-play a scene in which one of us is young and one is old, I can separate fantasy from reality, whereas if I thought there was any chance someone would hurt my kids, I would be one hell of a bitch to deal with.

LET IT FLOW

Probably the most common source of anxiety about desire is an anxiety of quantity — you've surely felt at some times in your life that you had too much sexual desire, and at others that you had too little. Well, Goldilocks, pull up a chair and eat as much porridge as you please. The truth is that however much desire you're feeling is probably just right for this time in your life. Everything you'll read in this book is an encouragement to be sexual, but to be sexual on your own terms. Keep in mind that sexual lust is just one aspect of an overall lust for life. Hormones ebb and flow, life situations change, but you are by definition a sexual being. You get to decide what that means to you.

> Sex is a part of who I am and not something I simply do. I remained myself and a sensual being just as much after kids as before.

COMMUNICATION

SE your words." We repeat this simple phrase constantly to young children as they learn to speak. We offer it up like a gift, knowing that words will help them move beyond frustrated tears to a place of comfort and understanding. And yet we who have mastered the art of language too often don't heed our own advice. We may not stomp our feet and throw tantrums, but we do the adult equivalent: We clam up when we're angry, hurt, frustrated, or just plain tired.

Good relationships—whether with lovers, friends, relatives, or children—are not possible without good communication. There's no denying that it's hard work; communication demands courage, empathy, and practice. When it comes to sexual communication, the challenges are even greater, largely because sex is a subject that has been off limits for most of our lives. But your success in sustaining an intimate relationship depends on your ability to both listen and express yourself effectively.

NOT TONIGHT, DEAR, THERE'S A BABY IN THE BED

Motherhood changes your life so profoundly that, particularly if you're in a long-term, coparenting relationship, your sex life can't possibly survive without clear, candid communication. Even if you and your partner see eye to eye on parenting decisions, you'll need to touch base on an ongoing basis about the impact these decisions have on your sex life. For example, you may both be philosophically committed to the importance of "family bed," but if one of you starts to resent the effect the little one's proximity is having on your sex life, you'll need to revisit the subject. How successfully you navigate potentially rocky terrain depends to some degree on how effectively you communicated before the baby was born, but you shouldn't feel limited by your past successes or failures. Many couples find that parenthood actually equips them with new tools that enable and enhance better sexual communication.

Growing Up

Let's face it, parenthood forces us to grow up. With a child's life hanging in the balance, we trade in our own childishness for responsibility and accountability. As this survey respondent so eloquently notes, many of the qualities required for good parenting also come in handy in the bedroom.

> To resolve sexual issues takes honesty, strength, flexibility, understanding, listening skills, and other attributes that are definitely important when being a parent.

> The day-to-day realities of parenting require a high level of communication, which makes for good practice when negotiating sexual concerns.

> Parenthood forced us to finally become really excellent communicators since we've had to settle so many conflicts over little and enormous things. A lot of sex issues between us have been resolved as a result of improved self-expression.

> Having to curb hotheadedness because there are children present leads some parents to adopt a more disciplined approach to communication.

> When we disagree now, the strongest effort is made to talk things out calmly and rationally with complete respect for the other's side of the argument. Emotions are controlled, shouting is nonexistent, and complications are smoothed over quickly (most of the time).

Finding Your Voice

Amid the cacophony of demands emanating from children and partners, many mothers learn how to speak up for themselves. This newfound assertiveness finds its way into the bedroom as well.

I'm bolder and more forward with what I want. As a mother I learned that so much of the attention was focused on the baby that if I didn't speak for myself, no one would.

I have stopped being a wimp because my happiness reflects directly onto my son's life. So if things are uncomfortable in our relationship (sexual or nonsexual issues), I have the motivation to stand up and speak out about it, instead of just shrugging it off. I find being a parent empowering.

We want to underscore the value of this self-advocacy, especially considering the cultural tendency to encourage passivity and submissiveness in women. The physical and emotional upheavals of motherhood can catch both you and your partner off guard. If you don't make a point of standing up for your desires, they'll all too easily get lost in the shuffle.

I am much more apt to say "do like this" or "let's try this" now than I ever was before. I feel so much more active. Being a mom has made me so courageous about a lot of things and this is just another. My husband has responded well even though getting used to it was shocking for him. He's been so much more supportive overall ever since I learned how to ask for things instead of waiting for him to give them to me.

Time Is Too Precious

Some parents explain that the frantic pace of their lives, coupled with the desire to maintain a peaceful environment for their children, forces them to deal with issues expediently.

I need constant communication. Even if it's too much at times, even if it just amounts to venting frustrations, it's completely necessary now. There is no time to waste being angry or having problems and not talking about them.

I think our communication has actually gotten better because we have more motivation for making sure our relationship thrives. We don't want bad vibes passed on to the baby.

Precisely because there is less time available to spend with a partner, some parents find that good communication enhances a long-awaited erotic encounter.

We have spent a lot more time talking about what we enjoy and what we would like to try than we did before the baby. We want to make the periods of time we have for sex the best they can be.

The Flip Side

We don't expect you to believe that parenthood has magically transformed every mother but you into an eloquent speaker whose every word is perfectly understood and whose every need is thereby fulfilled. Feeling exhausted and pressed for time and privacy can inhibit you from dealing with difficult issues at least as often as it inspires you to resolve them.

> My husband and I are both a little uneasy about talking directly about sex and our emotional relationship. The baby serves as an easy excuse not to confront issues.

> We are silent much more because we fear we will say something that may cause an argument and we both know we don't have time to fight.

Before the baby, you and your partner may have been able to intuit each other's thoughts, but your changing lives may now leave you somewhat out of sync.

> We used to think like one person, even finishing each other's sentences. Now we're on two different planets. The communication issues make it really difficult for me to feel intimate, and for me intimacy is a precursor to sex. He doesn't have this problem, but I know he feels unattractive and like I don't want to have sex with him.

Even if parenthood has taught us to grow up, to advocate for ourselves, and to make better use of our time, we may still be overwhelmed by the sheer number of issues that require discussion. When asked to name the most common challenges to their sex lives since becoming parents, our survey respondents most often cited lack of desire or desire discrepancies, body image, contraception and safer sex, conflicts over division of labor, sexual boredom, and difficulty negotiating sexual encounters. Take these examples:

- My husband doesn't understand my complete lack of desire.
- It is difficult with a new lover because of my poor self-image.
- It's hard for her to understand how tired I am.

- He's tired of me not being in the mood.
- He thinks I am not someone to be dating since I am a mom now.
- It has been difficult trying to explain why things have changed.
- He feels left out justifiably and I feel like I'm carrying the load on my own.
- I am afraid to tell my husband how little I care about sex.
- All he hears is me bitching.

All these frustrated women—and their partners—would benefit from applying a little more effort or a new approach to communication. Some of the issues implicit in these complaints (waning desire, poor body image) can't be resolved with a simple chat; we address these specific problems in more detail throughout this book. But every one of these issues is less likely to depress and demoralize if you can express your feelings and concerns effectively. Before we explore just how to communicate more effectively, let's examine the roots of our difficulty with talking about sex.

WHY WE KEEP OUR MOUTHS SHUT

Plenty of well-spoken people are speechless when it comes to sex. It may not appear that way at first blush—witness the talk-show host leering over sisters who sleep with each other's boyfriends, the lawyer eloquently prosecuting a sex offender, or a newspaper columnist making a case for porn's first-amendment rights. But listen closely to what's being said: You'll hear every emotion from out-and-out hysteria to clinical detachment, but no personal expressions of authentic sexual feeling. We see sexual imagery all around us, but when was the last time you told your partner everything about his or her body that turns you on? As a society, we are preoccupied with sex, but as individuals we are cowed by it. This disconnect between what we perceive and what we feel leaves many of us so confused that we are rendered mute when it comes to the subject of sex. How did we get this way?

Cultural Legacy of Sex-negativity

It's not easy to shrug off thousands of years worth of sex-negativity. We're all raised on a steady diet of stereotypes about sex: Nice girls don't have it, boys like sex and girls like romance, sex is either a reproductive necessity or a shameful pleasure. As a result, we live in a society of fairly ignorant and repressed sexual adults whose fascination with what has been hidden, forbidden, or denounced throughout their lives now drives a sex-obsessed economy. But this economy only reflects our collective checkered past and reveals the extent of our fundamental discomfort with sex. Although sex sells everything from cars to fast food to shampoo, you rarely see ads of any kind for sexual products (condoms, lubricants). Although TV shows and music videos depict kids dressing, acting, and looking mighty sexy, we balk at the idea of condom dispensers in schools. Sex rarely makes the news unless it topples a political figure or is the subject of an editorial on society's moral decay.

Where are the testimonials from individuals who have experienced firsthand the life-affirming, joyous qualities of sex? These women and men are out there, but given the jokes, threats, finger pointing, and condescension that would greet their testimonials, few have the combination of courage and thick skin it takes to stand up for sexual pleasure in our sex-negative culture. It's easier to keep quiet and, by default, perpetuate the notion that sex is something best not talked about.

Poor Sex Education

America's sexual dysfunction manifests itself most disturbingly in our inability to provide adequate sex education to our young people. Most of us received little more than a cursory lesson in reproductive biology during our youth; today's kids get bonus lectures in safer sex that contrast abstinence with dire alternatives (death, disease, despair). Kids are rarely taught about sexual responsibility, assertiveness, or technique, yet they are expected to mature into sexually fulfilled adults at an arbitrary age determined by their state, parents, or religion. The following quote underscores the fallacy of this notion, and the fact that learning to communicate about sex is a lifelong process.

> I'm thirty-eight and have been dating a bit. I swear, though, I feel like I'm an adolescent—I'm surprised at how much pressure there is to have sex, and how hard it is to speak up for myself and to stay clear about my boundaries.

No Role Models

Given that most of us were raised believing we *shouldn't* talk about sex, it's no wonder we find it a daunting task. Don't look to Hollywood for role modeling of sexual communication—when was the last time you saw TV or movie characters discuss contraception or pause a sex scene to say, "A little to the left, and not so fast!" Chances are your parents weren't exactly ideal role models, even if they had good intentions:

> My mother said she would be open to talking to me and my sister, yet she wasn't really. I never went to her because I could sense she was uncomfortable about it. I really hope to be easy for my daughters to talk to, so I

make a point of being there for my much younger sisters (nineteen, fifteen, and eleven) to talk to about sex and their relationships. I hope that by doing this I can be ready to talk to my own daughters.

This mom recognizes the value of modeling positive sexual communication. By participating in an open and honest dialogue about sex with the young people in her life, she is giving them the tools to do the same with future partners.

Lack of Sexual Self-awareness

Inadequate sex education affects sexual communication in another very fundamental way. If you are unfamiliar with your sexual anatomy or your own sexual responses, you will understandably have trouble telling a partner what pleases you sexually. Or if you have mistaken beliefs about what's sexually "normal," you may be too confused by or ashamed of your responses to discuss them. For example, we've talked to countless women frustrated by their inability to orgasm during intercourse. Many had no idea that the majority of women orgasm through clitoral stimulation — an area not typically stimulated during intercourse. Since girls are often not taught the correct names for their genitals, or are taught to regard them with distaste or disapproval, it's no surprise that they grown up into adults who aren't sure what an orgasm is or how to reach one.

If you could use a little Sex-ed 101, see the Resources section (page 340) for books and videos designed to help you better understand your sexuality. In addition, we recommend masturbation as the best way to learn about your sexual responses.

Language Barriers

Some people are unable to talk about sex because they're uncomfortable with sexual terminology. Perhaps you find words like "vagina" and "penis" too clinical, but words like "cunt" and "cock" too crass. Try to figure out which words you're uncomfortable with and why, and explain this to your partner. The two of you can choose to avoid certain words, make up new ones, or work on overcoming your aversion. Self-help books like *Talk Sexy to the One You Love* include lists of terms you can try. If you'd like to expand your comfort level with sexual terminology, try repeating certain words out loud by yourself when alone, which will make them more familiar and rob them of some of their awkwardness.

After my sister and I read [Eve Ensler's] *The Vagina Monologues*, we decided it was time to get over our shyness about anatomical terms. Now my sister will call me up and say, "Vagina, vagina, vagina" over the phone until we both start laughing.

Watch an erotic video or read some erotica in order to expose yourself to a range of sexually explicit language. Read up on the origin of the word as a way of finding something sexy about it—perhaps its etymology will inspire you. For example, "dildo" comes from the Italian *"diletto,"* which means delight. Now you have the option of using the sexy Italian version or merely delighting in the original!

Our Histories

Each of us brings our entire past to every relationship. Our unique approach to sexual relationships is shaped by a lifetime of social conditioning, religious upbringing, family values, and past sexual experiences. Sharing information about your past with your partner gives you both a valuable context for the issues that may arise in your sex life. For example, if this mom communicates about her past sexual abuse, she can provide her partner with crucial insights into how it affects her experience of intimacy and parenting.

> Before I was a mom, I was in deep denial about my past, but becoming a mother has put me face-to-face with my demons. Also, being the mother of a little girl has brought up a lot—I aspire to help her be strong and find her own voice so she isn't victimized as I was.

Fear

Perhaps the most frequently cited reason for poor sexual communication is fear. We're afraid of hurting, insulting, threatening, or displeasing a partner. We're afraid of embarrassing ourselves or of being rejected.

> It's very hard for us to communicate about the problems we've been having with sex, as it seems one or both of us get our feelings hurt when we try.

> Discussing sex with a partner can absolutely inspire emotional reactions that neither of you enjoy. But if you don't take this risk, you'll never get beyond whatever stalemate you're stuck in. Communication is the only catalyst for change, and if you follow some of the basic techniques we present in the next section, you can transform any initial awkwardness and hurt feelings into a new and greater understanding.

SAY IT LOUD, SAY IT PROUD

When it comes to communication, a little effort and a lot of patience go a long way. Try some of these basic pointers to start an ongoing dialogue about sex.

Make Time

One of the biggest complaints voiced by mothers is lack of time. With every hour of the day accounted for, intangible tasks like communication fall by the wayside.

> The children require 110 percent of everything: our time, attention, thoughts, worries. Everything else is shoved way down on the list, including our interaction with each other.

> We definitely have less time to communicate, and because of this, our different communication styles are more of an issue — and source of tension. This is a far greater change than any specific sexual issue.

If your partner is your coparent, you probably do most of your communicating on the fly. You need to supplement these communiqués by setting aside time for quality conversations that cover a wide range of topics. Couples often find that until they air and resolve differences about nonsexual issues, they have little motivation to deal with sex.

> If there are issues that really need to be resolved, I can't put them aside and have sex with the person I am angry with/at odds with. Needless to say, my husband is not happy with this situation, and we are trying to find ways to not let this happen. I have to find ways to talk with him before we're in bed, and he has to see to it that issues are resolved before he puts the moves on me.

The flip side is that good communication about day-to-day topics paves the way for a more fulfilling sex life.

> We never put sex ahead of communication. Even a tiny unresolved issue can put a damper on the sexual fires. We usually talk about our day — issues, concerns, etc. — just after work or before sex. We find that if we are comfortable with our lives and each other that sex is so much more intimate.

> The most important thing about prioritizing sex is to keep talking with your partner about your needs. They may not get fulfilled that minute, but if I make my needs known, they can be fulfilled sooner rather than later!

Make Sex Talk a Priority

Just as you have to plan for sex, you have to plan to talk about sex. Whether you're embarking on a regimen to get more comfortable with sexual subject matter (see the following section) or you have specific issues you need to discuss, you'll benefit from advance planning. Pick a time that's convenient for both of you rather than cornering your partner into a surprise talk. "Honey, could we set aside some time to talk about our sex life?" will be a more effective way to start the dialogue than "We need to talk about sex now because I'm miserable."

If you are disappointed or frustrated by your sexual encounters, avoid venting your feelings in the heat of the moment. It's hard to be rational, empathetic, and focused when you're reeling from a failed sexual encounter or a sexual rejection. Wait a day or two and then raise the subject. However, be aware that while time can bring perspective, it can also bring complacency and denial—make sure you address any issues that still bother you, rather than trying to convince yourself that they aren't really that important.

When the time comes for your sex talk, don't stray from your topic. Avoid switching midstream into an argument about who should pick the kids up from school. There will be overlap, because issues in your everyday life affect your sex drive; just keep the conversation relevant to your sex life. If you do find that your bottom line is "I have no energy for sex because I'm chasing the baby all day," make that clear and ask for help.

Get Comfortable with Sex as a Subject Matter

If sex was as easy to talk about as the weather, many of our sexual communication issues would disappear. Can you imagine this idle remark over coffee: "I'm thinking today is a mutual masturbation day." Or how about this one: "Gee, I liked last night's oral sex, but I think tonight my G-spot needs a workout." Perhaps if we practiced talking about sex more, we wouldn't be so reluctant to bring up the subject. By regularly engaging in conversations about sex, you become more comfortable with the subject matter, and you get to learn about your partner's views. Your sex life needn't be the focus of each discussion; in fact, less threatening subjects are probably easier to start with. Here are a few suggestions for steering the subject toward sex:

- Comment on sex-related issues in the news
- Bring up a subject from a daytime talk show (almost all involve sex)
- Share amusing sex comments from your toddler
- Share sex histories
- Relate messages you received about sex as a child
- Hum the tune from a sexy song; ask your partner to name some sexy music
- Describe your favorite sex scene from a movie
- Read a sexual enhancement book and share your findings
- Look at some erotic art together
- Share a favorite fantasy
- Read erotica together

Know the Issues/Be Prepared

Getting what you want is so much easier when you know what you want. Shopping is a cinch when you've got a list, a visit to the doctor's office is more productive when you can describe your symptoms, and a raise can be negotiated more effectively when you know what you're worth. So before you approach any conversation about sex with your partner, think about what it is you want or need, imagine how your partner might feel, and be prepared with specific suggestions.

If you're feeling vague dissatisfaction with your sex life, you need to pin down the specific source of your unhappiness. If it's physical—perhaps you don't orgasm when or how you'd like—stop thinking of the difficulty as all your partner's fault. Take the time to figure out what gives you pleasure during masturbation and partner sex, and you'll be able to tell your partner what stimulation works best for you. If you're experiencing emotional dissatisfaction, start by identifying what's troubling you. If you're feeling ignored, taken for granted, or angry, come up with specific examples to illustrate how your partner is (and isn't) contributing to your dissatisfaction, and think about what steps you could each take to address it. It may help one or both of you to seek therapy to get to the root of your problems.

Be clear about your own desires, but try to see the situation from your partner's perspective. If you can explore both sides of an issue before you discuss it, you may get a jump start on the empathy that's a prerequisite to constructive communication. Sometimes resolving what has seemed like a major source of tension is very easy; for example, this woman's partner simply needed reassurance that her fatigue wasn't a personal rejection.

> It was initially hard for my husband to understand how tired I was and that sex was literally the last thing on my mind. I had to convince him that I was not rejecting him and that it was a passing phase.

Be Direct and Clear

Forget the fantasy that the perfect lover will intuit all your sexual needs and supply you with orgasms till dawn. A good lover knows how to observe a partner's reactions and ask what feels good, but he or she can't read minds. Give your partner a hand by clearly explaining your needs. Instead of saying "I want more foreplay," be as specific as you can: "If you could spend more time kissing me, massaging my thighs, and whispering in my ear, I'd have a lot more energy to take you on with."

Similarly, when you're in the throes of passion, don't rely solely on nonverbal communication to express your pleasure or displeasure. Not everyone is adept at reading body language (especially if they're concentrating on what they're doing!), so offer a few verbal cues such as "Oh, that feels great," or "Don't move an inch," or "It feels best when you stop and start." Give your partner some appreciated encouragement and you'll enjoy a more satisfying encounter.

Make sure to define your terms. To you, "I just don't feel much desire these days" might mean that you don't crave lengthy sex marathons, but to your partner, it might sound like "I just don't find you attractive anymore."

> Sometimes I need to make it clear to my partner that it is not that I don't want sex with him, it's just that it is hard to relax knowing that our daughter might crawl into the room at any time.

Give as much information as you can about your feelings, and try to provide context. Rather than rejecting a partner's request for sex outright, take the time to explain what's affecting your loss of libido, what sorts of things can boost your sex drive, and how you would like to proceed. You may reveal something from your sexual history or current experience that helps your partner understand your position. Ultimately, your goal is to clarify your issues in order to negotiate a solution.

Directness serves you well whether you're entering into a new sexual relationship or fine-tuning an existing one:

> Now that I'm a mom and single again, I don't want any relationship other than physical, and I communicate that very openly.

> We found we had to be much clearer because spontaneity is so much harder. For example, on a Saturday night I might say to my husband, "Honey, tomorrow morning when Ruby goes down for her morning nap we have GOT to have sex!" This kind of directness was not as necessary before we were parents.

Minimize the Negative

No one responds well to the verbal equivalent of a finger wagging, so avoid attacking or blaming your partner. The best way to do this is to use "I" statements to convey your feelings. For example, the statement "I feel pressured to have sex" is a natural opening to a discussion of the many sources of pressures in your life (yourself, your partner, or your life), but the statement "You're always pressuring me to have sex" lays all the blame at your partner's feet. Similarly, trade in the criticism for some helpful suggestions, and be sure to use positive reinforcement when your partner makes an effort. You might think she gives a lousy massage, but instead of blurting out "That feels terrible," pick up a massage book and a bottle of oil, then try this approach: "I love it when you touch me, so I thought we could try learning more about massage. Would you be up for trying out a few techniques?" Finally, eliminate those negative absolutes from your vocabulary. Rather than saying "I *never* come when you suck my clit," or "You *always* rush through oral sex," how about "It feels best when you lick my clit, especially when you circle it slowly with your tongue."

Be a Good Listener

Expressing yourself well isn't enough—a successful conversation depends on your being a good listener. Listening may sound easier than it is; you'll want to hone several skills in this department. First and foremost, good listening requires that you stay present during the conversation (no daydreaming). You have to recognize when you're too tired to be fully present and postpone your talk as necessary. You may also find it helpful to practice what's known as "active listening." When your partner is through speaking, repeat what you heard and ask if you got it right. This approach ensures that you've registered and understood what your partner is trying to convey. Perhaps the most difficult aspect of listening is actually letting yourself hear the truth. Too often, our knee-jerk response is to defend a position or prove a partner wrong, and we don't stop to examine the legitimacy of his or her claims. Most people can accurately pinpoint how their partner's attitudes and behaviors could be improved, but have a hard time acknowledging areas for self-improvement. Learn from your partner, and don't be afraid to admit when he or she is right; this is an excellent catalyst for change.

Use Body Language

Busy schedules and needy kids may preclude long, leisurely lovemaking sessions, but you can regularly express affection without ever speaking a word. Affectionate touch can go a long way to reassure your partner, particularly during times of sexual drought.

> It is really important to communicate desire, even when physically too tired to act on it. When my husband is in the mood and I am exhausted, I let him know with gentle affection that I am too tired at the moment, but that I find him attractive and desire his affection.

Take a minute to think of the nonverbal gestures that delight and inspire you, then make a point of incorporating these into your daily routine. Here are a few suggestions:

- Make eye contact and hold it
- Make long, leisurely kissing a routine part of your hellos and goodbyes

- Touch gently during conversation—brush the arm, stroke the neck, rub the thigh
- Sit close together on the couch, or put your head in his or her lap
- Fall asleep in the spoon position
- Hold hands

Allow for Differences

You didn't choose your mate because he or she was a carbon copy of you (we hope), so don't try to turn him or her into one. Expect disagreement and respect your differences. While you can't force each other to change, the process of communication and compromise can lead to growth and change for both parties.

Communication issues were really rough the first three years after birth. He just wasn't as tuned in to the baby as I was, and I of course thought he did everything wrong. I had to ease up and let him find his way as a parent. We really had to sit down and talk about what we wanted family-wise and sexually. I had to make him talk and search his soul for answers when really he just wished I could decide everything and he could just follow.

Even as your communication skills evolve over the course of a long-term relationship, you'll always have to be willing to embrace the best and accommodate the worst elements of your individual styles.

My partner always gets me to explain my frustrations, and that helps resolve most issues for us. I yell at him sometimes, and he hates that, but we always "finish" a fight. We never leave it hanging there in the air. Because we have such an important connection now, and a very good reason to work things out, we really want to understand each other and "get along."

Negotiate

Communication won't be worth the energy you expend if you're bent on defending your position at all costs; you might as well be shouting at the moon. It's fine to disagree with your partner, but be willing to work out a solution that will satisfy you both. This is where the fine art of compromise comes into play. Throughout this book, we suggest ways to negotiate common sexual issues (see the Desire Revisited chapter, page 197), but for now we offer a fine example of the rewards of a little mutual backscratching.

We've agreed that it is too easy to "forget" to have sex, and that we are both equally responsible for making sure we both get what we need. If I want to get laid, I make sure the kids go to bed and then I dress in a favorite bit of lingerie and the rest is history. If hubby wants a bit, he either negotiates a blow job (I trade for an extra hour of sleep in the morning, which is what I really need) or he shaves, and kisses the back of my neck. We've been pretty good about not saying no when the other person has made the effort to ask in these ways.

Get Help

Don't feel you have to wait until you're at your wit's end to seek professional help. If you and your partner struggle with disagreements, standoffs, and a chronic inability to meet each other halfway, you could benefit from counseling. While many couples resist going into couples therapy because they see it as an admission that the relationship has failed (or is about to go down in flames), therapy can actually take your relationship to a deeper level of honesty and acceptance. A good therapist is an unbiased third party who can help you distinguish between projection, expectation, and reality and make you aware of the individual blind spots that are impeding your communication. We've listed some relevant professional organizations, along with some recommended self-help books, in the Resources section (page 340).

SEX IS COMMUNICATION

Sex is such an important part of our relationship, it's another road of communication for us.

We would be remiss if we left this chapter without pointing out the simple truth that sex *is* communication. Sexual intimacy allows us to express desire, love, vulnerability, and a host of other complex emotions. The language of sex cannot be adequately described with words or replaced with other types of conversation. We have used this chapter to promote communication as a requirement for good sex, but good sex becomes its own type of profound communication. Who needs more incentive than that?

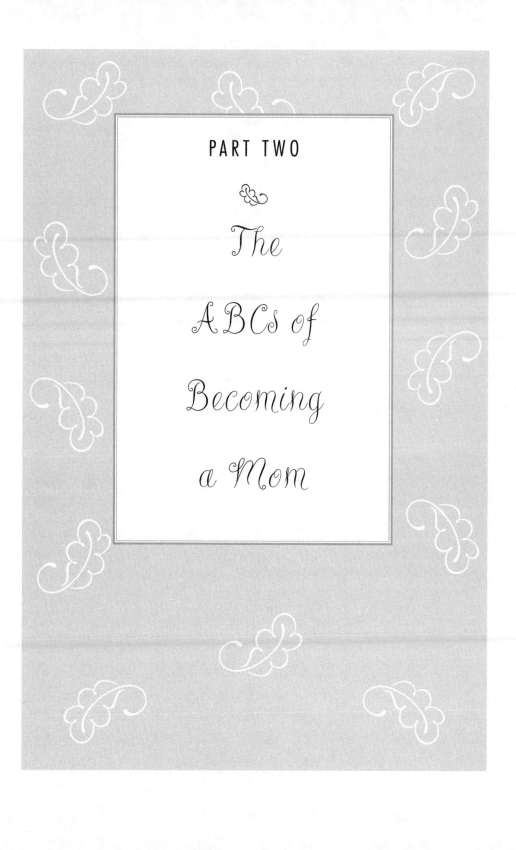

PART TWO

The

ABCs of

Becoming

a Mom

SEX AND CONCEPTION

WHERE BABIES COME FROM

YOU know the story, don't you? It's called "How Babies Are Made," and it usually involves a tender mommy and a gentle daddy who love each other so much that Daddy puts his seed inside Mommy to make a baby grow. Most sex information books for kids present procreation as the only possible motivation for sexual activity (Mommy and Daddy love you so much they were even willing to "do it" so you could be born). Given their innate and irrepressible sexual curiosity, kids quickly discover that there's more to having sex than making babies. Usually it isn't until we're adults that we discover the other half of the equation: Sometimes there's more to making babies than having sex!

While the majority of American babies are still conceived the "old-fashioned way," tens of thousands of women become mothers every year through donor insemination and a host of assisted reproductive technologies. Same-sex couples, couples dealing with infertility, couples who have medical reasons not to conceive a biological child together, and individuals who choose single parenthood are all exploring pathways toward conception that may or may not include sexual intimacy. And for the even greater number of women who become mothers through adopting, foster parenting, or joining blended families, sex has nothing to do with family building.

Some women become moms quite by accident; others spend years trying. Women who are trying to conceive, struggling with infertility, or opting to adopt are engaged in an emotional and physiological process that has a particularly acute impact on their sexual sense of self. Issues of self-image, self-esteem, and self-control arise during family building that are relevant to everyone who chooses motherhood, regardless of how it begins.

WHEN YOU WEREN'T EVEN TRYING

Women who have sex with men may well get pregnant without ever trying — in fact, the vast majority of our survey respondents under thirty reported that their pregnancies were the result of birth-control failures. Until that far-off day when birth control research gets as much federal funding as abstinence-based sex education programs for teenagers,[1] unintended pregnancies will be common. For women who had always wanted or planned to become mothers, these pregnancies can be happy occasions. Accidental conception can be strangely liberating — a stroke of fate that forces you to make a decision and stop awaiting some elusive optimal moment. And pregnancy can be a wake-up call to sexual self-awareness: You may feel a renewed sense of your body's power and potential, along with a heightened consciousness of the consequences of sexual activity.

> I didn't try to conceive in a conscious way, though I always wanted children. However, before becoming pregnant I did some risky things in the heat of the moment (and hence got pregnant) that I would normally avoid and tell others to avoid. Now that my daughter is born, I'm really aware of safer sex and I know I'll be more careful than I was in the year leading to my pregnancy.

But unintended pregnancy can also have a chilling effect on your sexuality. If you've been using contraception, pregnancy can seem like a cruel joke in which it's revealed that — even when you've done everything you can to be responsible — your body can let you down. When your plans for the future are derailed by pregnancy, it's difficult not to feel overwhelmed and helpless. In these situations, sex may come to represent an unwelcome loss of control that is simply not worth the risk.

> My son was accidentally conceived. Although I love my son, parenting is so hard and has really changed my life course. I had to leave school and give up my dreams to raise him. I'm so afraid of getting pregnant again (it was a birth-control failure — I am truly 100 percent careful and ended up being that 1 percent) that I try to avoid sex so it doesn't happen again.

If you're in this camp, we hope that what you read in this book encourages you to explore the variety of sexual activities that carry absolutely no risk of conception, and to cultivate compassion for yourself. A common way to cope with feelings of powerlessness is to point fingers—at yourself, your partner, that shoddy condom—because it can be more comforting to place, or even shoulder, blame than to face your own lack of control. The truth is that there will always be life circumstances that are completely out of your command, and it will stand you in good stead as a parent to accept this and develop flexibility. The process of family building is particularly resistant to the best-laid plans—personal preference has little to no influence over reproductive biology: Some women conceive who didn't want to, while others strive to conceive for years without success.

Of course, once conception does take place, every woman should have the right to decide whether to carry the pregnancy to term and whether to place her child for adoption. No one should ever be coerced into becoming a mom—while conception is not always planned, parenthood itself must always be freely and consciously chosen. All our cheerleading for women's sexual empowerment is nothing but pie in the sky unless women's inalienable right to reproductive freedom is recognized and protected.

TRYING TO CONCEIVE: THE BASICS

The methods of those actively trying to conceive (identified in the jargon of on-line chat rooms and bulletin boards as "TTC") run the gamut from heterosexual couples who put away the birth control and wait to see what happens to those pursuing donor insemination to those who turn to fertility drugs and assisted reproductive technologies when conception proves elusive. Before discussing how your individual journey to conception may affect your sex life, we want to review a few physiological basics.

Ovulation 101

If you've been trying to conceive for more than a couple of months, you probably know the drill. Conceiving is by no means as automatic a process as our collective experiences with failed birth control would lead us to believe! A woman is fertile for only a few days out of every menstrual cycle, right around the time of ovulation. In fact, so many ducks have to be in a row, biologically speaking, that even if a young man and woman have intercourse at her time of peak fertility, there's only a 25 percent chance of conception. Fertility declines as we age, and conception rates for women over thirty-five are approximately 10 percent per cycle attempt.

Conception can't occur unless the egg and the sperm meet in the right place at the right time. At ovulation, an egg is released from a woman's ovary, travels to her fallopian tube, and begins its journey down to the uterus. The egg must be fertilized by sperm soon after ovulation, while it's still in the third of the fallopian tube closest to the ovary. An unfertilized egg will die within twenty-four hours of ovulation, and the fertilized egg needs time to reach the developmental stage that allows it to implant successfully in the uterine lining (the trip down the fallopian tube takes about a week). So sperm should ideally be ready and waiting in the fallopian tube before the egg is released, which means you should have intercourse or inseminate prior to ovulation. You can fine-tune timing depending on whether you're using fresh or frozen sperm. The advantage of fresh sperm is that it can live for up to three to five days in a woman's body, so even if you have intercourse a few days before ovulation, there's a chance of conception. Frozen sperm only lives for up to twenty-four hours in a woman's body, so you would need to inseminate as close to the time of ovulation as possible.

In order to conceive, you'll need to learn the vagaries of your own individual cycle. According to the medical model, all women have twenty-eight-day cycles with ovulation occurring on day fourteen, at the exact midpoint of the month. In fact, women's cycles range from twenty-four to thirty-five days, and ovulation occurs twelve to sixteen days before the last day of any given cycle, rather than at its midpoint. Furthermore, your cycle can vary in length from month to month—stress, travel, fatigue, or illness can all lengthen or shorten the preovulatory period (however, the length of time between ovulation and menstruation will remain constant). We can't emphasize enough the importance of tracking your own cycle and getting to know your unique fertility signs. Don't be led astray by doctors, relatives, and well-intentioned friends who expect your cycle to fit into a cookie-cutter mold.

> We tried to conceive our first child for almost two years. I began to HATE sex. I would do it automatically and usually without desire for orgasm. Just to get the sperm. Ha ha, I was a sperm whore. My husband felt much the same. He was tired during that time from working on extra projects and work and was just performing a duty. The second time we took our fertility into our hands and were able to conceive in three cycles. Natural Family Planning made it possible for us to maximize our fertility where the outdated rhythm method we used with our first child (by advice of our doctor) had us missing my ovulation every month by two days!

So what *are* the signs of fertility? The most obvious and useful indication that you're about to ovulate is the presence of fertile-quality cervical mucus. Many a rapturous paragraph in fertility manuals has been devoted to cervical mucus, and it is, in fact, an amazing fluid. Distinctly different from your vaginal discharge or lubrication at other times of your cycle, fertile mucus is slick or slippery to the touch, clear in color, and so stretchy that it's commonly compared to egg whites. Generated by rising estrogen levels prior to ovulation, fertile mucus is designed purely to facilitate conception: It nourishes sperm, neutralizes the acidic vaginal environment that is normally hostile to sperm, and forms pathways that guide sperm up through the cervix. And as proof that Mom Nature is gently prodding you in the direction of procreation, your vagina feels especially lubricated (many women experience increased libido during their fertile time). Once you start paying attention to cervical mucus, you'll notice that it's present for a range of one to four days—its abundance does decrease with age. As soon as you ovulate, your fertile mucus will dry up and your chances of conceiving plummet.

Another staple of the TTC toolbox are ovulation predictor kits (OPKs)—these over-the-counter urine tests track the hormonal shifts that indicate ovulation is imminent. Some women find it helpful to chart the slight fluctuations in basal body temperature—your body's temperature at rest—that occur pre- and postovulation, though it can be very difficult to conceive by tracking your temperature alone; your "BBT" goes up perceptibly only *after* you've ovulated, so it's not an effective predictive tool. Other self-helpers whip out speculums to monitor the changes in their cervix—as you approach ovulation, the cervix softens and shifts to a higher position, and the cervical os perceptibly opens. You may be one of those women who notice distinct shifts in appetite or mood, or who experience midcycle cramping or spotting upon ovulation. Once you begin to track your fertility signs, you may be surprised that you hadn't identified your personal pattern before. Then again, your signs may be so subtle as to elude you completely—don't despair if you wind up feeling like an inadequate princess who simply can't detect that pea beneath the mattress. Some women are more responsive to the fluctuations of their hormones than others.

Depending on your age and your fertility, a little forethought and self-awareness may be all it takes to conceive within a six- to twelve-month time period. Or you may require some medical assistance. Women over the age of thirty-five should definitely be proactive and seek medical advice if they haven't conceived within six well-timed cycle attempts. Ultimately, some women are simply not able to conceive, for reasons that may have organic causes or may be unexplained. We'll discuss the stresses of infertility in more detail below.

Don't Forget the Sperm

Since women bear the physiological responsibility of pregnancy and often assume responsibility for managing the logistics of trying to conceive, they unconsciously tend to assume the responsibility for successful conception as well. The truth is that every good egg needs some good sperm, and if you've had well-timed intercourse for several months without conceiving, it would be a good idea for your male partner to have a semen analysis. A semen analysis is a very easy, affordable, noninvasive test—basically, the man ejaculates into a cup, and medical technicians view his semen under a microscope to evaluate sperm count and motility (the percentage of live, swimming sperm). There are many reasons for infertility in men; some are temporary, such as when fever or stress reduces sperm count, and some are permanent, such as when chemotherapy or testicular damage wipes out sperm production. With advances in reproductive technology such as ICSI (see the Alphabet Soup sidebar), male infertility is now highly treatable. Of course, many heterosexual couples choose not to undergo such an expensive and relatively new procedure, opting instead to pursue low-tech options such as donor insemination or adoption. If you're working with donor sperm from a sperm bank, the bank should be able to give you information on the sperm count and motility of every vial you purchase.

TRYING TO CONCEIVE: TAKE ADVICE WITH A GRAIN OF SALT

If you let people know you're trying to conceive, you will effectively open the floodgates to a torrent of unsolicited advice. Admittedly, this is good practice for becoming a mom, but we suggest you take everything you hear with a grain of salt. Folks tend to extrapolate from the ways in which they conceived to make recommendations that aren't necessarily grounded in science. If you spend time in on-line forums, you'll be overwhelmed by the sheer volume and contradictory nature of the tips and techniques. Here are some examples of the theories you may hear, along with our perspective on how well founded they are:

You will get pregnant if you have intercourse every other day. False. Unprotected intercourse can't result in conception unless you're in your fertile period. Intercourse needs to be timed with your peak fertility days. By all means, have intercourse throughout the rest of the month if you're enjoying the contraception-free sex—just don't burden it with unrealistic expectations. The "every other day" rule reflects the fact that it takes an average of forty-eight hours for sperm to regenerate in semen. If you want to optimize those ejaculates, give your sweetie sufficient time to replenish his sperm supply; if he's over forty or you have some other reason to expect his sperm count to be low, you should definitely time ejaculates strategically. Ask your doctor for more specific advice here.

You will get pregnant if you have an orgasm. Well, it sure doesn't hurt, and it may very well help. This theory has a lot of history. The second-century physician Galen believed that both male and female orgasm, as well as male and female fluids, were essential to conception—a belief that was widespread until the eighteenth century, when the microscope was invented and sperm discovered. Obviously, if every pregnancy required a female orgasm, ours would be either a considerably more satisfied or a considerably less populated world! However, some evidence suggests that orgasm can enhance chances of conception. When you approach orgasm, the uterus lifts up and the mouth of the uterus—the cervix—dips down into the vagina. The cervix will therefore be perfectly positioned to bathe in sperm, while the uterine contractions of orgasm may serve to propel sperm up the cervical canal. This theory also suggests an evolutionary rationale for why men reach orgasm before women.

If you're not pregnant yet, you must be doing it wrong. False. You can be doing absolutely everything right, and it can still take months to conceive. Remember, even well-timed intercourse has only a 10 to 25 percent pregnancy rate, while pregnancy rates from vaginal insemination with frozen sperm can be as low as 5 percent per cycle attempt.

You can control the sex of your child through timing conception. No guarantees. All the same, numerous entrepreneurs are making big bucks off parents who'd rather decorate the nursery in pink than blue.[2] If you visit on-line forums devoted to this topic, you'll learn about timing according to the Shettles method (popularized by the doctor whose book *How to Choose the Sex of Your Baby* has sold over a million copies), insemination according to the Ericsson method (a technique of sperm distillation invented by a cattle rancher), and "flow cytometric sperm separation," a sperm-sorting method patented by a genetics lab in Virginia which is still in clinical trials. None of these methods can promise success, although the sperm-sorting technique has been the most scrutinized by the medical community.

Both high-tech and low-tech methods of sex selection are based on the fact that sperm determines the sex of a fetus—there are sperm carrying X chromosomes which result in girls, and sperm carrying Y chromosomes which result in boys. X sperm is slow but hardy, and Y sperm is fast but fragile. Therefore, the logic goes, if you inseminate a few days before ovulation, the Y sperm will lose the tortoise-and-hare race to the egg, but the slow-and-steady X sperm will win the prize. Similarly, if you inseminate right before ovulation, the Y sperm will get to the egg first, while the X sperm lumber along behind them. Yet conception involves entirely too many unseen variables for these timing techniques to be reliable.[3]

You won't get pregnant if you use an artificial lubricant. It depends. Sperm is actually a fairly fragile organism that would rarely survive long enough to make it to the uterus were it not for the nourishing, alkaline environment of fertile-quality cervical mucus. During the rest of your cycle, the natural acidity of vaginal fluids has a spermicidal effect. Clearly, if you're trying to conceive, you wouldn't want to use any lubricants that contain spermicidal or detergent ingredients such as nonoxynol 9. However, it's less clear whether your basic nonspermicidal water-based lube would be problematic. Most fertility books err on the side of caution, primly advising heterosexual couples to put enough time into foreplay that they won't "need" lube (no help for those of us who simply don't generate a lot of vaginal lubrication even when aroused). If you're TTC with a male partner with no known fertility problems, a little lube shouldn't be a problem (especially if you apply it to the shaft, not the glans, of the penis). However, if your partner has low sperm count or you're using frozen sperm, your best bet is to skip the lube. And fertility labs recommend that you steer clear of saliva, which is loaded with bacteria that might contaminate the semen sample.

You will get pregnant if you "just relax." Oh, give us a break! The rationale behind this obnoxious axiom (the bane of every woman trying to conceive or struggling with infertility) seems to be that if you were just a "natural" woman, more in touch with your body and less cerebral, hey presto, you'd be knocked up in no time. Sure, it's true that the standard recommendations for stress reduction—getting regular exercise, quitting smoking, eating well, cutting back on caffeine and alcohol—are conducive to conception. But the greatest source of stress in the life of someone who's TTC is the fact that she's not yet pregnant, and all the uterine-toning herbal tea and yoga postures in the world aren't going to solve matters.

> We had a hard time conceiving, went on fertility drugs that eventually worked. Our sex life really sucked then. Every movement, touch, and eventual orgasm was in hopes of a baby. We both felt like machines. My suggestion would be NOT to listen to anybody who tells you to "just relax." Tell them to "just back off!" If there is another person who has been through it, or is going through it, they can be of some support. But it's still a very personal time between you and your partner.

Plenty of women conceive in situations of the utmost stress—think rape, war crimes, incest—and plenty of women, doing everything humanly possible to reduce their adrenaline levels, do not. Yes, we've all heard the stories of heterosexual couples who grapple with infertility for years only to conceive promptly after they bring their adopted baby home. In all likelihood, these stories make the rounds more due to their man-bites-dog novelty than the number of times the scenario actually occurs. Conception is a random event—no woman should ever be blamed when it doesn't come her way.

Some Enchanted Evening . . .

Folks sometimes generate excessive anxiety about the mood and setting they create for their conception efforts, fretting over whether they were making love with the appropriate degree of solemn joy, or remaining filled with pure positivity and light through the entire insemination. However intentional you try to be, it's worth remembering the lag time between doing the deed—intercourse or insemination—and actual fertilization. So while you might prefer to tell your son that he was conceived on a blanket beneath the stars, or to tell your daughter that she was conceived after you practiced creative visualization in front of your fertility altar, odds are that the physiological moment of conception took place a day or two later, while you were stuck in traffic. Don't beat yourself up over whether you were sufficiently "conscious" around the act of creating a new life, or feel cheated if you inseminated in a doctor's office—conception is a magical process whenever and however it takes place.

TRYING TO CONCEIVE THROUGH PARTNER SEX

Trying to conceive is bound to have an impact on a heterosexual couple's sex life. If you and your "dh" (that's "dear hubby" in chat-room-speak) are working on expanding your family, you may find that diving between the sheets with procreation as a goal is profoundly inspirational—then again, you may find it distressingly mood-dampening.

Switching Gears

When procreation becomes one of your motives for having intercourse, you may experience a certain cognitive dissonance. Women who've spent years of their reproductive life trying to keep bodily fluids at bay can have a difficult time switching gears and welcoming sperm deep into their bodies. Depending on one's point of view, pregnancy is either the greatest risk or the greatest reward resulting from sex with men—it may take a while to adjust your own attitude to your new circumstances.

> Having sex in order to conceive was stressful. Here I had spent half my life trying not to get pregnant, and now I wanted to get pregnant.

> We spend so much time preventing pregnancy early in our sexual lives, it's hard to get out of the mind-set when we feel truly ready to get pregnant. Give it time and enjoy it. Sex should still be fun, remember?

A Higher Purpose

Many of our survey respondents say they appreciated having a reason for intercourse that transcended "mere" sexual pleasure. For those whose religious or cultural upbringing leaves them susceptible to sexual shame or guilt, procreative intercourse can be a great way to make an end run around the lurking sensation that sex is sinful.

> I can say, however, that I was a lot more open to sex when I wanted so badly to get pregnant. I really enjoyed that "sex with a purpose." I think that's all tied in with the deep feelings of shame that surface now and again in the face of my own sexuality.

Needless to say, this method of guilt management tends to be short-lived unless you discover a spiritual component to sex that you can tap into thereafter, even when you're not baby-making.

> It was truly amazing to me. I had had an abortion at seventeen, and the amount of worrying about birth control I did thereafter RUINED my pleasure in sex. But when I decided that I wanted to become pregnant, suddenly sex became a very powerful, spiritual experience. Incredible. It changed the way that I looked at sex forever.

Plenty of people who don't experience sex as sinful nonetheless feel that procreative sex is imbued with a special dimension of spirituality.

> We ritualized our experience of getting pregnant. We used candles, incense, special fertility brews, and handmade "fertility pouches," with stones that increase your chances of becoming pregnant. It was very exciting and powerful.

This sense of purpose can manifest as a greater solemnity, or even prudishness, around sex.

> When trying to conceive, I would definitely say we made love, rather than having crazy sex. It just seemed odd to have life come from some "down-and-dirty screw." So I would say sex took on a more romantic, rather than a wild tone.

Or it can manifest as enthusiastic abandon. You may find that you become more sexually playful and adventurous during the time you're trying to conceive:

We got so turned on by the thought of making a person while we were trying that we had sex a lot more. My husband was wild. Trying to conceive increased my sexual desire. Gave me a higher purpose, I guess. And, because we weren't using birth control, allowed me to be more free with my sexuality.

Now that we are trying to have another child I get yelled at by my husband that "I don't want love, I just want sperm." All joking, of course, but it is mostly true. I am so baby-hungry that I know I should relax and all but it is hard. My desire level is very high right now and our sex life great because I am initiating it more.

At its best, conscious procreative sex can inspire a new level of honesty and disclosure.

When my husband and I decided to have a baby, it suddenly seemed that sex had a purpose, and because of this, I broke down crying one night and told my husband that I had been faking orgasms for years—for as long as I had known him. He took it very well and we talked about why I couldn't orgasm during intercourse. That was five years ago, and I'm really glad I "confessed."

Sex as a Chore

For every individual who appreciates the goal-oriented nature and spiritual possibilities of procreative sex, there's another who experiences "well-timed intercourse" as a total turnoff.

Trying to conceive actually killed our sex drive after the first two months. It did become more of a chore. Having sex for a purpose other than pure pleasure kind of spoiled it for me. I still liked it but I wasn't as into it.

I did not particularly enjoy sex when my wife and I were trying to conceive. To me, sex is and should be an end in itself, the physical expression of intimate friendship and love. Making a baby introduced this goal that I found disconcerting and anxiety-provoking.

While both women and men can have negative reactions to goal-oriented sex, men do seem to be more prone to complaining whenever intercourse involves something other than simply getting off. Some men are happy to chart along with their partners and wield a basal body thermometer with aplomb, but far too many take the attitude that conception is "women's work." Women do have more practice tracking their hormonal fluctuations than men or, at the most basic level, are aware that their bodies feel different at different times of the month. But that doesn't mean that men are physiologically incapable of reading a calendar!

> My husband hated the basal temperature charting. I think he was a little turned off by the mechanical aspect of keeping a chart, and he didn't like being told that we had to have sex on a certain day.

Admittedly, timed intercourse can be countererotic, but with a little imagination and a good sense of humor, there's no reason you can't make it work for you. For instance, why not imagine yourselves as actors in a porn movie? When the director shouts, "Roll 'em," porn stars have to put the rest of their day behind them and perform. At the very least, this tactic should give your fella a new level of respect for the overworked male stars of X-rated video. After all, there aren't any stagehands standing in the corner of your bedroom, tapping their feet and waiting for him to come on command.

> Sex-near-ovulation isn't so romantic — like when dh comes home from the midnight shift and wants only to sleep and I tell him, "Not yet, buddy, we've gotta do it first" — but sex at other times is the same as it always was. My advice is, don't lose your sense of humor. When you're trying to get it on with someone just for the sake of a few sperm, it's all you've got.

If you and your partner have been trying to conceive for some time, there's no question that timed sexual intercourse can become mechanical at best or grim at worst. Try to incorporate other types of physical intimacy during this time, so you're not always approaching each other with a specific physiologic goal in mind. Hey, it's okay to engage in sexual activities that don't even involve sperm! You'll both feel better about yourselves and each other if you make a point of including utterly frivolous sex in your routine as well.

> Sex was a mixed bag while trying to get pregnant. I'd been on the Pill, and it actually took almost two years to conceive. We'd expected it to be very easy, so sometimes sex was full of these feelings of sadness and desperation: Why haven't we conceived before now? What if we don't this time either? At other times, it was exciting: We're not using birth control! We might make a baby tonight! It was important to me to have sex during times when I was unlikely to conceive as well as when I was so I could still think of sex as something we enjoyed and did to connect with each other, as well as the way we'd make a baby.

Oh wow! I have had twenty-three pregnancies in sixteen years and only two (counting the one due next week) have gone beyond the eighth week. I know it's clichéd and everyone's heard it a million times, but the best thing to do when trying to conceive, especially if it takes a while, is KEEP YOUR SENSE OF HUMOR!! Also, learn as much as you can about your fertility cycle—that will mean that there's pressure only a few days each month, and the others can be spent on romantic times together instead of worrying about conception.

TRYING TO CONCEIVE THROUGH DONOR INSEMINATION

Intercourse with a partner isn't a conception option for all wanna-be moms. If you're a single woman, lesbian, or partnered with an infertile man, donor insemination may be the route you take to motherhood. While an estimated one million "DI" children have been conceived since World War II,[4] donor insemination is just beginning to be discussed as openly as adoption. Most women choosing DI purchase frozen sperm from a sperm bank or medical office (since the late 1980s, all licensed sperm banks have made it a policy to sell only frozen sperm, which can be quarantined for a six-month period while the donor is repeatedly screened for HIV and other STDs). Other women choose to inseminate with fresh sperm from a known donor, such as a close friend or relative of their partner.

While on one level DI separates the act of sex from the act of conception, inseminating does have sexual repercussions. After all, not only are you engaged in a process that involves your sexual organs, but issues arise around DI that can challenge your self-image. If you're a single heterosexual woman who has always assumed and expected you'd build a family with a loving partner, you may need to mourn this lost dream before moving on to embrace your identity as a "Single Mother by Choice."[5] If you're a heterosexual woman whose husband or male partner is infertile, both of you may be contending with feelings of disappointment and failure. If you're a lesbian, you may not relish the prospect of putting sperm in your body, and you may be unaccustomed to monitoring your reproductive cycle to the extent necessary for conception.

Donor insemination demands the same physiological self-awareness as other methods of trying to conceive, as well as a high tolerance for stress. If you're using fresh sperm from a known donor, you have the scheduling challenge of summoning your pal on short notice to come on over and masturbate in your bathroom. If you're using frozen sperm, which doesn't survive in a woman's body as long as fresh sperm, you're required to time your insemination attempts much more rigorously. Pregnancy rates tend to be lower with frozen sperm than fresh sperm, which means you can expect conception to take longer—not to mention that you're spending money with every cycle attempt.

You may find that trying to conceive through DI is a libido-dampening process (for some of the same reasons we'll discuss in the infertility section below). Or you may find that focusing on fertility is sexually inspiring.

> When you are thinking about insemination, you have sex on your mind a lot. I know I wish I had sperm so that I could make my partner pregnant.

Some women feel sexual activity is important to incorporate into their inseminations. Stephanie Brill of Maia Midwifery, who works with a largely lesbian clientele, comments, "Trying to be sexual around insemination can have the same forced element to it as when straight people need to have timed sex. It can take the joy out of it when you say, 'I'm going to be sexual for the next ten minutes while the sperm thaws.' But I've known people who have created amazing rituals around insemination that involve free sexual expression, whether through masturbation or with a partner." We doubt many women sustain the motivation to concoct elaborate rituals for more than one or two cycle attempts, but we certainly encourage you to find ways to incorporate simple pleasures into the process.

> I was inseminating as a single mom, so it didn't affect my sex life, really. I did have good orgasms while inseminating—for the cause!

If you're building a nontraditional family, prepare ahead of time for the curiosity your pregnancy will inspire. While heterosexual couples don't necessarily have to disclose that they conceived via DI, single women and lesbian couples often contend with a steady stream of nosy questions. Becoming a mother means you can expect to be treated as public property, and becoming a single or queer mother means you can expect your sex life to be the subject of public speculation. How you choose to respond to the speculation is entirely up to you—just keep in mind the value of preparing a response that is consistent with how you plan to explain his or her conception to your child.

THE IMPACT OF INFERTILITY

Over six million people in this country—about 10 percent of those in their reproductive years—are dealing with infertility.[6] In the majority of cases, infertility has organic causes and is treatable. However, if relatively low-tech treatments such as intrauterine insemination or fertility drugs aren't effective, women and men face dif-

Alphabet Soup

If you spend any time dealing with fertility issues, you'll need to get fluent in the acronyms of reproductive technology. Here's a short list of common lay and medical terms.

ART: assisted reproductive technologies. The loaded and inaccurate word "artificial" is thankfully out of use. After all, there's nothing artificial about a sperm fertilizing an egg, however and wherever it takes place.

BBT: basal body temperature. Your body's baseline temperature at rest. In most women, BBT goes up by several tenths of a degree after ovulation.

BD: baby dance. A particularly nauseating term for procreative intercourse used in the acronym-happy world of on-line forums.

DD/DS/DH: dear or darling daughter, son, or husband. Popular terms in on-line forums.

DE: donor egg.

DI: donor insemination. Replaces the term AI, or artificial insemination.

ICI: intracervical insemination. The medical term for vaginal insemination (doctors will go to ridiculous lengths to avoid saying the word "vagina"!).

IUI: intrauterine insemination. A method of insemination in which a catheter is run through the cervical opening and sperm is placed directly in the uterus. IUI must be done in a sterile clinical setting with specially prepared—or "washed"—semen.

ICSI: intercytoplasmic sperm injection. The latest trend in reproductive technology, in which a single sperm cell is injected into a single egg in a laboratory dish. Once fertilization has occurred, the embryo is transferred into the woman's uterus.

IVF: in vitro fertilization. Sperm and egg are combined in a laboratory dish. Once fertilization has occurred, the embryo is transferred into the woman's uterus.

OPK: ovulation predictor kit. An over-the-counter urine test that measures the rise in hormones that indicates ovulation is imminent.

TTC: trying to conceive.

ficult and expensive procedures such as IVF or ICSI (see sidebar). The emotional, physical, and financial costs of infertility can generate a staggering degree of stress.[7] Not only are you dealing with what feels like your body's betrayal, but you have to struggle for assistance from the health-care system and empathy from friends and family. Infertility can take quite a toll on your sex life.

Self-image

Pregnancy is seen as the ultimate "natural" condition, so it's equally "natural" for women who are unable to conceive to feel somehow defective or flawed. You'll spot pregnant women or stroller-pushing dads everywhere you turn, and become convinced that you're the only person on the planet whose body is out of sync with Mother Nature. This sense that your body is not "working" causes your self-esteem to plunge, which in turn leaves you feeling undesirable and sexually lethargic. And if you're constantly scrutinizing your body for fertility signs, you can begin to feel somewhat detached and asexual. If you spend half the month waiting to spot fertile-quality mucus on your underwear, and the other half waiting to spot a blue line on your home-pregnancy test, that doesn't leave much of the month available for sexual encounters. In fact, many women avoid sexual activity during the second half of their cycle out of a superstitious fear that they might somehow "dislodge" the embryo before it successfully implants in the uterus.

> Wow, six years of very intrusive (physically and mentally) reproductive procedures, scheduled intercourse, etc. pretty much reduced my sex life and desire to next to nothing. Pregnancy didn't much improve matters since I was at very high risk for miscarriage. My advice: Communicate, communicate, communicate with your partner.

Once you start taking medical steps to boost your fertility, you face a whole new set of challenges. Fertility drugs that hyperstimulate your ovaries to produce more egg follicles have some decidedly unpleasant side effects. Many women experience terrible mood swings, comparable to intense PMS, while on clomiphene citrate (a.k.a. Clomid, the most commonly prescribed oral fertility medication).

> When I was on Clomid, I didn't have the slightest interest in having sex. It took all my willpower for me not to smash my girlfriend's skull in, so getting cuddly wasn't really an option.

Injectable fertility drugs are less likely to cause mood swings, but they do cause bloating and discomfort — and giving yourself a shot in the butt every night will prove pretty antierotic to all but the most determinedly upbeat.

> Our child was conceived after three in vitro cycles, after six years of trying all kinds of things. We kept our sense of humor, our commitment to each other as a couple and a family — reassuring each other that we would have

a good life even if we could not have a baby. I cannot stress enough how important humor is. We were playing gigs with our band and my husband would be giving me shots of fertility drugs in the ladies' room of the bar and we would be laughing at the absurdity of the situation.

For those who move on to advanced technologies such as IVF, all the discomforts of fertility drugs are exacerbated by the anxiety of assuming a huge medical expense and the disappointment of losing control of the conception process.

We conceived our three sons by in vitro fertilization. Our sex lives were proscribed for us, and conception happened with my husband holding my hand and a relative stranger standing between my legs while I assumed the position. Not real sexy. Conceiving was hell. Simply hell. The drugs made me feel awful, the regimen was demeaning, and the outcome so uncertain and so very, very important.

One of the most disconcerting aspects of infertility is that what feels like a cast of thousands begins to meddle in your sex life. Your Chinese herbalist informs you that masturbation will hinder your ability to ovulate. Your kindly neighbor corners you in the elevator to suggest, "Just relax and drink some wine" before your next sexual encounter. Your husband has to come into a specimen cup in the cramped bathroom of your doctor's office and hand the semen over to a nurse who will ask him how many days it's been since his last ejaculation. If you are able to sustain your good humor and sexual joie de vivre in the face of these challenges, our hats are off to you.

Blaming Yourself

As we mentioned above, shouldering blame is sometimes more comforting than admitting to helplessness. When your reproductive life is beyond your control, you may be tempted to assume responsibility for your infertility by searching for a scapegoat in your own sexual past. This scapegoat may be purely illogical—*God is punishing me for that abortion I had at age eighteen.* Or it may have some relevance to your situation—*If I'd only been tested for chlamydia in my early twenties, I could have been treated before my reproductive tract was damaged.* Either way, we implore you not to default to internalized sexual shame and guilt. We tend to have such a tenuous grasp on sexual self-esteem that identifying our sexual "mistakes" as the ultimate source of our troubles is all too easy. Try to be conscious of your natural vulnerability about sex, and keep your perspective—infertility is not the price you're paying for being sexual any more than it's the price you're paying for shoplifting when you were in high school or taking a sick day when you're not really sick. Whatever else in your life does or doesn't go according to your plans, you will always have ultimate control over one thing — enjoying and asserting your birthright to a healthy sexuality.

Partner Issues

Infertility affects women and men equally and creates particular challenges in a couple's sex life. If you're attempting to conceive via intercourse, all the scheduling and medical scrutiny involved is guaranteed to make performing on cue difficult. If you're attempting to conceive in a clinical setting, you may have become so dispirited by the whole process that you lose desire for intimate physical contact with your partner. The infertile partner will often experience a profound sense of failure and inadequacy that inevitably affects how sexually desirable he or she feels. Maryl Walling-Millard, a psychotherapist specializing in infertility and adoption issues, points out that infertile partners are frequently "frightened that their partner might desire someone else who could give them a child. It just starts to erode the trust in the relationship. Obviously there are parallels in their sex life. Some people can compartmentalize and still think of sex as something they're entitled to, but most people can't."

In fact, whichever partner is infertile, both of you will be struggling — not only with guilt, sorrow, anger, and disappointment — but with each other's different styles of expressing emotions. One of you may be highly emotive and the other more buttoned down. One of you may be "protecting" the other from your true feelings — or both of you may be doing so.

> We had three miscarriages before this successful pregnancy. And to be honest, the miscarriages almost ruined our marriage. The main reason, LACK OF COMMUNICATION! We both wanted to "spare" the other our feelings and agonies, and it drove us further and further apart. So my big piece of advice would be to TALK! Neither of you is a mind reader, and there's nothing worse than feeling you are alone during hard times.

Communicating can be easier said than done. Discussing infertility is a lot like discussing sex — it brings up feelings of shame, resentment, embarrassment, and excruciating vulnerability. Your greatest challenge may be to find a way to negotiate the intense sense of powerlessness you're feeling without blaming each other. As Maryl Walling-Millard puts it, "At a certain point individuals can't tolerate their rage at their lack of control, and they project that onto their partners: Why can't *you* be different? Why can't *you* read the books on infertility? Why can't *you* go to the doctor? They have to feel like somebody could be doing something, rather than being stuck with a feeling of helplessness."

My husband and I fought like banshees each time I was in an IVF cycle. Even if they hadn't regulated our sex, we wouldn't have wanted each other then, anyway. Major life stressors tend to pull us apart as opposed to some couples who find themselves closer during such stress. Not to mention that I felt horribly unattractive and was so focused on achieving pregnancy that I ignored all else. Sometimes we wonder how we made it through those cycles without killing each other. Funny, it never occurred to us not to have a baby in the face of this horror. The baby seemed very right. The method seemed like torture we had invited on ourselves.

So how are you supposed to cope? Probably the most practical approach to sustaining your relationship and your sanity is to force yourself to take a break from the all-consuming project of trying to conceive. Get out of the house and spend some recreational time together—you could go to the movies, for a hike, to a ball game, or out of town for the weekend. You may be feeling too distanced from sexual feelings to have any interest in a romantic candlelight dinner, and that's fine. The point is to remind yourselves what you like about being together, not to feel pressured into sliding between the sheets. And who knows—simply sharing downtime may inspire you to get physical.

We'd just decide to forget it—forget looking at my temperature and all of that—and go away every now and then, so that we were out of our usual routine. We'd just try to refocus on ourselves and our relationship separate from the fertility issues. And it worked off and on.

Moving On

Your own infertility story may end with a biological child, an adopted child, a foster child, or the decision not to have children. If you have conceived, you may feel particularly cautious about your hard-won pregnancy and view any sort of sexual activity as potentially "risky." Then again, you may feel so liberated and exhilarated by your pregnancy that you experience a renaissance of sexual feelings. After months or years of struggling with uncertainty, both pregnancy and the decision to take steps toward adoption or fostering can feel hugely empowering.

We'd just been matched with our birth mother, and before our son was born, our sex life definitely improved. Spontaneity returned and things got active; there was a little rebirth. Now that he's three months old, we're too busy dealing with lack of sleep and energy to have any interest.

Some couples take the attitude that they might as well make hay while the sun shines.

> Before we adopted our daughter, our sex life was intense, if at times sporadic. We knew that life was about to change radically for us. The preadoption paperwork and razzmatazz wasn't that stressful.

Unlike the survey respondent above, many people report that navigating the bureaucracy of the adoption process can be stressful, and they experience their assessment by adoption agency employees and/or social workers as an intense invasion of privacy. Of course it's unpleasant to feel that your fitness as a potential parent is being evaluated by strangers, but you simply have to grin and bear it. Be prepared for the possibility that you'll be asked random questions about your sex life (such as how often you have sex and whether you're satisfied with your sex life) and answer these as briefly and politely as possible. There aren't any right or wrong answers, and you're certainly not going to be disqualified on the basis of having a sex life. On the other hand, it's probably a bad idea to display your favorite silicone dildo or erotic photography collection on the coffee table when the social worker comes by for a home study visit!

Once you bring your child home, you may be so filled with happiness and enthusiasm that your partnered sex life rebounds with ease.

> After my child was born, my sexual intimacy increased because I was sooooo happy to finally be a mom after nine years of trying and three years of waiting for the adoption.

Then again, it's perfectly understandable if your libido takes some time to resurface. When your child's an infant, you may put your sex life on the back burner, as so many parents do. If your partnered sex life has become nonexistent during the months or years of scheduled inseminations and fertility shots, you may feel awkward or unsure how to go about restoring sexual intimacy to your relationship. We'd encourage you to read the Desire Revisited chapter (page 197) for tips on kick-starting desire and meeting each other halfway.

RECONCEIVING MOTHERHOOD

Motherhood is so much more than the physical act of bearing and delivering a child. We assume that our readers represent the full spectrum of mothers — biological, non-biological, adoptive, foster, and step — but that you're reading this chapter because you or your partner have tried to conceive. If you've pursued conception, you may have found that other identity issues came up along the way. In our culture, being a woman is still inextricably interwoven with being a mother. We're defined by whether or not we have children, and becoming a mother is supposed to be the ultimate fulfillment of female identity. Obviously, this expectation can backfire.

> Think twice before you try to conceive. You may think that your family and life and femininity are "incomplete" without children. I don't feel any more fulfilled now than I did then.

Why not turn this model on its head? Rather than expecting that all women should become nurturing mothers, let's encourage all mothers to become outrageous women. Anyone who flouts conventional attitudes about mothers is doing her bit to expand the definition of what it is to be a woman, and all of us—with or without children—benefit.

> My partner and I found the whole pregnancy experience very sexy. We were way into each other and sort of on this big love trip. Being the nonbirth mom was hard on me. People would talk to my partner about the baby and talk to me about work. Some people even started calling me dad. Not to mention that the whole pregnancy experience is very heterosexual. I guess the best advice I have is this: The bad stuff passes. And then you have this little person in your life that doesn't care if you're the bio mom or not.

SEX DURING PREGNANCY

HONOR YOUR OWN EXPERIENCE

BECOMING a mother is probably the most intense invasion of privacy that you're likely to experience in your life. And we're not talking about coping with the family bed or visiting the bathroom with a toddler in tow. We're talking about the fact that you are now public property and that your friends, family, neighbors, the guy at the corner store, and the lady sitting next to you on the bus will feel blissfully entitled to attach their judgments, opinions, and biases to you as though you were a walking pin-the-tail-on-the-donkey game.

Every mom knows that it takes courage, ego strength, and a good sense of humor to weather the onslaught of public opinion. And every mom who's ever been pregnant has probably also figured out that pregnancy is a good crash course in cultural expectations. While pregnancy doesn't necessarily prepare you for *being* a parent, it does provide you with an excellent opportunity to practice asserting your individual reality in the face of a staggering weight of assumptions, superstitions, proscriptions, and sentimentality.

A pregnant woman is a lightning rod for a wide range of contradictory attitudes about sex and femininity. Depending on the audience, your swelling body could be read as that of a voluptuous earth mother, a luminous virgin queen, an out-of-control slut, a porn fetish, or an asexual incubator. Although there are plenty of men and women who find pregnant bodies extremely sexy and arousing, our culture as a whole does not view pregnant women as sex objects. Once you're expecting, you're expected to take on the baby's properties of soft, fuzzy sensuality.

> I felt very "desexualized" during my first pregnancy because the maternity clothes were so infantile. I remember standing in a maternity shop yelling, "I'm having a child, I am NOT becoming a child! Do you have anything without the little duckies or bunnies on it?"

By now, you're well aware of our own biases, and predictably, we think that every pregnant woman deserves to be viewed as the lush, sexy goddess she is, but how she chooses to enact her sexuality is entirely up to her. Pregnancy may be a time when having sex is the farthest thing from your mind; it may be a time of unbelievable erotic exploration; or your experience may fall somewhere between these two extremes. In any case, your body is undergoing enormous changes that are fundamentally sexual in nature, and you are engaged in a process that cannot fail to have an impact on your sexual self.

WHAT'S GOING ON IN YOUR BODY

Pregnancy is an elaborate symphony of hormonal and physiological adaptations in which your entire body expands to simultaneously nourish two human beings. Your heart pumps nearly twice its normal volume of blood, your lungs take in more air, and your digestive system processes nutrients more efficiently. The ligaments in your pelvic girdle stretch, and your uterus will ultimately expand to one thousand times its nonpregnant volume. Despite all this expansiveness, your body feels pretty darn crowded, and pregnancy is inevitably accompanied by some uncomfortable side effects. We're not just talking about the nausea and fatigue of the first trimester or the awkwardness of a growing belly. You can also expect to retain water (most commonly in your hands and feet); to suffer leg cramps and backaches; and to contend with constipation, heartburn, indigestion, hemorrhoids, and incessant urination. Doesn't sound very libido-enhancing, does it? But wait—there's more!

One of the transformations of pregnancy rarely discussed during prenatal visits is that your sexual organs are undergoing the same glorious expansion as the rest of your body. It's obvious to all that your breasts are expanding—the development of milk glands begins early in pregnancy, and your breasts will swell in size long before your belly does. What's not obvious to all is that your genitals are expanding too. By the second trimester, increased blood flow throughout your body is making its effects felt between your legs, where the erectile tissues of your genitals engorge with pooling blood and deepen in color. The increased level of estrogen in your body results in a distinct increase in vaginal secretions. Your clitoris is swollen, your labia are pulsing with extra blood, and your vagina is dripping with moisture—sound familiar? Yup, a pregnant woman's genitals bear a distinct resemblance to a highly aroused woman's genitals.

Most pregnancy manuals we've read grudgingly acknowledge that this increase in genital vascularity and lubrication can heighten sexual responsiveness, though the authors hasten to add caveats along the following lines: You may find your swollen genitals uncomfortable, your partner may be turned off by your blood-engorged vagina, you may both find the increase in vaginal secretions off-putting. The notion that a pregnant woman might feel like a raging sexpot gets short shrift, and "your clitoris may well puff up beyond your wildest dreams" never makes it onto the itemized list of physiological changes.

The truth is that you may feel like a raging sexpot some of the time, and then again, you may not. Every woman is different, and every pregnancy is different. Many women find that their sexual interest during pregnancy follows a bell curve, with desire decreasing during the first trimester, rebounding during the second trimester, and decreasing again for the final trimester.

> I desired sex less during the first and third trimesters, but that middle trimester was incredible. I wanted it all the time. It was our last hurrah!

> Oh, the second trimester, we chased each other around the house! The first tri, I was too tired, and the third I was too big, but oooh in between was fun!

Others may find that sexual desire steadily decreases throughout pregnancy, that it steadily increases, or that there aren't any discernible changes.

> I was too tired and sick for the first three months, had no sexual desire the second three months, and wanted it all the time the last three months. I was dramatically more interested in sex during my third trimester than at any other time, ever.

> During the first trimester, I had my usual interest in sex; during the second trimester, decreased interest; during the third trimester, no interest at all.

The individual variations aren't important. What's important is that you get the information you need and the encouragement you deserve to enjoy your pregnant sexuality without anxiety or self-judgment. Before we discuss the nitty-gritty physical details of sex during pregnancy, we'll review some of the emotional factors that play a big part in how you and your partners might feel.

WHAT'S GOING ON IN YOUR HEAD?

There's probably no time in your life when you'll be more aware of the complex inter-dependency of body, mind, and emotions than pregnancy. You're engaged in a total phys-ical upheaval, commencing a complete change in identity and lifestyle, and in the eye of a hormonal hurricane. Estrogen and progesterone, the same hormones that play a role in the emotional highs and lows of the menstrual cycle, are hard at work in your preg-nant body. Estrogen not only heightens libido, it makes you generally more sensitive, both physiologically and emotionally. Progesterone, produced in higher quantities dur-ing pregnancy than at any other time, has a relaxing effect on your central nervous sys-tem, which some women experience as "All's right with the world" and others as "I've never been so depressed." Dramatically higher levels of progesterone are responsible for the physical fatigue most women feel during the first trimester and the absentminded-ness and moodiness some women feel in the second and third trimesters. Hormone lev-els fluctuate throughout your pregnancy, so you can expect their effects to vary day to day.

Just as not every woman has emotional responses that correlate to the hormonal shifts of her menstrual cycle, not every woman will experience dramatic mood swings during pregnancy. But chances are good that you'll feel a wide range of emotions — pride, anxiety, excitement, ambivalence, elation, anger, fear — that will influence your self-image, self-esteem, and inevitably your sexuality during this time. We've summa-rized below some of the most common emotional issues related to sex. Rather than dismissing the feelings that may come up around body image and sex as "just the hor-mones talking," respect and attend to them. Your emotional responses during this life-altering time can shed new light on the feelings and attitudes you've always held about your sexuality — and they offer the possibility for some powerful transformation.

Everyone Knows I Had Sex

Pregnancy forces you to go public about your sexuality — after all, everyone around you assumes you must have had intercourse in order to get pregnant (if you got preg-nant through donor insemination, you have some choices about how public you wish to be). Public perceptions can be highly punitive if you're a teen mom; young women, while portrayed in popular culture as adorable midriff-baring fluffy sexpots, are often judged harshly if they actually have sex.

> Because I had my daughter when I was fifteen, I was automatically a slut in everyone's eyes.

> A nurse at the hospital cried because I was fourteen and still had braces and looked so young. Even though my parents had promised to be cool, they treated me like, and sometimes flat-out told me, I was a whore.

Boost Your Body Image

Pregnancy is a physically exhausting experience, and even the most "glowing" mom-to-be is unlikely to sustain an upbeat attitude about her body for nine whole months. When your hands swell, your feet throb, your back aches, and your stomach grows so large that you have a hard time getting out of a chair without assistance, feeling thrilled about the "miracle" of gestation can be difficult. But there is a silver lining. Many of us go through daily life without paying all that much attention to our bodies—a level of detachment that simply isn't possible when you're pregnant. Your body is forcing its way to the forefront of your consciousness, and if you accept this wake-up call to self-awareness, you stand a good chance of emerging from the experience with a heightened capacity for sensual pleasure.

Boosting your sensual self-awareness doesn't have to be complicated or highfalutin'—we're not suggesting you adopt a regimen of tantric exercises or compose erotic poems in honor of your swelling belly (but if that's your inclination, go to town). Any one of the following simple suggestions for dealing with pregnancy-related complaints is likely to improve your body image and, in turn, your sexual self-esteem. You can take your pampering into your own hands, or enlist the help of a friend or partner. Chances are your loved ones will be only too delighted to offer practical support and comfort.

Let your hair down. During pregnancy, your hair and nails grow faster, and often fuller, than usual (although some women find their hair also falls out faster). Invite a friend to give you a luxurious hair brushing, a stimulating shampoo, or a deluxe manicure or pedicure. Did you enjoy long grooming sessions with girlfriends or siblings when you were a teenager? Ever wonder why women so often stop touching each other in these casually intimate ways once we "grow up" and take lovers? Go ahead—exploit the fact that many people are drawn to touch pregnant women; simple tactile pleasures can go a long way to bring you into and awaken your entire body.

Celebrate your skin. Pregnancy hormones make some women's skin softer and other women's skin oilier than usual. As your pregnancy progresses, the skin of your abdomen can get quite itchy. You're also likely to develop stretch marks on all the parts of your body that are expanding the fastest: belly, thighs, and breasts. There's not much you can do to prevent these changes, but they provide an excellent excuse to rub oils or lotions into your belly, or let your partner caress you head to toe.

Love your feet. All that additional weight on your swollen feet and ankles makes them ache so badly that the pain can be hard to ignore. Whenever you have the chance, make a point of pampering your feet—wear good shoes, soak them in a cool foot bath, or ask your partner for a soothing foot massage. When you go to bed at night, prop up your feet on pillows and focus on the relief—sometimes the sheer absence of pain is nearly orgasmic in and of itself!

Worship your hands. It's not uncommon for pregnant women to experience tingling in the hands or the pain of carpal tunnel syndrome due to fluid retention in the extremities (the resulting swelling creates pressure on the nerves of your wrist). Help your hands feel alive—rub lotion into them yourself, or ask your partner to kiss, hold, and massage them.

If you're a teenage or unmarried mom, you'll appreciate this reminder from Ariel Gore, activist and author of *The Hip Mama Survival Guide:* "Jesus, as you may recall, was the son of one of the most revered unwed teenage homeless mothers in history."[1] Of course, Jesus' mother attained her revered status only by sacrificing her sexuality—and the Madonna/whore dualism still underlies twenty-first-century perceptions of women. For many centuries, women have only been able to redeem themselves for the selfish, unseemly act of having sex by trading in their lush maiden identity for a sexless maternal identity. Plenty of women who don't subscribe to traditional religious beliefs are still susceptible to a vague sense that motherhood and sexual self-expression are mutually exclusive.

Till about my sixth month, I was extremely sexually active with my son's father, but when I started to "show," I didn't even want to be looked at in that way. I was very self-conscious and thought there was something really wrong with my partner for even wanting me while I looked like that!

And women who have grown up with religious proscriptions against sexuality may find it's not easy to turn on a dime and discard the baggage that sex is the original sin—even married women, like the survey respondents below.

I was very self-conscious as a pregnant woman. I felt everyone looked upon me as a loose woman, that is, a woman who fornicated, and now everyone knew I had done the dirty deed. I grew up in a very Catholic family background. Proud and happy to be a mother? Well, yes and no.

I grew up Catholic. I wasn't supposed to be a sexual being before I became a mom. In fact, I still have problems allowing myself to be a sexual being and sometimes feel I can't admit to having sex, ridiculous and repressed as that may sound.

Meanwhile, there are religious traditions in which pregnancy is seen as not only an acceptable, but a blessed, time for sexual expression.

> My husband and I are Orthodox Jews who follow Jewish Family Purity laws, which means sex only two weeks out of the month, no physical touching during menstruation, and seven clean days after. So when I'm pregnant, it's heightened, 'cause we can do it any time we want!

The fact of the matter is that, once you're pregnant, there's no accounting for the widely disparate responses you'll inspire in others. For every raised eyebrow, there's an appreciative smile. For every man or woman who can't perceive you as a sexual being when you're eight months along, there's another who finds you erotically irresistible. Ultimately, how other people respond to your pregnancy doesn't matter; only how you feel matters. If you're uncomfortable with how pregnancy "outs" you as a sexual being, we can't order you to shrug off a lifetime of conditioning, but we can encourage you to look at the big picture and tease out those aspects of your changing identity that bring you a sense of power and pleasure.

> I felt like I was no longer the "ingenue," which was somewhat threatening to my sense of self. However, my sense of safety increased by a large measure. I felt safer for being the queen rather than the princess . . . more in control, less fearful.

Freedom from Birth Control

For women whose sexual partners are men, one of the most thrilling aspects of sex during pregnancy is that they can kiss birth control goodbye. This pleasure is familiar to women who have tried to conceive for some time, and an unexpected bonus for women whose pregnancies were the result of birth-control failures. Many women revel in a sense of freedom and abandon they've never enjoyed before.

> I felt more free, more juicy, more soft and sweet. I felt like I wanted to envelop my partner. I wasn't worried about getting pregnant, for obvious reasons!

> I had WAY more desire for sex during pregnancy. And the sex was much more pleasurable. It seemed like I was truly free to have as much sex as I wanted because I was always wet and sloppy and because there was no fear of pregnancy.

Passion and Vulnerability

You may find that having the enormous potential consequences of sexuality made manifest adds a greater sense of meaning and passion to your sexual encounters.

I would think about the baby during lovemaking and think: Wow, this is how he was created, through this kind of passion and love. It made the experience very personal and intense.

I wanted sex a lot when I was pregnant and it felt amazing, but I was also so emotional about it. I would cry after sex a lot, probably because I had so much going on in my heart and hormonally.

Sex before parenthood was very much self-centered, only about us. Now it feels like we made love and we changed the world!

This flip side of this passion is a vulnerability—both physical and emotional—that can make sex a more serious affair. Partnered women may feel a particularly strong intimacy and connection with their partner or their baby's father. Single women may feel particularly cautious about choosing sexual partners. And some women find that partner sex is simply too overwhelming or distracting and that they're most satisfied by solo sex.

I couldn't get enough sex during my pregnancy. Though the father and I were separating, I couldn't imagine being with anyone else except the father of my unborn baby—nothing religious, just my own personal choice.

I had an intense desire for sex, but was more careful about who it was with. I was very careful about what energy I would expose my baby to. I wanted her first experiences of sexual energy to be loving, safe, and pleasurable, whereas before pregnancy I was OK with sex being just a physical attraction. I was not interested in rough play at all during pregnancy.

During both my pregnancies I felt very sexual, but my sexuality turned inward—I preferred masturbation to actual sex with my partner. It was as if that was too much trouble—but I was turned on all the time. It was like being a young teenager in a way, with hormones constantly going. Partner sex was okay but I didn't want to take the time somehow, which isn't at all how I feel when I'm not pregnant!

Crossing the Gulf

First-time pregnancies provide the opportunity to begin integrating a new sense of self. Some women find that their maternal bodies give them an enhanced sense of their own womanliness and expand their sexual possibilities. Others find that the sexual responses they have during pregnancy challenge their preconceptions of what's appropriate for a mother to feel.

> I began to feel more liberated and more comfortable with my body, which may have been a result of finding that sex organs are for something other than just sex, i.e., reproduction and nourishment. I started to lose my sense of sex as dirty — and my modesty as well.

> In the second trimester, I actually had increased sexual desire. From that point on, though, it disappeared until about two years later. Even during my hypersexual phase in the middle trimester, I started to feel like it was a huge leap from pregnant woman to sexual being. Like there was an enormous gulf to cross to satisfy the two roles. I still felt the same about sex, but something about me having it seemed illicit. This feeling has remained.

> With my first child, it felt unmotherly to have sexual feelings — that started during the pregnancy. I went through the typical second-trimester horniness, but I would not ask my partner for sex because I felt embarrassed by the intensity of my sexual feelings. With my second child I felt fine about being sexual. I am ten years older now, and I'm just more OK about being a mom and a sexual being — in fact, being a mom has made me feel more sexual and powerful and good about my body.

As this last survey respondent points out, building a bridge between your maternal and sexual identities sometimes simply takes time. Most women find that their sex lives become truly fulfilling only when they are sufficiently mature and experienced to take charge of their own satisfaction and to relish the power and potential of their own bodies, regardless of imperfections. For many women, becoming a mother begins a process of self-acceptance and celebration that can be profoundly erotic.

Body Image

In our society, a lot of attention is paid to appearances, and looking young and slender is considered particularly desirable. Being pregnant subverts this ideal in spades: No matter what your chronological age, once you're pregnant, you're old enough to be somebody's mother. And once you're pregnant, you're not going to stay slender. Maintaining a healthy body image during pregnancy is challenging, especially if you have a pretty tenuous grip on your self-esteem to begin with.

> During pregnancy I just didn't feel like being sexual because I felt so enormous. It was more a body issue thing than feeling as if I was too big to move

around. Feeling too fat or ugly to have sex wasn't new—this time it was just because I was pregnant instead of because I was in my normal everyday body.

During pregnancy I wanted nothing to do with sex. I found myself undesirable (my husband disagreed, but I couldn't get past the extra weight). Keep in mind I have a history of depression, anorexia, and bulimia.

While plenty of lip service is paid to the glory of a pregnant belly, expectant mothers receive a near-constant stream of lectures from medical professionals and well-intentioned friends about the best ways to avoid putting on "too much weight" during pregnancy. Pregnancy manuals offer strict dieting guidelines, and popular magazines are filled with tales of celebrity moms who have returned to their personal Pilates trainers and recovered their pre-pregnancy figures within weeks of delivery. But most of us gain some weight during pregnancy, and these extra pounds don't automatically melt off even with breast-feeding, sleep deprivation, and the upper-body workout of toting diaper bags, car seats, and strollers every time we leave the house. Sure, it's important to stay in shape during pregnancy and postpartum—in fact, every woman should strive to eat nutritiously and get plenty of exercise throughout her life. But it's counterproductive to get co-opted into the pursuit of some unachievable goal. The truth is that it's possible to be physically fit and still wind up with cellulite thighs, stretch marks, and a belly that will never be flat. So? Welcome to the human race.

I went through a period of disappointment with my own body as everything altered. This has improved since I stopped looking at "women's" magazines and started looking at other real women.

The good news is that pregnancy can be a golden opportunity to kiss those old oppressive standards goodbye. Your body is being shaped by forces beyond your control, and the concept of staying petite via "willpower" is completely irrelevant. Many women find it quite liberating to expand in size and shape, and this sense of liberation can be accompanied by a burst of sexual energy.

I was very sexy. I felt older, and full of life because, well, I WAS full of life. Plus, my breasts were huge! I was floating in a sea of love (not from the father, but from myself) and it was rejuvenating.

I lost any previous inhibitions I had had about my body because it was just so PREGNANT that what could I do? I was incredibly horny too, and it was fun trying to figure out how to do it with that huge belly!

In the second and third trimesters my desire went way past anything I had experienced before, as well as my capacity for orgasm. As my belly blossomed, so did my body image and my relative self-worth, so I was less inhibited.

Maybe, like so many women in the Western world, you're sure you'd feel better about your body if only you weighed five pounds less. Maybe you're a butch woman who finds the sheer "femme-ness" of your pregnant body disorienting. It doesn't matter what your personal aesthetic has been up until now; once you're pregnant, your body will be larger and more curvaceous than ever before. The transformation is temporary, so why not enjoy "playing dress-up" in your new body? Take time to admire your lush proportions in the mirror, or celebrate your porn-star-sized breasts by lounging around in lingerie that features your assets. We tend to take our body image quite seriously — if you can cultivate a playful appreciation of your pregnant body, you may be able to sustain a more relaxed attitude postpartum as well.

Sex during pregnancy was great. I had really heightened sensation and we were so excited about the pregnancy, about being more of a family, that emotionally and physically it was tremendous. Try viewing yourself as all of these different people you never thought you'd be — every time your body changes it's like you're someone else and yet yourself. It's fun and can be great for fantasy for both partners.

Focus on your own experience of your changing body rather than fretting over what your partner might or might not be feeling toward you. As we'll discuss below, the partners of pregnant women are making their own adjustments to a life-altering event and may be grappling with fear, anxiety, excitement, arousal, or loss of desire — none of which necessarily has anything to do with your physiological transformation. You're the one who is discovering just what your body is capable of, and your loved ones can only bear witness. You can use pregnancy to cultivate a sense of acceptance about your physical appearance that will stand you in good stead throughout the rest of your life.

I loved sex during pregnancy. I felt free in my body for one of the first times in my life. I didn't worry about how thin or buff I was. I felt big, beautiful, and healthy, and I guess that did wonders for my sex life.

My sex life has gotten better since I was pregnant. I think due to heightened body awareness. I got more overtly into my womanliness. I think being bisexual and somewhat butch caused me to limit myself prior to motherhood. I now revel in my female sexuality, while still maintaining my old butch edge.

TWO TO TANGO

If you're in a relationship, many of your sexual concerns will be influenced by your partner's responses to your pregnancy, the changes you're going through as individuals, and the changes you're going through as a couple. You're both coping with feelings about becoming a parent and creating a family that are bound to affect your sex lives. Some of the issues that come up during pregnancy will be part of your emotional landscape for years to come. If your relationship doesn't have a strong foundation, choosing to have a baby together won't solve any of your problems — it may just speed up the relationship's demise. But if you're both committed to creating a relationship based on intimacy and trust, you're more than likely to weather the issues described below. After all, pregnancy provides you with plenty of opportunities to establish and practice good communication habits that will be invaluable as you raise a child together.

If you're single throughout your pregnancy, all of the topics addressed below will be relevant to your interactions with lovers. However, these issues will probably be less charged for you simply because you don't have a history of expectations and assumptions to overcome as you adjust to your new reality.

When You Need to Take the Lead

You may be wondering how you're supposed to love your pregnant body when you're convinced that your partner is turned off by it. First you'll have to determine whose issue this really is. Talk about your fears (see the Communication chapter, page 56, for tips on how to most effectively communicate about sex), and you may discover that you've been misinterpreting his or her reactions. Perhaps you've assumed that your husband is reluctant to touch your pregnant belly because it disgusts him, but he's really just scared of causing you discomfort. Maybe you think your girlfriend hasn't initiated sex because she finds you unattractive, when she's actually waiting for you to give her the go-ahead. In reality, many men and women find pregnant women utterly compelling and are highly aroused by this physiological transformation.

> I found it incredibly stimulating to be making love to a woman who was pregnant. The round curves, the firm belly, the shape. Absolutely beautiful.

> I felt very sexual while I was pregnant. My husband loved the way I looked and the way my belly got rounder and harder, so it was very easy to feel special and beautiful.

> I became a mom at age nineteen, and I was astonished how many men

came on to me because they thought pregnant women and/or nursing women were sexually attractive.

Don't underestimate the extent to which partners may need explicit encouragement that their sexual attentions are welcome and pose no danger to the fetus. We're all heirs to the Victorian notion that pregnancy is a "delicate condition," and this notion is reinforced in the twenty-first century by the increase in "high risk" pregnancies, as more women postpone childbearing until their thirties or forties. Pregnancy has become medicalized to such an extent that it's understandably difficult for partners to relax and do what comes naturally. They will need reassurance from you that physical intimacy feels comfortable — after all, they can't intuit what does or doesn't feel good to you, especially since this changes day to day — and they may want further assurance from your medical practitioner. In a normal healthy pregnancy and with a doctor's okay, there's no need to restrict sexual activity — we discuss those specific instances when it is advisable to abstain from intercourse and orgasm later in this chapter.

Concerns about sex can ebb and flow during a pregnancy. You and/or your partner may be hesitant to engage in sexual activity during the first trimester because you're afraid of somehow triggering a miscarriage. Although the medical professionals we consulted for this section could find no data that sexual activity causes miscarriages, it's common for pregnant women to feel particularly tentative about sex during the first months while they're riding out fatigue, nausea, hormonal overwhelm, or trepidation if they'd had a lot of trouble conceiving in the first place. As midwife Stephanie Brill comments, "The first trimester has a damper effect, and I truly think that any fears should be honored. If sex isn't appealing during the first trimester, whether it's because of fear or just because of feeling sick and needing to sleep — I think a woman knows what's going on in her body, and that needs to be respected."

Your partner may simultaneously feel genuine concern for your physical comfort and a certain amount of shock at your rapidly morphing body — face it, on a certain level you're no longer "the girl I married." Frequently partners become more hesitant about sex when the pregnancy progresses to the point at which the baby-to-be's presence is tangible.

I was one whose libido increased, but my hubby was afraid he'd hurt the baby, despite all the confirmations that he wouldn't! He only really began to be afraid when I started to show and the baby became more of a reality.

Partners can be totally turned on by your body, totally turned off, or simply too busy grappling with their own anxieties — about your health, finances, or their readiness to become parents — to feel particularly sexual. Just because your honey isn't going through a physical gestation doesn't mean that he or she isn't going through a psychological gestation.

> I had expected to be sexually turned on by having a pregnant and nursing wife — the woman I loved but with a very different and changing body. Oddly, I felt rather turned off. Part of this, I think, had to do with the anxiety I felt about becoming a parent (with pregnancy #1), or managing two kids (with #2).

> My husband had zero sex drive during my third trimester. It was a huge issue because I was horny and concerned that my great, loving, always supportive husband was grossed out by my largeness. He explained that he was slightly freaked out about the baby being "right there," about being a dad, and that he just plain didn't have the urge to screw. It worked out.

If you can avoid taking your partner's flagging libido personally, it will be easier for him or her to speak about it candidly and for the two of you to work on some coping mechanisms. Sometimes simply expressing anxieties helps them dissipate. If you're willing to be explicit about the specific factors inhibiting sexual feelings, the two of you can find ways to focus on the changes in your body that your partner finds arousing. Maybe he can't get past an irrational worry that intercourse will somehow hurt the fetus, but he is excited by the thought of burying his penis in your new cleavage. Maybe she finds your increased vaginal discharge puts her off oral sex, but she's eager to enjoy the sensual pleasure of massaging your firm, round belly and manually stimulating your protruding clitoris. It may be your libido, not your partner's, that is flagging — we discuss this situation below in "When You're Out of Step." Regardless of who is feeling a sense of sexual restraint, we'd encourage you to communicate honestly about your responses. The very fact that pregnancy is a transitional state could embolden both of you to identify what activities turn you on or off during this time, and you might discover erogenous zones that you'd never enjoyed before.

When Three's a Crowd

> Whenever we did have sex, I'd feel like all three of us were connected in some way, all three of us joined together in an act of pure love.

Maybe you, like the woman quoted above, relish the sense that the whole family is somehow participating in lovemaking during pregnancy. More likely, this thought makes either you or your partner a bit squeamish. It's fairly common for men, in particular, to be uncomfortable with intercourse during pregnancy because of a feeling that the baby is in on the action, which can manifest as fear that the fetus might somehow be injured by the penis, or even as embarrassment that the fetus is somehow witnessing the proceedings.

> My husband wasn't interested in sex while I was pregnant. I had assured him the baby couldn't be harmed. But he was consumed with the thought that his child was inside me at the same time he was.

> I had a higher level of desire while I was pregnant, but after the fifth month my husband didn't want to have sex. He couldn't get over the thought that there was a "person in there." Unfortunately, when I was already feeling unattractive and huge, his apparent lack of desire for me just made me feel worse.

In actuality, the fetus is extremely well protected by the uterus and well cushioned by amniotic fluid. The cervix—the entrance to the uterus—has only a small opening which is sealed off by a mucus plug until shortly before labor begins. No penis is going to poke the little peanut in the head. A fetus often responds to the uterine contractions of orgasm by kicking and moving about, but this is not the equivalent of a neighbor banging on your apartment walls and yelling, "Keep it down in there!" Your baby isn't watching through the keyhole.

But the definition of an emotional response is that it isn't rational, and if your partner feels uncomfortable having intercourse, logic isn't going to help. In fact, you may both simply be distracted by the increasing amount of space your baby-to-be is taking up, both literally and emotionally.

> I enjoyed sex throughout most of my pregnancy. But by the seventh or eighth month, the baby was the only thing I could think about and was at the forefront of my mind even during sex. My husband and I like positions in which we face each other, and there was a feeling of having a third party involved in our lovemaking, which felt weird to us. Now that we're parents, we have sex in bed with our sleeping baby. So it's not so much the baby's presence, but the feeling of having someone literally between us.

There's certainly nothing wrong with forgoing intercourse during this time period. Heck, we think heterosexual couples should get outside the box of vaginal intercourse whether or not they're pregnant. But if you find yourselves uncomfortable with any type of sexual activity—intercourse, oral sex, manual stimulation, mutual masturbation, or erotic massage—it's a good idea to sit down and talk about what's going on. We're not saying that you must have sex during pregnancy even if neither of you is feeling desire, but it's crucial that you communicate what you're feeling, or you risk creating misunderstandings and resentments that could linger long after the baby's born.

When You're Out of Step

Pregnancy is a time when desire discrepancies loom large for many couples. The stereotype is that of the pregnant women who is completely uninterested in sex and either endures the unwelcome advances of an insensitive partner or becomes so unavailable that the partner takes leave emotionally.

> During my pregnancy, I didn't always feel well and was tired a good deal of the time. My husband was not sensitive to my needs and demanded the same frequency of intercourse as before the pregnancy. I had had a lot of trouble getting pregnant, including surgery and a year of trips to the doctors for all kinds of invasive stuff, so when I finally did conceive, I felt protective of my body and the baby. Because of my husband's lack of sensitivity to my needs, I felt like he was invading me much of the time we had sex. Needless to say, my sex life went downhill at that time.

However, we have heard just as often from women who were frustrated by their partner's lack of desire during their pregnancy.

> I was extremely ready for sex all the time, but it was a very lonely time sexually because my husband couldn't understand my need for sex and connection. He experienced a real decline in desire during my pregnancy, which was stressful for both of us.

During pregnancy, both partners have a lot to deal with, both physically and emotionally, so there's no way to be in perfect sync. Instead, focus on identifying your own yearnings and anxieties so that you can explain them to each other. As a pregnant woman, you're obviously contending with the greater physiological upheaval; however, your experience is by definition the main event, and your partner may feel a little left out—or even put out—at being relegated to a supporting role. You're both contemplating a major life change that is equal parts exhilarating and debilitating, which is bound to affect your libido. A little compassion can go a long way. Too often when couples aren't feeling the same level of desire at the same time, they become antagonistic, defensive, polarized, and ultimately distanced. If you can accept that you each have the right to your individual feelings, you will ultimately nourish your intimacy far more than if you hold out for some unachievable goal of simultaneous desire, arousal, and orgasm. Pregnancy reveals the utter impossibility of this goal—a pregnant woman is going through sexual, emotional, and hormonal fluctuations that her partner simply can't share—so it can be a good time for a couple to practice getting comfortable with their differences.

We believe that couples should encourage each other's sexual expression without judgment, but we don't have much patience with pregnancy manuals that advise women to make a point of satisfying their husband's "needs" even if they themselves aren't "in the mood." Sometimes you may not feel particularly amorous, only to become pleasantly aroused if you're willing to follow your partner's lead. And sure, it's great to be willing to give pleasure without keeping score or expecting immediate reciprocation. But if you're thoroughly uninterested in sex, providing a conjugal blow job for the sake of some retro notion of keeping your man happy is only likely to leave you feeling resentful and angry.

Your right to be uninterested in sex, however, doesn't mean that you have the right to feel hostile to or betrayed by your partner for his or her sexual drive. Too often the partner who's not feeling amorous takes offense at any overt expression of sexuality, and a couple drifts apart like this survey respondent and her husband:

I didn't like having sex when I was pregnant, especially when I got further along. During my pregnancy, when I didn't feel like having sex, my spouse got heavily into pornography, which has completely turned me off. And we didn't have as much time to reconcile afterwards.

As another survey respondent demonstrates, if you take the attitude that neither partner's feelings are wrong and adopt a lighthearted approach to differing desire levels, your relationship will ultimately be stronger.

After my daughter was born, I just felt that she needed me more than my husband did. I gave him a stack of porn magazines and told him to have at it for a few months and I'd be back soon enough. He was great.

If you can respect and appreciate your partner's sexual desires rather than being threatened by them, you're likely to sustain intimacy regardless of whether you're sharing every sexual experience. In our society, we tend to approach sex from the standpoint of scarcity, not abundance. All too often the equation becomes: "If my partner is masturbating, watching porn, enjoying sex chat on-line, or fill-in-the-blank, there won't be any sexual energy left for me," as though sexual energy is a finite resource when, in fact, it's endlessly renewable. Similarly, your partner can turn his or her sense of scarcity into the equation — "If we haven't had sex in three months, we're never going to have sex again" — and either badger you for attention or withdraw completely. The bottom line is that it's definitely countererotic to feel guilty, pressured, or abandoned, so if you can empathize with each other, you stand a better chance of being met halfway in some sensual encounters. A healthy self-esteem and a good sense of humor can go a long way to help a couple navigate their inevitable sexual ups and downs.

> Pregnant sex is a toughie, everyone has to be patient and understanding. And lovers have to remember that they can never understand how weird it is for you to be pregnant so pressure will get them NOWHERE. They should learn to beat off, go with the flow, and make the most out of what they can get.

Just Connect

Everyone who's ever been in a long-term relationship has experienced a sexual dry spell at one time or another. Pregnancy itself can be a dry spell, or it can be the rains that end the drought. Couples who have struggled for a long time to conceive, or who have used assisted reproductive technologies to conceive, often become so stressed and demoralized by the process that their sex lives suffer. Once your sex life has slowed to a standstill, it can be very intimidating to jump-start physical intimacy again — a host of assumptions and hurt feelings conspire against you. For couples who aren't sure how to re-create sparks, the sexy side effects of pregnancy — the genital blood flow, the wet dreams, the expanding breasts — can be a welcome wake-up call. Even if you or your partner aren't feeling turned on by your pregnancy, the sheer momentum of this body-centered time can inspire physical encounters — massages, foot rubs, or just lying together and stroking your belly.

> Being tired inhibited some sex drive. But we made ourselves connect — I think one can commit to pushing through inertia and it can really be invigorating, to commit to keeping all those parts of yourself alive.

When you're pregnant, prevarication becomes next to impossible. You can't ignore or dismiss the process your body is going through. Women often find that being pregnant enhances their self-respect, which in turn inspires them to communicate with greater authenticity about their physical desires.

> If you are pregnant, listen to your body. Any other time in your life you can give in to sex from your partner even if you're not really in the mood, but while you are pregnant don't do it. It will make you resent your partners and feel as if they don't care as much about you and your baby. Talk to your part-

ner at length about your sexual feelings: your wants, needs, or your lack of them. For nine months you get your body in this wondrous state—don't compromise it for a second!

WHEN TO PROCEED WITH CAUTION

As noted above, sexual activity doesn't pose a threat to a normal, healthy pregnancy. However, under certain circumstances, you may need to avoid any form of vaginal penetration or even orgasm. If your medical practitioner tells you to abstain from sex during all or some portion of your pregnancy, ask for more specific guidelines. Doctors receive little training in human sexuality and can use imprecise language (referring to vaginal intercourse as "sex") or make inaccurate assumptions (lesbians don't have penetrative sex). You may need to apply a little gentle persistence to determine what specific activities are or aren't off limits and for how long (see the How to Get the Information You Need chapter, page 159, for tips on talking with your medical professional about sex). The following are some reasons to abstain from sexual activity during pregnancy. However, every pregnancy is different, and you may want to get your doctor's go-ahead even if you don't have the risk factors below.

Vaginal Bleeding

Many women have spotting during their first trimester, especially around the time they would be menstruating if they weren't pregnant. And throughout pregnancy, many women spot as a result of penetration, since the cervix and vaginal tissues are softer, more elastic, and filled with more blood than usual. You can make adjustments to the angle and depth of penetration to avoid bumping the cervix and to minimize spotting. While this kind of bleeding is not necessarily cause for alarm, you should discuss it with your medical practitioner; if you repeatedly bleed after penetration, he or she is likely to recommend that you avoid intercourse for the duration of your pregnancy.

Heavy bleeding could be a sign of far more serious problems—including an impending miscarriage, an ectopic pregnancy, premature labor, placentia previa (see below), or placenta abruptio (a condition in which some or all of the placenta separates from the wall of the uterus, threatening the life of both mom and fetus). If you experience heavy bleeding—especially accompanied by pain, cramping, nausea, or fever—you should contact your medical professional immediately.

Risk of Miscarriage

A miscarriage is the loss of pregnancy before twenty weeks' gestation—approximately 80 percent of miscarriages occur in the first trimester. An estimated 15 to 20 percent of clinically confirmed pregnancies end in miscarriage, but the actual miscarriage rate per conception is even higher, since many women miscarry even before they know they're pregnant. Miscarriage rates go up for women in their late thirties and forties.

Most miscarriages occur for physiological reasons over which we have little to no control. The most common cause is some type of chromosomal abnormality, and less common causes include uterine, cervical, or hormonal abnormalities; immune disorders; or infections. If you have a history of miscarriage, or your medical practitioner has determined that you're currently at risk, you will be instructed to abstain from penetration and orgasm for at least the first trimester. Many of the doctors and midwives we spoke to acknowledge that there's no conclusive data supporting a restriction on sexual activity to prevent miscarriage—they and their patients simply prefer to err on the side of caution. Given that any ban on sexual activity is usually lifted once the woman has reached her second trimester, most women choose to follow doctor's orders. However, should you miscarry, keep in mind that it was *not* because you were sexually active, no matter how many orgasms you may have had.

Risk of Premature Labor

Premature labor is labor that occurs before the thirty-seventh week of pregnancy. If you have a history of premature labor, or your medical practitioner has determined that you're currently at risk, you'll be instructed to abstain from intercourse and orgasm in the last trimester of your pregnancy until you reach thirty-seven weeks. A related risk factor is the condition given the unflattering medical term "incompetent cervix." In some cases, a woman's cervix dilates under pressure from the growing uterus midway through her pregnancy, putting her at risk for previable delivery. When diagnosed, her cervix is usually stitched closed in the second trimester, and doctors tend to recommend a ban on penetration and orgasm throughout the remainder of her pregnancy.

The restriction on vaginal intercourse and orgasm is based on the possibility that strong uterine contractions might trigger premature labor. Semen contains prostaglandins, and prostaglandins cause uterine contractions and soften the cervix (a preliminary to labor). Obviously, the male partner could wear a condom, and his semen wouldn't contact the pregnant woman's cervix, but other factors are involved. Oxytocin—a hormone released during the uterine contractions of orgasm—also initiates the contractions of labor. In the early months of pregnancy, the uterus is relatively insensitive to oxytocin, but sensitivity increases as you get closer to term; that's why synthetic oxytocin, or Pitocin, is sometimes used to induce labor. When a woman is due to deliver, her doctor or midwife may recommend intercourse or orgasm as a way of bringing on labor.

Again, these precautions reflect a certain amount of erring on the side of caution. After all, many women report having orgasms in their sleep during pregnancy.

Because I have an incompetent cervix, I was banned from having sex or orgasms during pregnancy. I tried to block sex from my mind, which was hard because I felt very sexy. It also backfired because I had orgasms in my dreams. All three of my children were full-term anyway.

As one obstetrician we interviewed remarks, "I have patients who I tell not to have sex or orgasms because they're at very high risk, and they come in saying, 'You know I was asleep and I had this orgasm, and it was really strong because it had been a while.' So yes, the uterus contracts. With female orgasm, the uterus contracts. But the uterus contracts all day long, off and on, and I'm not aware of any facts that would tell us that a certain amount of contraction is okay, but twenty percent more isn't."

The ban on orgasm may be somewhat arbitrary, but we're by no means suggesting that you ignore doctor's orders. Even if it's only a possibility that uterine contractions would trigger labor, why tempt fate? You have only nine months to be pregnant and the rest of your life to enjoy as many orgasms as you please.

Placenta Previa

The placenta usually attaches itself to the upper wall of the uterus, but in placenta previa (which occurs in fewer than 1 percent of live births), the placenta grows on the lower wall of the uterus, partially or completely covering the cervix. This condition is usually discovered during either a routine ultrasound at twenty weeks or in the third trimester, when women with placenta previa often experience vaginal bleeding. If you're diagnosed, you'll be advised to restrict vigorous physical activity and avoid any form of penetration in order to prevent dislodging the placenta, which could result in heavy bleeding and premature labor. In most cases, the placenta moves away from the cervix by the third trimester, but when it does not, the baby is delivered via cesarean section.

Ruptured Membranes

Once the membranes around the amniotic sac rupture (also known as your water breaking), the fetus is very vulnerable to infection. Under no circumstances should you insert anything in your vagina after your water has broken. If your membranes rupture several weeks or months prematurely, you'll most likely be put on bed rest—with no penetration whatsoever until after delivery, and no orgasms until you reach thirty-seven weeks.

Risks from STDs

And now, just a reminder from your friendly sex educators that pregnancy is no time to give up on basic safer-sex precautions. Sexually transmittable diseases can jeopardize both your pregnancy and the health of your child. Chlamydia, which is often symptomless, has been linked to miscarriage and premature labor. Viral infections such as herpes can be dangerous to the fetus if you experience an outbreak (particularly your first outbreak) during pregnancy or childbirth. Please make a point of requesting a thorough screening from your medical practitioner either before you attempt to conceive or early in your pregnancy. You can be treated for any bacterial infection—such as chlamydia, syphilis, or gonorrhea—with antibiotics, and you can be monitored for any viral infection—such as hepatitis, herpes, genital warts, or HIV—in order to reduce the risk of transmitting the virus to the fetus or newborn.

A proactive approach is essential to your child's health and well-being: untreated HIV-positive pregnant women have a 25 percent chance of transmitting infection to their child, but transmission rates are dramatically decreased for women who are on a course of antivirals during pregnancy (cesarean-section births and bottle-feeding may also be recommended to reduce chances of HIV transmission). Women who are positive for hepatitis B risk transmitting it to their newborns, a risk that can be averted if the newborn receives an initial immunization shot within hours of birth. Hospitals now routinely recommend hepatitis-B shots for all infants, but you should still determine whether you're infected, in which case you'll need to ensure that your baby is immunized.

Safer sex is all about preventing contact between bodily fluids—blood, semen, vaginal secretions, and breast milk—and the mucus membranes of the mouth, vagina, and rectum. You can practice safer sex by using latex or polyurethane barriers—condoms, gloves, or dams—to avoid transmission of viruses or bacteria. Check our Resources section (page 340) for more information on safer sex and the impact of STDs on pregnancy.

Other Common Infections

Bacterial vaginosis (or BV) has been linked to miscarriage and, according to some studies, is found in up to 30 percent of pregnant women. Although it's actually an imbalance of the natural bacteria of the vagina, BV is sometimes grouped with bacterial STDs because it can be transmitted from one partner to another. If you're diagnosed with BV, you and your partner should be treated with antibiotics.

Yeast infections, another overgrowth of unhealthy bacteria, are very common during pregnancy. No, the white, milky discharge you have throughout pregnancy probably isn't yeast. If your discharge becomes thick and yellow or green in color, smells bad, and is accompanied by itching or soreness, odds are good that you have an infection. You can be treated with antibiotics, but resign yourself to the fact that infections may recur. Since you can transmit yeast to a partner, you should avoid receiving oral sex or having intercourse during this time—not that you're likely to feel so inclined!

I didn't really want sex a whole lot because I had a horrible yeast infection
for most of my pregnancy. So I was more itchy and crabby.

Urinary tract infections (or UTIs) are quite common during pregnancy, and while
these don't qualify as an STD, they are exacerbated by sexual activity, and you will be
advised to abstain from intercourse while you're treating the infection with antibiotics.
UTIs can be asymptomatic but would be diagnosed during your routine urine cultures.
Symptoms include the urge to urinate (which is pretty much a symptom of pregnancy
in general), a burning sensation when you pee, fever, and sharp abdominal pain.

If you're requesting medical attention for any sexually transmissible infection,
please make sure your provider knows that you are pregnant. You'll want to make sure
you're not taking medication that could be harmful to your fetus (some antibiotics are,
some aren't).

STAYING SAFE: MYTHS AND REALITIES

We have no quibbles with legitimate medical reasons for limiting sexual activities during pregnancy, but general cautions are sometimes interpreted in ways that don't have
much to do with science. As a public service, we've itemized some of the warnings we
came across during our research. Can you guess which are true and which are false?

Don't use dildos during pregnancy. False. Because the vaginal tissues are more
elastic and blood-engorged during pregnancy, some folks suggest that pregnant
women could injure themselves with dildos or insertable vibrators. Hmm, that's
funny, no one ever suggests that women could injure themselves with a penis. This is
a classic example of sex-toy discrimination (as former vibrator saleswomen, we're all
too familiar with the syndrome). If your pregnancy is low-risk and you have your doctor's okay, there's no reason not to enjoy penetration with whatever pleasure tool floats
your boat. Some common sense precautions: Keep your toys clean, use lubricant, and
adjust the angle and depth of insertion to avoid bruising your cervix and your tender
internal tissues. Guess what? Those same precautions apply to your beloved partner's
fingers or penis.

Desire for intercourse went down for both of us. I was HUGE, and I think
that affected my hubby, although he'd never admit it. I used my dildo every
single day, though—I was very into that.

Superintense vibrator-induced orgasms may cause premature labor. False. An
orgasm is an orgasm is an orgasm. If your medical professional has advised against

orgasm, that's because she or he feels that any uterine contractions might trigger labor. We could find no scientific data identifying a specific danger zone on the Richter Scale of orgasms, and in any case, there's no way you could consistently aim for an orgasm of a specific intensity. For one thing, how would you control the orgasms of your sweet dreams?

> My desire went through the roof! Being pregnant with twins, with all that blood flow to my pelvis area, made even just walking a wonderful experience! I could not have sex because of premature labor, so my brain took care of it by having wet dreams practically every other night! I was hooked to a home monitor, and the nurses would get such a kick out of my orgasmic/contracting uterus the following morning!

Superintense masturbation-induced orgasms may cause premature labor. False. Geez, if we were heterosexual men, we'd get a bit of a complex from reading pregnancy manuals. The subtext seems to be: Gals, the powerful orgasms you give yourself are capital-D dangerous, but those wimpy little orgasms your hubby gives you are nothing to worry about!

Don't have anal sex during pregnancy. False. Anal stimulation is well worth exploring at any time. The anus is an erogenous zone loaded with nerve endings that practically cry out to be caressed lovingly, and many folks enjoy the erotic pressure and fullness of anal penetration. You may find that anal penetration is a great way to make an end run around any anxieties you have about vaginal penetration. Pregnant or not, you should always follow three basic rules for any kind of anal sex: relaxation (you can learn to relax your external sphincter muscles, and you should never force anything into your anus); communication (let the receptive partner be in control of the action); and lubrication (use plenty of lubricant because, unlike the vagina, the rectum produces none of its own). Hygiene, always an important consideration in anal play, is crucial during pregnancy, when your swollen genital tissues reduce the distance between anus and vagina and you're generally more susceptible to vaginal infections. Never transfer a finger, penis, or sex toy that's been in your rectum to your mouth or vagina without a thorough cleaning, or you run the risk of transmitting bacteria from feces. You'll find that condoms and gloves can simplify matters, and it's definitely advisable to use a latex barrier for oral/anal contact.

If you're suffering from the hemorrhoids that are common to pregnancy, you probably don't want to insert anything in your rectum, but gentle external anal stimulation could result in increased blood flow and a relaxing of your sphincter muscles that would be downright beneficial.

If someone blows into your vagina, you could die. True! You will find this warning in just about every pregnancy manual ever written, and, by golly, it's true. Because of the way blood flows from the uterine wall into the placenta, if your partner was to blow directly into your vagina with sufficient force, the air could conceivably make its way up through your cervix, underneath the edge of the placenta, and into your bloodstream, thereby causing a potentially lethal air embolism. Phew! We were unable to find any statistics on how often this has actually happened, but apparently there is clinical literature to support its occurrence. But, we hasten to add, provided your partner isn't huffing and puffing directly into your vagina, oral sex during pregnancy doesn't pose a risk.

SOME SEXPERT ADVICE

Many women enjoy sexual activities that get nary a mention in mainstream pregnancy manuals. The most diligent search between the lines won't turn up any guidance for the reader seeking bondage safety tips. And although we dream of the day when "vibrator" appears in the index of any and every book related to women's health, we stopped holding our breath long ago. Doctors and midwives aren't always much more help. Even if you get up the nerve to ask medical practitioners about the safety of vaginal fisting or S/M play, they simply may not know what to tell you. Herewith, some advice that will hopefully fill in some of these blanks.

Is it safe to use my electric vibrator during pregnancy? There's been some controversy in recent years over whether EMFs (electromagnetic fields) increase the risk of miscarriage and fetal damage, and we've been queried more than once by expectant moms who want to know whether vibrator use could be generating a harmful force field. After all, it's a minor inconvenience to give up that electric blanket, but a considerably greater sacrifice to tuck yourself into bed night after night without that Hitachi Magic Wand to soothe your restless body to sleep. The good news is, at least one study indicates that EMFs do not have any adverse affects on pregnant women.[2] If you're not reassured by science, you can always pull the plug on your electric vibe and turn to a battery-operated model.

Is S/M play safe during pregnancy? If you're someone who usually enjoys rough-and-tumble sex or likes to incorporate aspects of power play (bondage, discipline, dominance, and submission) into your partner sex, you will want to make some adjustments to your routine. Even when your body feels great and you're on a hormonal high, you need to keep some common-sense restrictions in mind. Don't overexert yourself at a time when your back muscles and pelvic ligaments are particularly susceptible to strain. Don't let your partner strike your breasts or abdomen. Avoid bondage, particularly later in pregnancy, as you will be much more prone to stiffness or painful cramping due to constricting circulation. Of course, you can continue to enjoy the psychological aspects of power play, but many women report that they feel too vulnerable and self-protective during pregnancy to be so inclined.

Is vaginal fisting safe during pregnancy? Vaginal fisting is the term used for inserting an entire hand into the vagina, an activity favored by women who enjoy a sense of internal fullness and pressure. Fisting involves gradually coaxing the vaginal muscles to accommodate your partner's hand—it's not about having a clenched fist slammed inside you. During pregnancy, the tissues of the vagina become so blood-engorged that you may feel like you don't have as much room as you're used to, and you may not be particularly interested in penetration. Your soft tissues are likely to bleed should you engage in such vigorous penetration. But is fisting during pregnancy dangerous? Needless to say, there's no clinical data on the subject. We spoke to one midwife who firmly discouraged fisting, as she had seen a correlation in her practice between fisting and second-trimester miscarriages. Two other medical practitioners felt that fisting is safe provided you follow the same precautions as with any other type of penetration—i.e., avoid causing trauma to the cervix, and be gentle.

What should I do about my piercings? Some pregnant women have to deal with a wedding ring that no longer fits over swollen fingers, and some have less traditional jewelry to worry about. If you've got a navel ring, remove it early in the pregnancy, as it's likely to tear under the force of your expanding belly. For genital piercings, we'd advise removing your jewelry in early pregnancy, before your genital tissue swells around them. Some women do keep their labia rings in throughout labor, but as Ariel Gore notes, "There's going to be plenty of action down there without having to worry about additional metal and holes."[3] And yes, you will have to remove those nipple rings when you're breast-feeding.

THE NITTY-GRITTY: SEX WILL BE DIFFERENT

Let's talk about sex! Sex in all its slippery, sweaty, tissue-engorging, exhilarating glory. One fact of life that you can't learn soon enough in your pregnancy is that sex as you knew it is history. How could it be otherwise? Your body is undergoing a rapid sequence of changes that affect your sensory experience from head to toe. You may find the transformations of pregnancy to be purely positive:

My desire level increased and sex was more delicious — before parenthood, sex was still nutritious, yet when I was pregnant, sex was a gourmet banquet!

Or you may feel decidedly downbeat about the whole thing:

My desire level was close to nil while I was pregnant. I didn't like sex at all — it was very uncomfortable no matter what position we tried.

Your experience of sex during this challenging time could reflect the physiological vagaries of your own unique pregnancy. However, odds are good that it also reflects your comfort level with any sexual change of pace. Most of us are more set in our erotic ways than we might realize. We tend to get comfortable with reliable forms of stimulation — a certain position, touch, fantasy, or beloved sex toy — and we don't want to mess with success. This is just one more way in which the prevailing culture of sexual scarcity has a chilling effect on our sex lives: We'd rather have our customary orgasm than risk having no orgasm at all. This don't-rock-the-boat approach can work just fine until something comes along to tip your boat right over — something like pregnancy.

In her essay "Egg Sex," author Susie Bright gives a typically straight-shooting account of how unnerving it can be to discover that your body is changing in the most intimate of ways:

I was unusually sensual and amorous, and yet, twenty weeks into pregnancy, I found I could not successfully masturbate the way I had been doing since I was a kid. I was stunned and a little panicky. My engorged clitoris was different under my fingers; too sensitive to touch my usual way, and what other way was there? That's when it hit me. The experts all say that it is a mystery why some women get more horny when they're pregnant while others lose interest. I'll tell you something — no one loses interest. What happens is that your normal sexual patterns don't work the same way anymore. Unless you and your lover make the transition to new ways of getting excited and reaching orgasm, you are going to be very depressed about sex and start avoiding it all together.[4]

We touched briefly on some of the physiological changes of pregnancy above, but here's a more detailed blow-by-blow of their potential repercussions.

Don't Touch Me There!

In early pregnancy, your breasts may feel like they've been taken over by evil forces beyond your control. For one thing, they no longer look the same. As the milk glands begin to develop, your breasts inflate seemingly overnight. As blood flow increases, they become crisscrossed by protruding veins and highlighted by larger, darker areolae. Unobtrusive they are not. You may find it quite arousing to have morphed into a hyper-buxom version of yourself, or you may find it somewhat cartoonish and antierotic. And your partner's perceptions may or may not jibe with your own.

> With my second pregnancy, I was aroused all the time, but my husband was turned off by my body. I told him, "Enjoy these breasts now, 'cause they won't be this big or feel this good ever again," but he chose to pretend they didn't exist.

More to the point, your breasts no longer *feel* the same. Most women find their breasts painfully sensitive and sore early in pregnancy. This extreme tenderness usually passes by the fourth or fifth month, but some women find breast stimulation thoroughly unpleasant throughout pregnancy. After all, stimulation causes additional blood flow that can make their already swollen breasts feel excruciatingly tender.

> My breasts were ultrasensitive from the moment of conception and I didn't want my husband anywhere near them.

> My breasts were extremely huge and uncomfortable early on, so I could only take really gentle brushings of fingertips.

Others find the increased size and sensitivity of their pregnant breasts a sensual boon and discover a whole dimension of sexual pleasure in having their breasts fondled, sucked, rubbed, tweaked, and otherwise worshiped.

> I loved the increased sensitivity of my belly and breasts (especially after that first trimester when my breasts were sore all the time). I could practically come just by having my partner play with my nipples.

By your third trimester, you're starting to produce colostrum, the fluid that precedes breast milk, and you might leak some when your breasts are stimulated. While one popular pregnancy manual kindly suggests that you "refrain from breast play" if you're uncomfortable with the leaking, you'll be better off trying to adjust your attitude. After all, if you go on to breast-feed your infant, you'll discover that all kinds of sexual and emotional stimulation will induce a milk "letdown." That term sounds quite gentle and almost passive, doesn't it? But there's nothing passive about the spray of milk that shoots out of your nipples upon arousal. So go ahead and make a mess.

Because breast stimulation releases the hormone oxytocin in pregnant women, it's sometimes recommended to induce labor (or forbidden if you're at risk for premature labor). The uterus grows increasingly sensitive to oxytocin throughout pregnancy, so the oxytocin released from breast stimulation can kick-start the uterine contractions of labor. The best-case scenario is that you'll launch childbirth with an erotic interlude. Then again, you may feel like you're back in high school, parked in a car, while some well-meaning partner twiddles your nipples.

> I had heard that breast stimulation could start labor, so my partner and I gave it a try since I was a week overdue. We had a good laugh about it, but I was so nervous and stressed, I couldn't really enjoy myself. I just felt like we were trying to trip the right switch.

Who Turned on the Faucet?

Pregnancy is a slippery time. The increased estrogen in your system and the increased blood flow to your genitals result in increased vaginal lubrication, which has a heavier texture and a stronger odor and taste than usual. You may love feeling all juiced up, or you may wish you could turn off the waterworks. Either way, do yourself a favor and stay away from douches or the scented oils that some retro manuals recommend you use to mask your natural scent (to not offend your man's delicate sensibilities). The last thing your sensitive, yeast-prone genitals need right now is anything that might tip the pH balance of your vagina in the direction of an infection. If you're feeling overwhelmed by fluids, you can wear panty liners or wash your vulva more than once a day with unscented soap. And if you're uncomfortable with the heavier scent of your vulva, try adjusting your attitude. Susie Bright describes a woman's pregnant genitals as smelling "like a big cookie" — maybe you can come up with some positive associations of your own.

The Big O

All that blood flow to your genitals is bound to have an impact on your physiological experience of orgasm. Sexual arousal is a combination of muscular tension and blood flow — your pelvic muscles contract, and your erectile tissues become congested with blood. On the most fundamental level, orgasm is an involuntary series of muscular contractions that discharge built-up tension and release blood from the engorged genital tissues. Many women find that the increased vascularity of their pregnant labia results in a greater excitement phase (so many more blood vessels flooding their erectile tissues) and more intense orgasms (a much greater sense of release). Some women experience their first orgasms or multiple orgasms during pregnancy.

Before I was pregnant, I found it difficult to experience orgasm and rarely found sex pleasurable. During my pregnancy, I experienced intense and wonderful orgasms. Now it seems easy to enjoy sex.

On the other hand, some women find that as their pregnancy progresses, this increased vasocongestion can become somewhat frustrating. Their blood-engorged genital tissues remain in a state of semiarousal that orgasm is insufficient to resolve (resolution can take even longer when this pregnancy is not your first). You may orgasm over and over again without achieving a sense of completion, or you may find the release of orgasm seemingly just beyond your reach.

Orgasm changed a lot for me. It was harder to achieve, and it was duller and less satisfying. Whereas before pregnancy I was so sensitive postorgasm that I couldn't even stand to be touched, when I was pregnant (and for a while afterwards), as soon as I came it was like nothing had even happened.

We've had sex much less than we did before pregnancy, but those times are kind of stellar and emotionally intense — though actual orgasm is harder for me to come by and somehow muted in my hyperhormone state.

If you continue to achieve orgasm throughout your pregnancy, you'll notice one physiological response that women aren't always particularly conscious of otherwise: the uterine contractions that accompany orgasm. These grow stronger during pregnancy as your uterus becomes more and more sensitive to the oxytocin released during orgasm.

I had very intense orgasms during pregnancy. I was very sensitive to touch and highly aware of the physiology of orgasm with the contracting muscles.

The uterine cramping was a little disturbing and distracting at first. But the overall sensation was great. It was wonderfully intense. The vaginal wall swelling that started towards the end of my second trimester helped a great deal with the overall sensation.

Midway through pregnancy, many women start experiencing Braxton-Hicks contractions, an involuntary flexing of your uterine muscles in a warm-up for labor. You may find that your orgasms sometimes segue into a series of these contractions, and that the accompanying tightening of the uterus has an erotic component.

It was really cool how hard my uterus would get when I had an orgasm—solid solid solid! Whenever I came, my belly would just become hard as a rock!

By the end of your pregnancy, your contractions may become more intense and last for a longer period of time—from ten minutes to half an hour. For some women, these contractions are a thrilling ride; for others, they are painful enough to be a reason to avoid orgasm entirely. As long as you're not at risk for premature labor, you needn't be concerned about the contractions, and you can rest assured that your baby is enjoying the ride.

I found sex during pregnancy to be the most intense, most remarkable, most deeply moving experience of my life. My orgasms during pregnancy made all that morning sickness and general discomfort worth it. They seemed to roll over my entire body and I could feel my uterus bunching up in ecstasy. Each baby would lie very still for several minutes after orgasm and then begin to move and kick and dance inside me as if to say they enjoyed the experience, too.

Expect the Unexpected

In order to relax and enjoy your pregnant sexuality, you (and any partners) should learn to accept the fact that your moods will be utterly unpredictable. Between the hormones, the physical overload, and everything that's on your mind, your interest in sex will probably never again swing so erratically from full-bore to forget-about-it.

My sex drive fluctuated a lot during pregnancy. Sometimes I was tearing his clothes off before he got through the door, and other days I didn't want him to come near me. Before, my drive would shift, but never so dramatically.

It was SO erratic! There were days all I could think about was eating Ben and Jerry's Phish Food and having sex. Then there were days that I was so tired and sore and sick that I didn't even want to be touched.

And it's not just your physical interest that ranges all over the map. Many women say their pregnancies are distinguished by an unprecedented intensity and variety of sexual fantasies. Pregnancy is the biggest hormonal overhauling your system has had since puberty, and you may well find yourself time-traveling to a zone of polymorphous perversity in which your erotic desires can't be neatly compartmentalized. One midwife who works primarily with lesbian and bisexual women comments, "Lesbians are often surprised by the fact that they want to have sex with men — they don't necessarily follow through on it, but it's a very common desire." Heterosexual women can find their fantasies wandering over the fence as well.

> During this time, I first became really curious about having sex with other women, and fantasized about it often. I have no idea why, but I'm still curious to this day, although not at the same level as when I was pregnant. I'd say my desire level was at a peak very similar to that of my teenage years.

> I was so horny when I was pregnant I could barely see straight. I couldn't dream straight, that's for sure. My fantasies included men I'd never considered as partners and plenty of women too.

You may find it particularly unnerving to have hard-core fantasies during pregnancy, the time when you're supposed to be fine-tuning that warm, fuzzy, cookie-baking persona. Yet our most powerful fantasies are rarely sugar and spice and everything nice — taboo themes such as rape, incest, domination, and submission are staples in many a fantasy cupboard. We can't emphasize enough the importance of giving yourself permission to fantasize about anything and everything that gets you off. There's absolutely no evidence that fantasizing about a particular scenario means you want to live it out in real life. As the quotes above would indicate, some fantasies are compelling precisely because they involve activities outside your realm of experience.

Fantasies aren't merely harmless, we hasten to add, they can be downright healing. Your sexual fantasies may provide an outlet for some of the anxieties that inevitably accompany the huge life change you're going through. Psychotherapist Jack Morin has identified four "erotic cornerstones" that commonly fuel sexual arousal: power, ambivalence, anticipation, and prohibition.[5] As an expectant mom, you grapple with these themes on more than one level. Even the best-planned pregnancy involves a loss of control or power: You're probably ambivalent about the more carefree lifestyle that's about to end; anticipating your baby's arrival; and juggling an unprecedented array of do's and don'ts, many of which revolve around whether it's really okay for you to be sexual at this time. It makes sense that sex becomes a loaded experience — a way to simultaneously generate anxiety and relieve tension. Paula Bomer describes this well in her essay "Knocked Up, Getting Off":

> As someone who's always enjoyed the naughtiness of getting slammed, this bad-girl pleasure only increased during pregnancy fucking. The books and

your obstetrician will tell you that sex during pregnancy is safe. But it doesn't feel safe, and that weird sense of danger charged me with a kind of breathless, almost adolescent excitement.[6]

Whether your pregnant fantasies are filled with sensuous waterfalls or sleazy gang bangs, try to appreciate them all without censorship. The appeal of any individual fantasy is bound to ebb and flow depending on how useful it is at a given point in your life. If you grant your erotic imagination the same respect you're showing your body during this time, you'll gain access to a powerful tool for understanding your sexuality over the long haul.

Who's on Top?

Though authors of mainstream pregnancy manuals take only the most minimalist stab at the topic of sex, they will always include a paragraph or two about intercourse positions, encouraging readers that with a pillow here and a little gymnastic effort there, you can enjoy the same old moves. Many of our survey respondents mentioned their desire for more details on positions ideal for each trimester. But when you get right down to it, there's not that much to say on the subject. Perhaps the real issue behind this interest in negotiating positions is a nostalgic yearning for reliable pleasures—for sex to feel like it used to. We suspect that some folks focus on intercourse positions because of a certain resistance to and resentment of the inevitable changes pregnancy brings to partner sex. On the most basic level, this resistance is fueled by embarrassment at reliving the type of physical awkwardness most of us thought we'd left behind in adolescence. Suddenly your suave moves aren't landing you in the same places anymore. You have to put thought into what you're doing instead of operating on automatic. The truth is that the physical adjustments required are quite minor compared to the attitude adjustment. If you're willing to let go of that James Bond complex, you'll find that a lot can be said for bringing humor and a spirit of compromise into bed with you.

> The last trimester, sex was great, but I was so big that I laughed at myself when I caught a side glimpse in the mirror, and then my husband and I couldn't stop laughing.

> After my belly began to grow, the old positions didn't work, but we had fun trying new ones and developed a few new favorites. We also tried anal sex, which worked once or twice when nothing else would.

> Not every woman wants to have intercourse, or wants to have intercourse during

pregnancy. But if you do crave penetration, the following tips are equally applicable whether your partner's slipping a penis or a dildo between your legs, or whether you're enjoying vaginal or anal intercourse.

Cautions: Truth be told, your belly is not likely to be an impediment until about your fifth month, and for much of your pregnancy you can safely enjoy any position — just make sure your partner never puts his or her full weight on you or applies pressure directly on your uterus. In the second half of pregnancy, you should avoid lying flat on your back or on your right side for prolonged periods of time; you'll probably notice some dizziness and discomfort if you do. The weight of your uterus reduces the flow of blood returning to your heart through the vena cava (raising your blood pressure), and will also reduce blood flow to the placenta — neither of which are good things! You can easily adapt to this state of affairs by reclining on pillows in a semi-upright position.

Partner on top: You don't need to give up the full-body contact and face-to-face intimacy of the so-called missionary position just because you're pregnant. As you get larger, you will need to fine-tune this position by shifting slightly so that your abdomen is off to the side, not directly beneath your partner's body. If you and your partner scissor your legs, penetration is still possible. Alternately, you could lie on your back at the edge of the bed with your partner kneeling or standing on the floor between your feet.

You on top: Some women particularly enjoy being on top of their partners because of the opportunities the position provides for mutual stimulation and because they can control the depth and angle of penetration. Others find later in pregnancy that this position takes too much effort and they'd rather just be lying down.

> In my second trimester, I was horny all the time and loved having sex in kinky positions. I especially liked being on top and seeing my newly larger breasts bouncing around.

> We have always tried different positions, so finding a comfortable one wasn't hard. I found that I no longer enjoyed being on top after a point because I found my size made it hard for me to move how I wanted.

Rear entry: A common favorite, rear entry provides the opportunity for your partner to reach around and stimulate your clitoris and breasts. The position is good for G-spot stimulation and is a practical way to avoid jostling your pregnant belly. You can either kneel on the bed with your upper body propped on a pillow or kneel on the floor with your upper body supported on the bed.

During pregnancy I was more interested in sex than usual, but I gained weight quickly, so my husband and I had to be much more creative with positions. Rear entry and (believe it or not) anal sex were most comfortable for me.

Side by side: Side-by-side positions are excellent during pregnancy since neither partner has to support the other's weight. You can link legs face to face, or "spoon" with your back tucked up against your partner's chest. The beauty of these positions is that they are comfortable, provide full-body contact, and allow you to stimulate each other's genitals or caress each other's bodies with ease.

Enhancers: Pillows can be your best friend. You can surround your belly with pillows to make it more comfortable to lie facedown; prop yourself upright on pillows; kneel on pillows; or position pillows beneath your hips to take pressure off your back. And speaking of best friends, don't forget that you can either hold a vibrator against your clitoris or slip it between you and your partner in every one of these positions!

WHEN YOU'RE HOT

And now a few words from our sponsors—the moms who took the time out of their jam-packed schedules to complete our sex survey. We've organized some of their erotic memories of pregnancy into common themes. Do bear in mind that these quotes are from women who enjoyed sex during pregnancy. There are plenty of women who don't; every woman's experience is different, and every individual pregnancy is different.

Fringe Benefits

Pregnancy forces you to pay attention to your body, which can liberate you to pay attention to sexual sensations.

> My desire level is at its highest during pregnancy. I think about sex a lot, which is kind of emancipating, actually. How wonderful to be preoccupied with sex instead of trivial and unpleasant things. The level of enjoyment is different and higher for me because I come faster and more intensely than usual.

> During pregnancy, my sex drive skyrocketed. As I started prioritizing motherhood in my life, I think sex became different because having a new body to explore and new miracles inside me made my body that much more appealing.

Pregnancy sex was the best ever. We were both so enraptured by the biological events and their visible effects. I was physically more sensitive, emotionally more relaxed, socially more confident than ever before.

Try a Little Tenderness

Many survey respondents report that they craved a more gentle touch than usual during pregnancy, due to heightened physical and emotional sensitivity, and that they appreciated partners who were willing to focus on foreplay.

> I had some wonderful sex during pregnancy. I stopped worrying about how my body looked and paid more attention to how it felt. My partners had to be very gentle and loving to avoid hurting me, but they were, and that gentleness felt great.

> I wanted to have less "crazy sex" while I was pregnant due to my ever changing feelings about my body. Sex during pregnancy (when I let him near me) was soft and sweet.

> We had a lot of stress at first—it was an unplanned pregnancy, and we immediately moved in together and were dealing with trying to cram a few years' worth of togetherness into nine months. We spent more time trying not to focus so hard on intercourse. He'd rub my belly with lotion and oil and brush my hair. Sweet, tender things like that.

Plenty of women enjoy rowdy and ribald sex during pregnancy, and so they should. The bottom line is that during pregnancy most women find themselves more sensitive to the mood being created during sex than they might otherwise—and this heightened awareness can be a valuable addition to their sexual bag of tricks.

Different Strokes

Women who enjoy sex during pregnancy tend to be those who don't give in to despair when their old turn-ons cease to do the trick; instead, they adopt a spirit of exploration. These are often the same women who are experiencing a surge in libido during pregnancy—their willingness to experiment is fueled by heightened sexual desire.

> I did a lot of sexual experimenting during pregnancy. I found penetration to be totally unsatisfying and even annoying, and learned a lot by seeking different forms of stimulation.

My desire changed subtly, too. I found things arousing that I generally don't when not pregnant. That was the one time in our marriage that my husband and I experimented with X-rated movies. We decided that we would "go with the flow" and enjoy whatever whims came along.

One of the side effects of a surging libido that you (and your partner) might enjoy is a willingness to initiate sex more often.

I was turned on all of the time. My partner would come home and I would attack him at the door. Previously I had been fairly timid and this changed. I initiated more sex. I took a very active role during sex.

Sweet Dreams

Maybe nature rewards you for putting up with the stresses and strains of pregnancy — this is one time when it's common to orgasm while you're sleeping!

While I was pregnant I frequently had such intense sexual dreams that I orgasmed in my sleep. I joked with my husband that I didn't even need him anymore and I looked forward to falling asleep.

I had some of the most amazingly vivid sexual dreams when I was in the second trimester. So vivid I couldn't be sure it hadn't happened when I woke up.

And the dream fantasies I had were great also. It was the only time in my life I experienced full orgasm while dreaming.

Masturbation

We were especially pleased that solo sex helped many of our survey respondents maintain their sexual sanity during pregnancy. Whether you're interested in partner sex or not, masturbation is a great way to keep in loving contact with your body and to take the edge off your mounting tension. The demand-free aspects of masturbation can be particularly soothing to women in the late stages of pregnancy.

After the first two months, my clitoris throbbed! I couldn't wait to touch it or have it touched. My best friend became the removable shower head in my bathtub. It became a big joke with my husband and me. I wanted sex up until I became too big, then I just masturbated alone pretty much right up until my son was born. I didn't really feel "sexy" after my sixth month, so masturbation alone was all I was interested in.

Sex during pregnancy sucked—I just wanted to sleep or be massaged. Then again, I did masturbate plenty. It made my womb feel good and released a lot of tension. I just didn't want my partner touching me.

WHEN YOU'RE NOT HOT

Fair's fair. We'd like to give equal time to those women who don't experience pregnancy as a sexual wonderland. Maybe yours is a particularly difficult, high-risk, or medically complicated pregnancy, or maybe your libido simply can't override the cumulative effect of pregnancy's myriad discomforts.

Sex during pregnancy was pretty bad for me: In the first trimester, I was too tired; in the second trimester, my natural lubrication became very watery and sex was physically irritating; in the third trimester, the belly of the whale kept getting in the way, and my vagina kept getting smaller and smaller as my tissues swelled.

Some women find that the mere concept of sex during pregnancy does not compute. Their focus is on the baby growing within them, and sex now seems at best irrelevant and at worst dangerous.

During my pregnancy, I felt much more modest about sex. I believe the whole hormonal process that happens during pregnancy and afterward is nature's way of protecting the unborn and of keeping the energy focused on the life inside the mama. After birth it's about nurturing the newborn past the fragile first months. I had almost NO desire while pregnant. I think I was so obsessed with my little science experiment that I really saw my body as a protective wrapping for my baby.

When I was pregnant, I was so focused on the development, and later, the movement of the baby, that sex seemed like something that would be enjoyable but just wasn't a priority. It was like I felt that I have the rest of my life to have sex, but only just this moment to enjoy a certain movement or feeling. Also, after my third month of pregnancy, I started spotting a lot after each time we had sex, so then it became a concern to us and we didn't have intercourse again until two days before the baby was born.

Other women are facing stressful and libido-dampening events during their pregnancies. If you're focusing on getting clean and sober, dealing with the death of a relative or loved one, or struggling with the demise of a relationship, losing interest in sex would be natural. Pregnancy can also trigger memories of sexual trauma, such as abuse or rape, that complicate your responses to desire.

> Early in my pregnancy I went through some dramatic changes. I actually wanted sex more, but at the same time I had to deal with issues of sexual abuse I had experienced as a youngster. I learned to take each day as it came and not to stress myself about things other people had done to me.

We've got no bone to pick with any woman who simply chooses not to be sexual during this intensely demanding time. But be aware that any hiatus from sex that starts during pregnancy is more than likely to extend onward into the postpartum period. If you simply don't have the energy or the inclination to engage in partner sex, it's best not to "do your duty" anyway.

> I had no sexual desire during pregnancy, and as the pregnancy progressed sex became uncomfortable and a chore. I would do it anyway for my husband and then get resentful. I never once enjoyed sex while I was pregnant.

But if you're partnered, keep the lines of communication and the possibility of sexual encounters open, or you could jeopardize the quality of your relationship. Partnered or single, continue to treat yourself to sensual encounters — from foot rubs to new haircuts to masturbation sessions. As a mother, you won't be receiving much societal support for keeping your sexual self alive, and it can be all too easy to lose touch with that vital part of yourself.

Every Pregnancy Is Different

We wouldn't want to leave this topic without reiterating that every single pregnancy will be a different experience. Not only are hormonal and physical responses unique to each pregnancy, but you're at a different point in your life with each pregnancy.

> During my first pregnancy, I was pretty horny for the first few months (so much so that I orgasmed during masturbation for the first time), then my interest waned. During my second pregnancy, I just never wanted to have sex, though I did lend a hand to my husband. My third, I was horny all of the time, but only wanted to masturbate — which I did, frequently.

With my first child I lost total interest in sex—no cuddling, no hand-holding, no kissing—I was obsessed with my body's function as an incubator and was offended by the mere mention of sex. With the second, I was a sex kitten and couldn't get enough sex to save my life.

With my first pregnancy, sex was always very wonderful, soul-bonding kind of stuff. We were thrilled that I was pregnant, and just terribly in love and content and pleased with ourselves. I wanted to make love all the time. The second pregnancy, I was feeling very tired (chasing around after a toddler) and felt almost apathetic at times about sex. But it was still enjoyable and helped us, I think, to maintain a feeling of closeness. I was also much more comfortable with my body and less self-conscious the second time around. Like "This is it, I have nothing to lose from here on out. Might as well go for it, and let it all hang out." Maybe that's why my husband thinks I'm sexier now, because I was so nonchalant and mellow about it!

BE PREPARED: SEXUAL TRAINING

Although you may feel like you're going to be pregnant forever, by your third trimester, the good news is that the end is in sight. The not-so-good news is that, unlike any other endurance event, crossing the finish line requires even more physical stamina than the marathon that's gone before. But take heart—if you want to prepare yourself for child-birth, sex provides some of the best conditioning around.

Kegels Revisited

Yes, it's true—you're not going to get out of this chapter without a pep talk on the importance of doing your Kegels. Kegels are simple exercises that involve tightening and releasing the pelvic floor muscles, which play an important role in sexual response. But your medical practitioner probably didn't recommend Kegels out of concern for your sex life. Nope, you're advised to do Kegels during pregnancy in order to tone the muscles that will play such a big part in labor and delivery; you're advised to do them postpartum to recover strength in your pelvic floor, abdomen, and back. Weak or strained pelvic muscles can lead to reduced vaginal sensitivity, urinary incontinence, and lower backache—inconveniences that can be easily overcome by incorporating exercises into your routine only a few times a week.

What About Circumcision?

As part of your preparation for childbirth, please take the time to determine whether or not to circumcise your son, so that you can clearly communicate your desires to your doctor before you deliver. The United States is the only country in the world where the majority of newborn boys are circumcised, and until quite recently the procedure was routinely recommended by pediatricians. In 1999, the American Academy of Pediatrics withdrew its previous recommendation and acknowledged that circumcision is painful and should not be performed without anesthesia.

Circumcision became the norm in this country after World War II largely due to two obsessions: the peculiarly American obsession with hygiene and the peculiarly Victorian obsession with masturbation. A circumcised penis was considered a "cleaner" penis, and for years the received wisdom within the American medical establishment was that circumcision reduced rates of penile cancer, cervical cancer, urinary tract infections in infants, and the transmission of STDs. In fact, penile cancer is extremely rare; there's no proven link between circumcision status and cervical cancer; behavior, not anatomy, is the more likely determinant of an individual's risk for STD transmission; and, although the risk of developing a UTI in the first year of life is lower for circumcised boys, the risk for uncircumcised boys is at most 1 percent. Our Victorian ancestors embraced circumcision as a useful weapon in their war against masturbation, assuming that a circumcised boy would be less inspired to masturbate since the glans of the penis is less pleasurably sensitive without its protective foreskin.

We believe that everybody deserves all the sexual sensitivity they're born with, so our own bias is against circumcision. If you have religious or cultural reasons to circumcise your boy, we wouldn't presume to argue with these, but if you're simply falling sway to the knee-jerk desire to have your son look just like his daddy, think again. The worry seems to be that if Sonny-boy notices that he has a foreskin and Daddy doesn't, psychic scarring will ensue. Meanwhile, countless Sonny-boys have been able to cope with the fact that Daddy has pubic hair and they don't. Circumcision rates are falling fast in this country, so your sons (and daughters) inevitably will come into contact with both cut and uncut penises throughout the course of their lives. Don't let your own squeamishness at the prospect of discussing genital anatomy with your children lead you to subject your son to an unnecessary and painful procedure.

After childbirth, mild urinary incontinence (the old sneeze and oops, my pants are wet) became an unwelcome presence. But they include Kegels at my Jazzercise class, and it's all but taken care of the problem.

Bear in mind that the value of Kegels is not merely to tone and tighten — it's to gain awareness of vaginal muscles. Too often, people take a "hard body" approach to Kegels and focus all their attention on contracting their muscles, when it's equally crucial to learn to relax them. After all, your vagina needs to expand considerably during childbirth. Developing confidence in your ability to voluntarily contract and release your vaginal muscles will stand you in good stead when that baby's on the way. And cultivating genital self-awareness is undoubtedly preferable to enduring the techniques that social anthropologist Sheila Kitzinger describes seeing in an Eastern European hospital:

In one university hospital when I asked what women were taught about awareness and conscious control of their pelvic floor muscles (those that need to open up for the baby to be born and that need to be well toned afterwards), I was led downstairs to the basement. There I saw women sitting in rows, their white hospital gowns drawn up to their waists, knees spread, while opposite them, men in rubber suits aimed hoses of ice-cold water between their legs! As they gasped, they involuntarily contracted their pelvic muscles.[7]

We review the how-tos of Kegels in more detail in the Sexual Self-Esteem chapter (page 22), but we'd like to take this moment to review the whys. Kegels seem to be one of those pregnancy prescriptions that inspire a lot of passive resistance. In a 1999 survey of over one thousand women on the Babycenter.com Web site, over 50 percent reported that they mustered up the energy to do Kegels only "once in a while." And one of the midwives we interviewed confirms, "People hate Kegeling and hate being nagged about it." We're talking about a simple exercise that you can do anywhere, at any time, that has the pleasant side effect of being mildly arousing—doesn't it seem more fun than sit-ups?

Maybe the resistance to pelvic exercises is precisely because they do heighten genital awareness. If women are feeling pressured about having sex, anything that focuses their attention on sexual sensations — even in such a minor and benign way — could irritate. And maybe it's because of the cultural opposition we have toward being intentional when it comes to sex. We're more comfortable investing time and energy in looking so good that a partner will want to sweep us off our feet than we are investing time and energy in feeling good and being knowledgeable about the specific stimulation we enjoy. Pelvic exercises are one way to develop and assert your sexual power—we'd like to see women incorporate these into their life-long self-care repertoire.

About Your Perineum

Your medical practitioner may or may not suggest exercises, along with Kegels, that are designed to prepare your perineum for the intense stretching required during vaginal delivery. The perineum is the inch or so of skin between your vaginal opening and your anus. While it's naturally quite elastic, the perineum doesn't always stretch sufficiently to accommodate the head of a newborn, and this area commonly tears during delivery. When women receive an episiotomy—a surgical incision designed to enlarge the vaginal opening—the incision is made in the perineum.

If you're working with a midwife, she'll encourage you to let nature take its course and to tear if necessary rather than to have an episiotomy, because an episiotomy may take longer to heal. There's some evidence that a surgical incision is more damaging to muscle and nerve fibers than a tear would be. If you're working with a doctor, she or he will probably encourage you to keep an open mind about having an episiotomy if it seems indicated, for instance if the natural tear might extend into the urethra or rectum, or if the delivery has complications. You should definitely talk things over with your medical practitioner to find out if he or she has any strong biases that you disagree with (some doctors just prefer episiotomies because they're easier to stitch up). You have a right to participate in a decision that affects a portion of your anatomy that plays a big part in your sexual sensation.

Some midwives recommend "perineal massage" techniques which they believe can condition perineal tissue in preparation for childbirth. Perineal massage involves relaxing the perineal area with compresses and warm-oil massages, then pulling down on the vaginal opening until there's a slight burn or stinging sensation. The logic is that if you can get accustomed to the stretching and stinging sensation that accompanies delivery, you'll be better prepared for the real thing. To us, the more pressing logic would be: Why do anything that doesn't feel good? There's no evidence that perineal massage has any effect on whether or not you will tear during delivery, since the elasticity of the perineal tissues seems to be hereditary—you can't train or bully the tissues into becoming more stretchy.

We're not suggesting that you avoid doing any kind of perineal preparation for childbirth. By all means, apply warm compresses and lots of loving energy to that precious area between your legs. Do your Kegels and discover the control you have over your pelvic region. But skip the goal-oriented "Let's see how wide open I can get" approach in favor of relaxation and release.

IS CHILDBIRTH A SEXUAL EXPERIENCE?

"Start with the premise that birth is the biggest sex act you will ever take part in, and everything will flow from that," advises Susie Bright in her essay "Egg Sex."[8] Sheila Kitzinger writes lyrically that "in a strange way the energy flowing through the body in childbirth, the pressure of contracting muscles, the downward movements of the baby and the fanning open of soft tissues can be powerfully erotic."[9] Research psychologist Niles Newton is frequently quoted for her 1973 article, in which she compares childbirth with sexual excitement, noting that in both cases women experience accelerated breathing, rhythmic uterine contractions, and "a tendency to become uninhibited."[10] How's that for academic understatement? Certainly vaginal delivery involves your entire body — and most exquisitely your genitals — in a way that is as utterly compelling and absorbing as great sex. And in our wet dreams, every one of our readers would have had labors that were deeply sensual experiences. However, if your experience of labor was too overwhelming, medically complicated, frightening, moving, or just plain painful to be sexual, rest assured that you're not alone. Childbirth tends to be over-hyped as the defining peak experience in a woman's life, and we wouldn't want you to burden yourself with yet more expectations of this event. Whether you've had childbirth experiences that were empowering, alienating, or both, the birth is just a beginning — a lifetime of peak experiences as a mother lies ahead.

THE FOURTH TRIMESTER:
SEX AND THE POSTPARTUM MOM

ONCE you bring your baby home, the proverbial glow of pregnancy is swiftly replaced by a haze of exhaustion. Not only are you coping with a new set of physiological and hormonal challenges, but you have an extremely high-maintenance new housemate on your hands. If you already have older children, you'll be juggling their competing demands on your attention. You may be one of the many mothers who puts her sex life on the back burner during her child's infancy, or you may resume sexual activities within a few weeks or months of childbirth. Either way, you can expect the first postpartum months to be a hair-raising roller-coaster ride that is emotionally unpredictable and physically exhausting. Whether you experience more highs or lows has a lot to do with compassion—how much you have for yourself and, if you have a partner, how much the two of you have for each other.

PHYSICAL CHALLENGES

Let's face it. Even the smoothest childbirth in the world is physically debilitating. Once the initial euphoria wears off, you're left with a body that feels unfamiliar and a little unsteady, an aching back, a jelly belly, bruised genitals, a sore perineum, and strained pelvic muscles. Your breasts are initially swollen to the bursting point, and any suckling or nipple stimulation triggers intense uterine contractions as your uterus shrinks back down to its pre-pregnancy size (while the painful contractions shouldn't last for more than two weeks, the entire process of involution takes about six weeks). Now that your placenta is no longer pumping out pregnancy hormones, you're dealing with a dramatic postpartum decline in estrogen and progesterone levels and an increase in the hormone prolactin, which stimulates milk production. These hormonal shifts, which can exacerbate your fatigue, do serve a purpose. As nurse-midwife Cheri Van Hoover explains, "The hormone prolactin that makes milk is a natural tranquilizer, and most new mothers must get used to having this in their bodies before they can even begin to drag themselves out of the house. This is almost certainly the way nature planned it."

If you had a cesarean section, your abdominal wound will be painful at first and may limit your mobility for several weeks. If you had a vaginal delivery that resulted in a tear or an episiotomy, the wound may be visibly healed in as little as two to six weeks, but it may continue to hurt or feel tender for anywhere from three months to a year. Even with no tear or episiotomy, there will be plenty of small abrasions in your vagina and perineum that initially make it unnerving to pee, let alone contemplate genital stimulation.

I felt like a virgin all over again. Even when my husband just wanted oral sex (me as recipient), I cried. It's only been four weeks, I know, but I'm pretty frightened to have sex, and worried that our great sex life won't come back.

Most couples get sent home from the hospital with instructions not to have sex for at least six weeks. In this case, "sex" means vaginal intercourse, and the reason for the precaution is that until your uterus has completely healed, penetration could lead to infection. When the lochia, or postpartum bleeding, has stopped, it's an indication that the uterus has healed. This can take anywhere from a few days to six weeks. But there are plenty of ways to be sexually intimate without intercourse, and many couples are inspired to share some form of sexual contact before the arbitrary six-week bell has sounded.

I didn't expect it, but I wanted sex again right after childbirth. Things were so right, and I felt so much joy and satisfaction, that I wanted to celebrate. It was a huge release. Then, after a few weeks, I was just too dog-tired.

During the initial postpartum time, my entire body felt like this sacred temple. We had sex two weeks after our daughter was born, and I think that was some of the most delicately loving sex we have ever had. There was this increased sense of respect for my yoni.

It's also common to experience an initial, exhilarating surge of sexual desire that fades away by the time you've endured six weeks of sleepless nights.

I remember after my daughter was born, during the latter half of that six-week abstinence period, I REALLY wanted to have sex every day. Then, when I could, I wasn't remotely interested.

During the first six weeks after birth, when we weren't supposed to "do it," I was horny as hell. After that I was too tired, and all I wanted was to find a minute in the day when a male wasn't grabbing my boobs.

On the other hand, you may find that the all-consuming responsibilities of mothering an infant render sexual encounters irrelevant at best and intrusive at worst. You're now engaged in a relationship that has the potential to provide all the sensual gratification you can handle. Cheri Van Hoover points out, "There are a lot of different reasons why people have sex. Part of it is the thrill, the pleasure, the orgasm, but part of it is having flesh-to-flesh contact with another person, just touching and being intimate. A mother with a new baby has almost continuous flesh-to-flesh contact with another person twenty-four hours a day."

Breast-feeding

If you're breast-feeding your baby, you've probably discovered that certain libido-dampening effects persist even when uncomfortably full breasts and cracked, sore nipples become a thing of the past. Breast-feeding suppresses your ovarian estrogen production; a decrease in estrogen leads to a decrease in vaginal lubrication and a possible decrease in your general sense of well-being. Instead, you're flooded with the hormones prolactin and oxytocin, both of which have a physiologically calming affect. (If you nurse for many months, these hormonal effects will level out—your prolactin surge will be less extreme, and your ovaries will resume producing estrogen.) But, as always, hormones are only part of the story. Every woman's experience of breast-feeding is affected as much by her attitude, emotions, infant, and support system as by physiology. If you breast-feed more than one child, you can expect each experience to be unique.

> For the entire year my first baby nursed, I could not stand to have my nipples touched and experienced what I think of as "affection overload"—I had nothing to give after taking care of him. But for the year-plus of nursing my second baby, my nipples were an amazingly sensitive erogenous zone and I had huge sexual desire.

For some women, breast-feeding is basically a chore.

> Since I was breast-feeding and all my daughter did for the first three months was nurse, I felt like a walking, talking cow. My breasts hurt and they leaked all the time. It was definitely not attractive or sexy, in my opinion.

Others find breast-feeding pleasurable but more than enough to satisfy their desire for physical contact, leaving them "touched out" and uninterested in partner sex.

> At three months, sex seems too much like another chore to do it much. After having a baby physically attached to my body all day and nursing and sleeping in the same bed at night, I feel like I need my own space.

There's a psychological component at work as well. Some women feel that sexuality is inappropriate when they're in nursing mode. They need to feel secure that the sexual and maternal functions of their breasts don't overlap in any way.

I didn't like having my breasts touched at all for a while. They had to be either for breast-feeding or sex, not both, it was too weird.

My breasts used to be a great source of sexual pleasure for me and my husband, but now that I'm breast-feeding my daughter, I no longer want my breasts to be "sexualized." I feel like they belong to her right now, and I'm comfortable with that. It's just going to be different for a while.

It's fine to issue these proclamations, but the truth is that your maternal body is inexorably intertwined with your sexual body. Breast-feeding involves both an erogenous zone—your breasts—and an erogenous hormone—oxytocin. Humans release oxytocin in a wide range of situations involving emotional or physical intimacy, from stroking a beloved's arm to hearing a hungry infant's cry to experiencing orgasm.[1] Sensuality and sexuality exist on a continuum, and a woman's reproductive life can't be disentangled from her sexual life. Certainly your infant isn't making any arbitrary distinctions and will happily play with his or her genitals while nursing. Many women discover that breast-feeding can be an erotic experience in and of itself.

Breast-feeding continues to be a powerful reminder of my sexuality. I'm amazed by these seemingly innocent organs, and the way my milk flow is stimulated by my son's cry, a short absence from him, and his feedings. Nursing is satisfying and sexual in a way I hadn't experienced before.

I was surprised at how erotic and physically stimulating breast-feeding was— my desire to have my husband fondle or chew my nipples abated completely, as it was a pale imitation of the real thing.

Meanwhile, a taboo is a taboo is a taboo, and you have every right to establish your own boundaries between giving milk and getting down. You may be a survivor of child sexual abuse who needs to keep sex out of the picture while negotiating your infant's demands on your body. You may feel more comfortable putting your sexual identity on the back burner while you're nursing an infant, or you may find it easier to access your sexual identity if you make clear distinctions between your roles as a mother and a lover.

We live in a society that is a minefield of mixed messages about breast-feeding. Women are encouraged to breast-feed their infants, but they're generally expected to do it behind closed doors so that nobody else has to be reminded that breasts are designed for something other than wet-T-shirt contests. And the discomfort you can expect to generate in bystanders rises in direct proportion to the age of your breast-feeding child—a babe in arms is more likely to elicit warm murmurs of approval than a toddler who marches over and yanks up your shirt. Basically, you will have to contend with a lot of big babies when you're breast-feeding—not merely the one who's suckling.

> Breast-feeding in public was interesting because I felt as though some people saw me as actually having sex in public. Their only possible interpretation of a bare breast was as a sexual object.

> I'm still nursing a two-year-old, so I deal with a lot of hypersexual awareness and prudish glares on the part of onlookers. But now that I'm a mom and no longer a "chick," I get far fewer leers from the male world when NOT nursing.

Your partner may also feel sexually inhibited by your new talents. He or she may feel awkward about "sharing" your body when you're nursing—either out of a sense of having been displaced, a desire not to overburden you with demands, or just a preoccupation with adjusting to your new identities as parents.

> I nursed both of my sons and just loved the feeling. I also enjoyed sex much more than I ever had before. Unfortunately, my now ex-husband could not get over the fact that his sons also had access to my breasts. So, while I was feeling so wonderful and empowered, he was withdrawing and becoming turned off by the thought of sex with me.

You or your partner could be intimidated by the fact that your lactating breasts will leak milk whenever you're sexually stimulated, and that milk can spray out of your nipples upon orgasm. If you're not used to generating a lot of fluid during sexual activity, adjusting to the messiness factor can take a while. As we noted in the last chapter, some pregnancy manuals primly suggest that you try to control those leaky breasts by avoiding nipple stimulation or by wearing a nursing bra to bed. An attitude adjustment and a couple of strategically placed towels will probably be more useful to you in the long run. You can also reduce the fountain factor by nursing before you have sex so your breasts aren't so full. Plenty of couples are not only comfortable with, but titillated by, the opportunity to incorporate a new fluid into their lovemaking.

> Nursing made it wild, you know the squirting milk thing. Again, nursing your kid and your mate is primeval.

> I loved breast-feeding. I like a man that suckles my breasts.

If you do choose to breast-feed your child, we hope you feel free to explore as much of its sensual potential as you please. And if you don't breast-feed—or don't do it for long—we hope you won't let anyone bully you into feeling inadequate as a mother. Despite the current emphasis on breast-feeding's benefits, it's simply not for every woman. Sure, breast milk is an amazing fluid, but millions of babies never taste a drop and still grow up healthy and happy.

EMOTIONAL CHALLENGES

The physical and hormonal challenges of the postpartum months are just the tip of the iceberg. You can also expect to confront challenges to your self-image, self-esteem, and emotional equilibrium that often send your sex life packing.

A Changing Self-image

Caretaking of an infant is emotionally demanding, calling on all your reserves of patience, flexibility, and stamina. Self-sacrifice becomes the name of the game, and one of the first "indulgences" you may jettison is sexual activity. Many first-time moms find that adjusting to their new role can make them feel somewhat detached from their sexuality.

> My sense of self has changed drastically. In fact, right after the girls were born, I spoke to my husband about how I needed some time to get used to my "new" self; I explained to him that it was like going through puberty again in many ways. Everything about me had changed, the way I look, the way I look to other people, and it had changed quickly.

> I don't feel like a sexual being anymore, I feel like a nurturing being. Intellectually, I know I will feel again like putting on fishnets and stilettos, but right now all my energy is going into a different kind of love. The nurturing I feel is for my husband as well as my son. I think my husband feels this to some extent. I can see it in his eyes as he watches me breast-feed our child, but he still asks me to help him wash his motorcycle nude (and I've humored him), so I don't think I've become ALL mom to him.

If your delivery was frightening or physically traumatizing, you may need time to process feelings akin to those of sexual assault. And if your delivery required medical intervention, you may feel a sense of disappointment and failure, blaming yourself for a birth experience that wasn't what it "should" have been. This sets up a nice double whammy in which you may come to feel you "deserve" the pain you're in and, by extension, don't deserve any physical pleasure. Given the nerve damage that can occur with an episiotomy or other types of obstetric intervention, genital stimulation—especially penetration—can be painful for up to a year postpartum. Don't let anyone dismiss this pain as "all in your head"; it's very real. See below for suggestions on minimizing pain and maximizing pleasure during sex.

> I had a C-section and expected some soreness, but after a few months went by, and the pain lingered, especially during sex, I began to shy away from sex or anything sexual. The pain is very mild, but a constant reminder that my body didn't work right during labor and birth. I'm still trying to shed these feelings.

Recovering from a sense of loss can also be difficult. During pregnancy, you are the focus of your family's and friends' concerns and caresses, and your body is lush and fertile. Postpartum, all the attention goes to your baby. You're expected to assume a nurturing role while simultaneously getting back to "normal" as soon as possible so you won't inconvenience those around you. Meanwhile, your body is unlikely to bounce back to its pre-pregnancy state as quickly as you might like. Instead of being round and taut, your belly is slack and stretched out. Varicose veins, hemorrhoids, and stretch marks may all contribute to a distinct drop in your physical self-esteem.

> After my first child was born, at first I felt like a milking blob, despite the fact that my husband loved the fact that I was lactating. All I could see was my porridge belly.

> My self-esteem went down due to bad stretch marks. I feel more inhibited and embarrassed. I used to be outgoing and crazy (would do it in broad daylight in a field)—now it's got to be in the complete dark or by candlelight.

Others take justifiable pride in their new bodies, battle scars and all.

> Any illusions of modesty are shattered during the birthing process, and in my case this was a good thing. After having my son I found that I just didn't give a shit anymore what others thought about my body. Sure, I had extra rolls where I never had them before, psychedelic stretch marks, and weird pigmentation, but my body had given birth, and that was pretty incredible!

> I have to say that since giving birth, I have never been more confident or assertive with my husband. I know I have a stretched-out body with some

Survivors' Issues

All mothers discover that having a child inspires strong memories of their own childhood. The hormonal changes of pregnancy and childbearing can be a particularly powerful catalyst for memories, perhaps from other hormonal transition times such as puberty. If you're one of the many women who were either sexually abused as a child or sexually assaulted as an adult,[2] this visceral experience of remembering can evoke emotions and sensations that are a challenge to integrate with your new maternal role. Even if you've worked hard on recovery, feelings of anger, rage, grief, guilt, and shame can engulf you all over again.

> I was raped four years before I got pregnant. I had dealt with a lot of the issues right after the abuse, but when I got pregnant a whole bunch more came up.

Survivors may experience pregnancy as a frightening invasion and loss of control over their bodies. Perfect strangers feel free to touch your belly. An interchangeable cast of medical personnel examines you. Ideally, you'll be able to control as much about the experience of pregnancy as possible. You'll want to trust your medical professional to respect your feelings and decisions regarding prenatal care, labor, and delivery. Survivors can experience an acute dread of pain during delivery; being in a position of genital pain while being "managed" by those around you can provoke flashbacks. Others experience childbirth as profoundly empowering.

> I had major sexual issues when I got pregnant with my son, due to childhood abuse. My sex life went way downhill when I became a mom, because of the traumatic abuse flashbacks I experienced during labor. Once I had worked through these with therapy, however, my sex life improved a lot, and eight years down the road, I am very comfortable with my sexuality!

Breast-feeding, which requires "servicing" another creature on demand, is not an option for some survivors. Others develop coping mechanisms. Rather than sleeping with or breast-feeding your infant in bed, where you will be repeatedly woken from deep sleep by groping hands and mouth, you may want your baby to sleep in a bassinet by the bed. It can also be helpful to get up, turn the light on, and pull on some clothes in order to retain a sense of control while breast-feeding.

All mothers are overwhelmed with both love and anxiety at how vulnerable and defenseless their infants are. This recognition is particularly painful for women whose own childhood vulnerability was so cruelly exploited.

After the first few months of being completely absorbed by my daughter, feelings, memories, and impressions of my childhood sexual abuse became intrusive and very problematic in terms of having a sex life at all. My daughter's infancy really brought it all to the surface. I think I reacted so strongly because of how vulnerable she was, which made me realize just how innocent and trusting and defenseless children are, and I was.

As a survivor mom, you may have a natural tendency to be overprotective or painfully aware of every worst-case scenario that might befall your infant. Reach out to other mothers—both survivors and those who aren't—to talk about your fears and put your anxieties in perspective. Pregnancy and parenthood can be fruitful times for therapy, and becoming a mother can set you on the road to deep healing and a newfound integration of your sexuality.

I made peace with my sexuality as I went through pregnancy, and as I became a mom. Having been a victim of sexual abuse and rape as a young teenager, it was a very healing time for me. I had already done much work in past years to get over that one, but motherhood brought me back full circle.

SCARY stretch marks and a little more weight on my ass, but I know now what this body is capable of and I'm proud of it. He thinks it's great too.

As the following survey respondent suggests, coming to terms with your changed body and changed identity can simply be a matter of time—and a little creative self-love.

Because I gained a lot of weight with my first pregnancy, I felt for a while that I wasn't somehow entitled to a sex life. To be frank, I sometimes felt like a drudge. Images of new mothers in the media seem to be these women who look like their prebaby selves, carrying around a perfect infant or toddler. I had spit-up on my clothes, uncombed hair, etc. I wasn't able to hold everything together. After a pregnancy in which I felt like a goddess, I was suddenly someone I thought no one could possibly find attractive. The big change came when I pierced my nose. I did this exotic, totally decorative thing that had nothing to do with the baby or the size of my hips, or anything other than the fact that I wanted to be noticed in my own right. It was very painful. It was transformative. I didn't feel like I was denying my own motherhood, but denying a kind of motherhood that had nothing to do with me and reinventing myself as this other, stronger person. I found that very sexy.

Changing Priorities

Nurturing a newborn—especially if you're the primary or sole caretaker—doesn't leave a lot of room on your dance card for recreational activities. And sleep deprivation is nobody's idea of an aphrodisiac. You may well choose to prioritize taking a shower (alone) over partner sex during this time.

> After my second child, sleep deprivation and breast-feeding haven't affected my level of desire, but have affected how I prioritize what to do with the little time I have. Sex comes pretty low in the list, probably due to the energy required! Sad, isn't it?

> I wasn't very interested in sex for the two years I was breast-feeding. After I stopped, sex was better than ever, but I wouldn't have traded great sex for breast-feeding ever. I plan on having great sex for the rest of my life but I can only breast-feed my babies for so long.

Same Old Fear

Most women have a healthy aversion to the idea of getting pregnant again within the first year of their child's life. If you have a male partner or have had birth-control failures before, you may be avoiding intercourse because you're afraid of conceiving again.

> For the first five years after I started having babies, my sex drive was somewhat inhibited by a fear of pregnancy. After I had a tubal ligation I began to find my center sexually.

> After trying to get pregnant for two years, going back to birth control while lactating is a challenge. I have a teenager's fear of getting pregnant again right now, and it does have a negative effect on my sex drive.

It's imperative that you reestablish birth control as soon as possible postpartum. You may ovulate again as soon as a few weeks after delivery, and you'll ovulate *before* your first postpartum period, so you do need to be prepared. Despite what you may have heard, breast-feeding is not a viable method of birth control: It will only help prevent ovulation if you're nursing on demand and if your infant is receiving no other food or fluids — but it is not a surefire contraceptive.

Some women may avoid intercourse postpartum because their birth-control options seem so uncomfortable and/or invasive. In the first couple of months after delivery, condoms are probably your best bet for birth control (though you'll want to use plenty of water-based lubricant to prevent irritating friction on your delicate genital tissues). If you used to wear a diaphragm or cervical cap, you'll need to be refitted, as there will be some changes to the shape of your cervix and vagina. Similarly, you should not have an IUD reinserted until your uterus has fully recovered. You will need to wait until your periods are regular again before recommencing oral contraceptives. Depending on your sensitivity to hormones, you may find that birth-control pills reduce your libido. Try different prescriptions until you hit on the combination that works best for you.

> Physical problems from childbirth and the wrong type of birth-control pill, plus being really tired, put our sex life on hold for a while. Just recently, I changed birth-control pills and have been pleasantly surprised to want to have sex again.

Depression

Baby blues — in which you feel overwhelmed, emotionally vulnerable, and depressed for the first couple of weeks postpartum — are very common and are usually explained as the result of hormonal shifts, exacerbated by sleep deprivation, an overwhelming new responsibility, and social isolation. An estimated 50 to 80 percent of mothers experience these blues.

> The first week after the baby was born I wanted to cry. Not from joy or fatigue, but because I needed to process the whole mind-boggling, body-ravaging labor experience. I hadn't realized how much I'd just "toughed it out" when going through it, but afterwards it was like I felt each contraction emotionally!

A minority of women (perhaps 10 percent) experience more serious, long-term postpartum depression that requires clinical treatment. If your "blues" persist for longer than a few weeks and your symptoms include panic attacks, inability to cope with daily activities, inability to concentrate, changes in sleep and appetite patterns, or fears of hurting your baby, you should definitely consult with a medical practitioner. You can get help from any combination of therapy, antidepressants or other medications, support groups, or practical assistance with parenting. Certain antidepressants are safe to take even if you're breast-feeding. Don't go through this experience alone; you deserve to be helped.

Nonbiological or adoptive mothers, as well as fathers, can also experience postpartum depression. Becoming a parent is comparable to a major life crisis in terms of the stresses involved. Overnight, your habits, environment, schedule, and sense of self change. You become defined in terms of your relationship to a dependent being and have to fight to retain your own identity. As more and more women with postpartum depression step forward to combat the stigma and lack of information on the topic, treatment options will multiply. One common side effect of depression is reduced libido. Unfortunately, this side effect is equally common with some antidepressants. If you're taking antidepressants, you should consult with your doctor to find the type and dosage that wreaks the least havoc on your sex drive.

> I had a really bad birth experience, and a horrible episiotomy that was repaired poorly. This really impacted our sex life in two ways: It hurt like hell for the first year to have sex, and then I was really depressed, so I went on Prozac. No libido, no sex. I've since gone off Prozac and my libido has kicked in with a vengeance!

Imperfection

Once you become a mom, you're under a lot of scrutiny — not just from busybodies around you, but from yourself. When you're pregnant, you're taking care of your baby without even trying. Once you've delivered, you may feel like you have myriad opportunities to screw up on a daily basis. Anxiety can be distinctly antierotic. Give yourself a break. Trust us, you will have plenty of opportunities to cultivate your talent for self-sacrifice from here on out. Now's the time to cultivate your talent for self-care.

> I'd suggest that other moms-to-be make sure they feel good. I was so busy trying to be the perfect mom that I didn't let myself feel anything other than my perfect infant's lips on my nipple. Let your partner touch you. Feel the water when you shower. Taste the juice in fruit. Close your eyes and feel yourself.

Incorporating regular treats into your routine can work wonders. Get a massage. Order takeout. Buy yourself some flowers. Take daily walks with another mom. Enlist the aid of friends and family to help with chores and baby-sitting so you can get some rest. Masturbate. Indulge yourself in the pleasures of the senses, and the Sleeping Beauty that is your sex drive just might wake up.

TAKING THE PLUNGE

At some point, you're going to want to reach out for sexual contact with a partner. You may desire intimacy and long to be treated as a sexual adult within a few days of your child's birth, or it may take you months to arrive at the point when you're ready for that kind of connection again. A postpartum drought in your sex life is quite common, which is why one midwife we know counsels all her partnered clients not to expect to resume their sex life for ten or eleven months: "Then they can celebrate if they are pleasantly surprised." If you're partnered, you and your sweetie may want to think of your sex drive not as having vanished but as having taken a brief leave, while you focus your energies on achieving some degree of competence in caring for your infant. Once you adjust to your new routine, you'll probably remember why you wanted to create a family together in the first place.

> Our sex life changed instantly—I had a new love besides my husband and I couldn't even focus on anything else. Eventually (four months later), I realized that I wasn't married to my son, and my husband and I resumed having sex.

Partner Perceptions

It's a safe bet that your partner has as many conflicting fears and desires around sexual intimacy postpartum as you do. He or she is probably just as uncertain about how to integrate sex and parenting, just as sleep-deprived, and just as overwhelmed by your lifestyle change as you are. Your partner may be reluctant to pressure you into a sexual encounter for fear of causing you pain, or may be itching to jump back in the sack regardless of how you feel. Both of you will need to summon up all your self-awareness and communication skills in order to avoid falling into ruts, developing resentments, or establishing stalemates that can linger long after your child's out of diapers. Here are some anxieties and misunderstandings that commonly derail a couple's sex life postpartum.

Childbirth is a messy business

The theme that a male partner might be irreparably traumatized by witnessing childbirth is sounded depressingly often in pregnancy and parenting books. One popular guide even suggests that a laboring mother strategically position her husband by her head during delivery in case the horrifying sight of his wife's distended vagina renders him incapable of ever attempting intercourse with her again. Give us a break! Sure, there may be some men who are so attached to an airbrushed ideal of women's genitals that the realities of labor will come as a shock, but not only will they need to grow up fast to cut it as a parent, they probably aren't the kind of fellas who'd even be in the delivery room to begin with. Perpetuating these stereotypes of squeamish men is bad enough, but acting as if there's any reason to coddle and accommodate such attitudes is even worse.

A partner who has witnessed the physical impact of labor and delivery might be reluctant to treat you as a sexual being until you're healed and rested. (One father we know described feeling like his wife had been in a car wreck.) Your partner may be feeling too anxious and protective to respond to you in an erotic way right now. Then again, he or she may be processing feelings of great awe and admiration!

> I went through a period of feeling like my husband thought I was disgusting, because he witnessed both births, and although it is easy to romanticize birth, it is in reality a messy, smelly business, and not what I would consider conducive to sexual excitement. I finally 'fessed up to what I was feeling, and my husband responded by telling me he thought the whole birth thing had shown how powerful I was and what amazing things my body could do. He wasn't turned off—quite the contrary. I was reassured.

Many partners find the experience of witnessing childbirth liberating and inspirational.

> When your partner sees you go through labor, it certainly changes perceptions of what "those bits" are for! But once we resumed lovemaking at about six weeks postpartum, my partner made it very clear to me that he found me even more attractive since participating in the birth. For him that was a very sexual moment, the birth, as well as emotional and parental. Of course there are many layers to an experience as intense as birth and one of them is sexual. He thought I was a goddess.

> Labor and delivery made me into a goddess. My husband actually got an erection watching me deal with contractions. He said I was getting all shimmery.

> We are wilder now. Delivering together busted down the last bastions of prudishness.

I'm not sexually appealing anymore

As we discussed above, pregnancy and the postpartum state can leave women struggling with issues of body image and self-esteem. When you're run-down and bedraggled, feeling sexually desirable is difficult. And when you're not feeling sexually desirable, it's practically impossible to believe that anyone else would think you were.

I don't feel very sexy anymore, and I don't think my husband perceives me that way. We have not really had uninterrupted nights since the birth of our daughter, which contributed to this. My figure is gone, and the idea of resuming our sex life is embarrassing to me. He has been sympathetic and polite, but I know he doesn't feel attracted to me the way he did when we were childless.

Who knows whether this husband truly is having difficulty finding his wife attractive or whether he's simply fatigued, insecure, or anxious about her condition? Who knows if the wife is simply projecting her own disinterest in sex onto her husband? If it's true that he's no longer attracted to her, he's probably as worried about this fact as she is. Either way, they're more likely to experience empathy for each other — rather than guilt and mistrust — if they try communicating about their concerns.

All my partner wants is sex

A partner's jealousy of a biological mother's bond with her infant can take many forms. The classic scenario is that of the jealous male who resents feeling like he's being made to take a number and get in line.

Instead of her being there for me whenever I wanted to have sex, I now have to wait until she's finished doing the maternal stuff and then it's my turn.

Well, boo-hoo. We have a hard time mustering up much sympathy for any guy (or gal) who can't handle the fact that nurturing a newborn might take precedence over dishing out a hand job. On the other hand, mothers are sometimes their own worst enemies when it comes to claiming the space and demanding the support that is their due — and that would allow them to get back in touch with their own sexual desires. Our cultural model is still that of a selfless Madonna who nurtures her child in a perfect self-sufficient love bubble. It's not surprising that partners sometimes feel excluded, or that they might act out just to get your attention. You may consciously or unconsciously feel that no partner would (or should) be as competent a caretaker as you. Mothers who can't accept or ask for help risk feeling martyred, resentful, and put upon; and they frequently take out their resentment on their partners.

I feel that refusing sex when I'm too tired in some ways gives me back a little control of my body, as my son demands it as his night and day. I can't really handle having someone else wanting it too, when even I don't get it to myself.

I felt angry and confused while nursing my first son. It seemed that his demands and my partner's demands were just too much; one male or another wanted to have access to my body more or less all the time, it seemed. And I felt bad about feeling that way.

For the survey respondents above, refusing sex is a way of retaining a sense of control. While their physical overwhelm is understandable, they might feel different about their partner's physical "demands" if they were being offered—or had requested—a home-cooked meal, a leisurely massage, or a soak in the tub. See the Desire Revisited chapter (page 197) for more on negotiating differences in desire with your partner.

Like a virgin . . .

Sex after childbirth is frightening: on a physical level, as you deal with pain, discomfort, and the sense that your body is no longer familiar to you; and in terms of the emotional vulnerability you might feel.

> For the first year after my daughter's birth, I was always completely overwhelmed by my emotions during and after sex. I would say that I felt very emotionally raw.

> It was hard to get started again because of the pain. They had had to pull my baby's head out of my birth canal, so I was bruised, and since I hadn't had sex in almost three months, I felt almost like a virgin.

Sometimes you simply have to throw yourself into the water to discover that the swimming's fine (see below for some practical tips on enhancing the experience).

> I felt really bad about my looks, even though my husband was still very attracted to me. We refrained from having sex, entirely my doing, for nine months after Angel was born. Once I finally said, "Let's do it" (not exactly in those words), it was incredibly wonderful and relaxing for me.

Rock-a-bye baby

Couples often have trouble figuring out the logistics of being intimate when they're sharing their home—and their family bed—with an infant. Babies seem to have a knack for sensing when there's love in the air, and you may be inhibited by your own child's unerring radar.

> Many babies wake up as soon as you're about to have an orgasm. Kids are energy sensors. I think, at a certain point, my daughter's alarm would go off because she'd sense that I wasn't paying psychic attention to her.

> A sense of humor is invaluable—it's relaxing and releases tension. If the baby's cry deflates an erection or short-circuits your orgasm, you might as well learn to laugh

it off. And maybe you can turn the uncertainty about when you might be interrupted into a source of inspiration rather than a source of performance anxiety.

> We don't always like the distraction of listening for the baby, but it's kinda fun to be making out on the couch like teenagers!

See the Surviving Scarcity chapter (page 175) for tips on creating and maintaining the privacy necessary for your sex life to flourish.

Put Self-love First

Before you engage in partner sex, spend some time masturbating. We're not saying you should pull out all your sex toys and see how many orgasms you can rack up while the baby's napping (though that *is* one way to make nap time fly by!). We are saying that you deserve to take the time to acquaint yourself with the changes in your genital geography and sexual responses — after all those months of monitoring your pregnant body for the sake of the baby's health, you owe it to yourself to take stock in a purely self-centered way. You'll gain the information that can reduce whatever fear of genital stimulation you might be feeling, and the confidence that will make it much easier to relax in the company of a lover. Look at your genitals in a hand mirror and locate any tears or episiotomy scars. Gently touch your entire vulva, perineum, and vaginal opening to determine where you feel tender or bruised and what type of touch feels pleasurable. If you do masturbate to orgasm, you may be disappointed to find that it takes longer to become aroused or reach orgasm and that your orgasms feel muted or less intense than before. This effect can last anywhere from a few weeks to a few months as your genitals return to their pre-pregnancy state.

While these negative sexual side effects are temporary, childbirth does permanently change your reproductive organs. Your uterus and cervical opening are a little larger than before, your vaginal walls are more relaxed, and your pelvic muscles are looser and more supple. We're all painfully familiar with the stereotype of a postpartum vagina as being "stretched out" and no longer as appealing to a male partner. Certainly the loss of vaginal muscle tone can reduce a woman's pleasure, as well as reduce her sexual self-esteem.

> I was saddened to discover that birth loosened my vaginal muscles. It took about a year to return to the same level of pleasure from intercourse as before.

> I hate to admit this, but as empowering as natural childbirth was and as much as it made me feel like a stronger woman, I feel desexualized now. Vaginally, I feel changed and not always for the better.

However, any woman can retone her pelvic muscles simply by incorporating regular Kegel exercises into her routine (see the Sexual Self-Esteem and Sex During Pregnancy chapters, pages 22 and 94, for more about Kegels). The recovery period may take some time, but you can count on improvement.

> My orgasms are more intense and complex, and I feel like my vagina is tight and flexible, rather than listless — as we all hear happens after childbirth. In fact, I feel tighter than before (must be all those Kegels).

During this time, you might want to shift your attention to other, more positive changes in your sexual physiology — many women develop new vaginal awareness or a heightened orgasmic response after childbirth. Extra blood vessels grew during your pregnancy, which means that you'll have the capacity for more blood flow to the genitals than you did before. This increased genital vascularity can result in more dramatic sensations during arousal and orgasm.

> I have often thought it was the process of giving birth that made me more sensitive internally to my G-spot.

> It feels to me like after the baby my clitoris has dropped lower, actually making sex more enjoyable.

> Now I have better orgasms, but less sex. A fair trade in my mind.

The Nitty-gritty

When you are ready for partner sex, try acting as though you're experiencing a completely new sexual activity. After all, you are rediscovering your erogenous territory together. Before you embark on any sexual activity — whether oral sex, genital massage, or penetration — make your partner aware of all your genital trouble spots. Perhaps you have painful scar tissue from a tear or episiotomy at the base of your vagina or perineum, or a tender or bruised area deep inside your vagina as a result of torn ligaments or lacerations. Resist the temptation to just grin and bear discomfort rather than communicate. Sometimes women can get so concerned about hurting a partner's feelings that they act in self-defeating ways. You're not rejecting or failing your partner if you experience his or her touch as painful or frightening. If either of you had a sore back or sprained ankle, you'd both feel perfectly comfortable communicating about accommodations during sex. Try to adopt the same attitude about your postpartum aches and pains.

Before any kind of vaginal penetration, remember the importance of relaxation, lubrication, and communication. You should be in control of the moment of entry, and your partner should wait for your vaginal muscles to relax and welcome in the finger, penis, or dildo rather than forcefully penetrating you. In fact, you might want to start small with a finger or slim dildo before having intercourse. Penetration may feel scary, uncomfortable, or painful at first, so you should feel in control and able to call a halt to the activity at any time. Experiment with positions that allow you to control the angle and depth of penetration. Use a water-based lubricant for any genital stimulation; not only would unlubricated friction be hard on your tender genital tissues, but if you're breast-feeding, you will be experiencing a dramatic decrease in your production of vaginal lubrication.

> Hormonal changes can cause crazy insecurities. After the birth of our son, it took much longer for me to become wet. My partner thought I hated her. Thank heaven for the book *Susie Sexpert's Lesbian Sex World.* It addressed the issue of hormonal changes and the need for lubrication, and my partner felt better after reading that.

Whether your sex life suffers postpartum, or whether it is the beginning of a new level of eroticism, you'll weather the transition best by being kind — to yourself and to your partner.

> We are tired. That is our biggest challenge. And my partner is just coming out of a long depression. We're learning to start small, massage oil is great, even if you stop with the massage. Kindness is a wonderful aphrodisiac. We're both much gentler with each other now.

YOU'RE DIFFERENT NOW

A woman's experience of sexuality incorporates the physiological changes of a lifetime. Some biologists argue that women's relationship to their bodies is as much defined by menstruation, pregnancy, labor, lactation, and menopause as by sexual activities with a partner. In other words, pregnancy, labor, and breast-feeding are just as much sexual events as intercourse is. Whether or not this rings true to you, your experience of sex has probably been changed by your experience of pregnancy and childbirth. Some of the purely physical changes — such as increased orgasmic capacity — may be welcome, and others — such as a tummy that will never be flat again — not so welcome. Similarly, some of the emotional changes (an enhanced capacity for intimacy and love) may be welcome, but not others (some uncertainty about your right to be sexual).

I remember putting on lingerie the first time. It felt silly, like I had become a different person after childbirth.

Ultimately, the pride and confidence that comes from having weathered this challenge can have a profound effect on your sense of self, freeing you to be — and be seen as — the lush, sexy goddess you are.

My husband says I'm sexier. One day I was getting ready to go somewhere, hadn't showered or put on makeup, hairy armpits and legs, bags under my eyes, some thrown-together hippie get-up. I said, "It's a far cry from when you met me, isn't it!" He said, "Yeah, but you're sexier now." I said, "How do you figure that?" He shrugged and said, "I dunno, you just are," and went back to reading his paper. That's my sweet husband. I've gained quite a bit of weight with my pregnancies, so I don't get attention on the street anymore. Male friends don't flirt with me anymore. But I *feel* more sensual. I feel very connected to the earth, I feel very spiritual. This has affected my sexuality immensely. I guess that's what my husband senses.

HOW TO GET THE INFORMATION YOU NEED

BECOMING a mom, particularly a biological mother, adds a new urgency to your interactions with medical practitioners. Unless you've been dealing with long-term illness or disability prior to motherhood, this is probably the first time in your life that you've needed medical care so regularly, or craved straight-shooting medical advice so desperately. Inundated with a torrent of wholesome facts about conception, nutrition, pregnancy, breast-feeding, and infant health, you may find it difficult to interrupt the flow for a personal question about sexual desire, activity, or safety. Medical professionals don't necessarily volunteer sex information, and patients are frequently too intimidated to ask explicit questions.

You, like many women, may choose to turn to friends, family, word of mouth, and the Internet for the answers you seek. While these resources can be invaluable, the sex information we get from peers and professionals alike inevitably comes tricked out in attitudes, expectations, and assumptions that make it hard to sort out "just the facts, ma'am." Once you equip yourself with a healthy skepticism and a willingness to stand up for your own experience, you'll find that enlightening advice is well within reach.

WHAT TO EXPECT FROM HELPING PROFESSIONALS

While you can count on your doctor to have an understanding of anatomy, physiology, human biology, and medicine, you can't assume that she or he is equally well informed when it comes to sexual desires and activities. For one thing, unless doctors have a personal interest in exploring human sexuality, they won't be any better educated than the average Joe or Jane. Medical schools in our country don't currently offer any comprehensive, standardized program of sex education, and training in this area is hardly prioritized. In California, for example, state licensing requires only twelve hours of training in human sexuality.

Furthermore, medicine is a problem-solving profession, and doctors are much better equipped — by training and sometimes by personality — to diagnose a condition and propose treatment options than to discuss the gray areas of human behavior. Once you're in a clinical setting, it can feel incongruous to express concerns about matters as difficult to quantify as a fluctuating libido or changes in orgasmic response. Doctors themselves aren't necessarily comfortable responding to "unscientific" queries. Given their focus on a very specific area of expertise, specialists aren't always adept at dealing with the interplay between physiological and emotional concerns. If you've ever had to pursue fertility treatment, you're probably well aware that specialists such as reproductive endocrinologists don't necessarily put a high premium on people skills!

> I really had some doctors say some pretty ridiculous things during my infertility treatment. I was doing Clomid, which is a low-level fertility drug, and feeling like a maniac, like I was going to kill someone, and my doctor said, "Well, maybe you're just finally feeling the way that women who have *normal* hormone levels feel."

Of course, plenty of doctors (including reproductive endocrinologists) are warm, caring, and sensitive to their patients' emotional concerns. But a general practitioner is likely to have more experience and be more fluent discussing sexual issues—which blend physiological, hormonal, personal, and emotional factors—than a specialist. You can expect health-care professionals such as nurse practitioners, nurse-midwives, family practitioners, and physicians' assistants to have a more holistic approach and a greater awareness of sexual issues. Midwives won raves from many of our survey respondents for their philosophy of female empowerment and education, as did many individual OB/GYNs, physicians' assistants, and nurse practitioners.

Acknowledge the inherent power dynamic in the relationship between patient and medical professional. After all, your medical practitioner is in the driver's seat as you steer your way through the health-care system: He or she affects what care you get and when you get it. Let's not forget that, when it comes to pregnancy and childbirth, we're also talking about *pain management*, a reality that only exacerbates the power imbalance. Pregnant women seem to inspire a particularly high degree of well-intentioned fascism from their practitioners, whether your midwife is instructing you to lay off the sugar and get cracking on those Kegels or your doctor is insisting on certain obstetric interventions. Faced with natural anxieties as to whether you're going to be a fit patient, let alone a fit mother, it's not always easy to hang on to the self-assurance you need to raise questions related to a topic as delightfully selfish as sex. But you can do it, and reap the rewards, by following these few tips.

Demand Good Care

Doubtless your health-care options are restricted by your medical coverage and your budget. But whether you're getting prenatal care from a local women's clinic, an HMO, a major medical group, or working independently with a midwife, the bottom line is that you should shop around. In America, we approach medical care with the same scarcity mentality with which we approach sex—"Better to settle for what I can get than to make waves." The truth is, you can be a good consumer. Research what medical options are available to you in your area, as well as what nonmedical support—such as childbirth assistants or doulas—you can afford.[1] And select your practitioner with care.

Sure, practitioners in clinics and HMOs are busy, busy, busy. But you still have the right to expect that certain basic requirements be met. Remember the old *Highlights* magazine (a staple of pediatricians' waiting rooms) and the comic strip about the two brothers Goofus and Gallant? Goofus always did the wrong thing, like slamming the screen door in his mother's face while her arms were filled with grocery bags, while Gallant always did the right thing, like carrying the groceries in for her. Well, here's what a Gallant medical professional looks like:

- Dr. Gallant spends time with you (during which you are sitting up and able to make eye contact, not simply lying on the exam table with your feet in the stirrups).
- Nurse Gallant asks if you have any questions and offers you a pad and pen to write answers on.
- Physician's Assistant Gallant tells you if he doesn't know the answer to a question and either refers you to someone who does or makes arrangements to research the answer and follow up with you later.
- Midwife Gallant treats you as though you're well informed about your own body and works to help you take control of your health.
- Every single one of these Gallant professionals responds to your questions about sex without smirking, shuffling papers nervously, or leaving the room.

And you, Ms. Gallant patient, will reward their professionalism by thanking them for their time, giving them appreciative feedback, recommending them to their superiors, referring them to your friends, and generally doing what you can to provide positive reinforcement. You are more than likely to run across Goofus professionals, but you don't have to stay under their care. Flex your consumer rights.

Be Realistic in Your Expectations

Sometimes we make the mistake of expecting too much from one practitioner. If you're in a relationship, you've either already learned (or will have to learn) that your partner can't satisfy all your needs for love, stimulation, and companionship—that's why you have friends, colleagues, and family. The same logic applies to your relationships with professionals. Be realistic about the limitations of their roles. Don't expect your fertility doctor to be warm and fuzzy; expect him or her to know the latest research and provide you with up-to-the-minute advice. Don't expect your midwife to sing the praises of epidurals; get some other perspectives on the subject. Keep in mind that obstetrics is a surgical specialty, so not every OB/GYN will be as focused on natural childbirth as you might be; make sure that yours respects and understands your birth plan, and prepare to be good and grateful for those surgical skills if you need them.

Get Their Cards on the Table

Medical professionals are people too, and they have their own biases and anxieties about sex. They have a right to these biases, and you have a right to full disclosure. If you conceived, or are trying to conceive, through donor insemination, you know how important it is to find a doctor who supports you through the process. Members of the medical establishment can be stupefyingly paternalistic, issuing edicts such as: Married couples should not use known donors; single women should not have children; lesbians should not have children; or even, women should not conceive mixed-race children through DI.

You need to communicate your situation honestly in order to determine what judgments your practitioner does or doesn't have. In big cities, it's reasonably easy to find medical professionals who are comfortable working with single and lesbian mothers, but if you live in a small town, you might need to either travel some distance to find a congenial doctor or be proactive about care from direct-entry midwives or family-planning clinics. Keep in mind that medical professionals are required to uphold confidentiality regarding anything discussed in your appointments.

Disclosure is equally desirable in your interactions with mental-health professionals. Although clear boundaries between client and therapist are essential to a successful therapeutic relationship, you're not violating these boundaries by requesting information about your therapist's philosophies regarding sex and parenting. That way, you'll have a context for assessing the feedback you get about your sex and parenting life, and you can take the insights that are useful to you and discard those that aren't.

> My therapist thinks I shouldn't have sex in my home while my son is sleeping—I see this as mom bias.

When you're pregnant or postpartum, it can be helpful to know what your medical practitioner's personal experience of pregnancy and child raising has been, if any. Surely you know by now that many people use their own pregnancy, labor, and postpartum experiences as a point of reference when dishing out the advice. Maybe your mother didn't breast-feed, so she not so subtly discourages your own efforts. Maybe your best friend had great sex during pregnancy, so she can't understand why your libido has disappeared. Maybe that nice old lady who rides the elevator with you spent two days in labor and thinks you got off a little too easily with twelve hours. Despite their professional perspective, doctors aren't completely exempt from this syndrome, so find out how long Dr. Gallant's wife breast-fed their twins or whether Nurse Gallant's labor was induced. Sometimes your practitioner's experience is reassuringly similar to your own, and sometimes not—either way, you benefit from being aware of what expectations might be influencing your care.

> I have not been able to talk to anyone but my doctor about my total loss of libido. She told me it took her six months to have sex after her first child was born. That made me feel better.

Put Your Own Cards on the Table

You may be hesitant to bring up sexual matters with your practitioner because you have a lot of history together, and you don't want to risk saying something that would embarrass either one of you. Your voice may tremble the first time you utter the words "Gosh, Nurse Gallant, I was just wondering if there's any medical reason not to have anal sex in my third trimester," but keep in mind that yours is not the only inquiring mind out there. There is no sexual activity you could possibly get up to that thousands of others haven't enjoyed and wondered about, just like you. If Nurse Gallant doesn't have an immediate answer for you, it will only be to her future patients' benefit for her to get the facts. And if your reluctance to speak about your own sex life is just too acute to overcome, you can always fall back on those old standbys: "A friend was asking me if . . ." or "I heard something on TV that made me wonder if . . ."

As we discussed in the Sex During Pregnancy chapter (page 94) medical professionals are just as liable to be lax or imprecise in their sexual terminology as laypeople. Every time you ask Dr. Gallant to clarify just what she means by refraining from sex for six weeks postpartum, you score a point for improved communication about sex in society at large. If you can be persistent and specific in your questions, you'll get the advice that allows you to make your own informed decisions rather than languishing in anxious uncertainty. The good news is that practitioners in the field of gynecology do hear from many patients about sex and relationship issues, and often develop a big-picture perspective that can normalize your immediate concerns.

> My doctor was incredibly helpful once I opened up to him about my lack of desire. There are so many options—like switching my birth-control pill—that I never knew about!

My doctor has been my best resource. I went to her for depression because I felt so overwhelmed with parenting and as if nothing was fun anymore, and when we talked about sexuality she pointed out that all of my intimacy needs were being met through my mothering. I felt less like a failure when I thought about it this way. More like it would change with time.

Your Future Is at Stake

None of us are getting any younger, and the time to become proactive around health care is now—or maybe yesterday. All the skills you cultivate as a mom—learning to shop around for caregivers, seeking more than one opinion, taking professional biases into account—will be useful throughout your lifetime. Women need to be active agents in their own health care, especially on reproductive and sexual matters. Bear in mind that centuries of medical "wisdom" asserting that a woman's brain and womb are uniquely interdependent have bequeathed us all a doozy of a double bind: On the one hand, a woman's mental health and well-being are linked to the health of her womb, but on the other, any ill health of the womb is dismissed as "all in her head." Even modern medical professionals can make the mistake of ignoring or dismissing physical problems that are all too real.

Until I gave birth, I didn't realize how problems connected to the reproductive organs can affect seemingly unrelated parts. An example of this is my uterus, which has been crooked since the posterior birth of my son and has caused increased UTIs, painful intercourse, and even back pain. It took me five years to find someone to explain it.

If reproductive organs aren't being ignored, they're being glorified as integral to true womanhood. Women who aren't able to conceive may feel like failures as women, and women who face hysterectomies may fear a loss of female identity. While hysterectomies are certainly overprescribed in this country (pretty much at the drop of a uterine fibroid), and every woman should seek several different opinions before engaging in such major surgery, a hysterectomy doesn't have to signal a death knell to either your womanhood or your sexuality. However, it *is* important that you discuss your sexual responses with your doctor before making a decision to proceed with surgery. If uterine contractions play a key role in your experience of orgasm, you may want to pursue treatment other than hysterectomy. If you get particular pleasure from vaginal penetration, you can request a supracervical hysterectomy (in which the cervix is left intact), so there's less impact on the nerves and muscles of the vagina. Ultimately, as this woman testifies, being freed from pain can have a liberating effect on your sexual responses.

> One of the biggest positive changes in my sex life was my getting a hysterectomy. I know other women who've had the same "side effects." We're extremely vaginally sensitive now, have easier orgasms and heightened libido.

Women are all too prone to toughing it out when it comes to physical discomfort, especially when the discomfort is related to reproductive biology. One British study of over eleven thousand postpartum women found that while nearly half developed health problems they'd never experienced before, with some symptoms lasting for months or even years, many never mentioned these to their doctors. Why not? Among the reasons given were: the symptoms didn't seem serious; they were too infrequent to warrant treatment; and they were assumed to reflect a "usual female problem."[2]

Start speaking out now about the interplay between health, well-being, and sexual pleasure—your future happiness as a strong, sexy old woman is in your hands. Hormones, physiology, and health all play a role in your sexual energy and desire, which will only become more apparent as you wend your way through menopause. Medical practitioners need to be reminded that sexual health is a crucial component of overall health, and we encourage you to emphasize the relationship between the two on every possible occasion. But first and foremost, you need to remind *yourself* that you deserve both, then pursue your own path to sexual well-being.

> I wish I'd treated my postpartum sexuality as an overall health issue from the beginning. I just dosed up on antibiotics and Advil and kept on feeling lousy. I finally saw an acupuncturist and talked about my whole experience and now I see that I have different options.

SPECIAL-NEEDS ADVOCACY

In certain circumstances it takes extraordinary persistence for a woman to assert her rights to be both sexual and a mother. Women with physical disabilities face an uphill battle, not only in gaining societal acceptance and support for their becoming mothers, but in even being *visible* as such. Although an estimated eight million American families have one parent with a disability,[3] many able-bodied people find the concept of disabled people having active sex lives so impossible that they often disregard the plainest evidence.

> I am tired of having to explain that my son is not adopted. It is entirely possible for women in wheelchairs to have sexual desire, intercourse, and children.

Medical professionals are just as likely to hinder a disabled person's path toward parenthood as to pave the way. One research study of disabled women found that half of those who had mobility problems (requiring crutches or wheelchairs) had had their doctors offer to terminate their pregnancies, the assumption being that these women wouldn't be able to handle the demands of child-rearing.[4] If you're disabled, you already know the importance of steadfast self-advocacy. You'll need a team of medical professionals you can trust to give you accurate, nonalarmist advice on the possible effects of your pregnancy on your disability, the possible effects of your condition and/or medication on the fetus, and what arrangements to make for the delivery and postpartum. You'll also need to ensure in advance that you have adaptive child-care devices in place: cribs, car seats, strollers, etc. Many resources and valuable networking opportunities are available on-line (see our Resources section, page 340).

Mothers who live under the threat of illness, such as those who are HIV-positive, encounter similar societal attitudes. Yet advances in controlling HIV infection have allowed many HIV-positive individuals to enjoy years of good health. The risk of transmission to infants can be greatly reduced when mothers are treated with anti-virals during pregnancy, deliver via cesarean section, and choose bottle-feeding over breast-feeding. While any mother who is contending with a life-threatening illness will need to make contingency plans for the care of her children should she die or become unable to care for them, the truth is that every well and able-bodied mother should do the same.

ADVOCATING FOR YOUR CHILD

When your children are young, you are responsible for safeguarding their sexual rights, and there are times when your child's sexual health may be jeopardized by well-intentioned but potentially harmful medical attitudes and interventions. You can be proactive in ensuring your child's ongoing sexual health by choosing a pediatrician who shares your values, as well as familiarizing yourself with some potential sexual health issues that your child might face.

Finding a Sex-positive Pediatrician

The best time to interview pediatricians or potential health-care providers is before your child arrives — once you're busy with child care, that first appointment will sneak up on you before you know it, and before you've had a chance to prepare. You should expect the same level of disclosure and courtesy that you do from your own health practitioner. Most parenting guides give you a laundry list of things to discuss with your child's provider, but rarely do they address sexual concerns. During your interviews, ask for an opinion on circumcision, advice on children's genital hygiene, and views on masturbation. If the answers don't meet with your approval, by all means shop around. Your primary-care provider may have recommendations for you, and other parents can be an excellent source of referrals.

Ideally, you're trying to cultivate a trusting and comfortable relationship between your child and his or her provider, so that your child will be able to articulate questions and health concerns — sexual and otherwise — later in life. Your daughter might one day seek birth control from her nurse practitioner, or your son may confide his fears of an STD to the family doctor, rather than approach you. A key ingredient in establishing this mutual trust — and one that you'll notice early on in your visits — is whether your practitioner possesses a kid-friendly bedside manner. This makes all the difference in getting your child to relax and cooperate. Once you've found a practitioner whose values and attitudes you admire, you'll be better equipped to address any of the following issues when, or if, they arise.

Circumcision

Many parents don't give much thought to circumcision until they find themselves confronted with the issue immediately after giving birth. Do yourself and your child a favor and research the issue beforehand. See our discussion of circumcision in the Sex During Pregnancy chapter (page 94) for details as to why we don't recommend this unnecessary procedure.

When Your Child's Genitals Don't Fit the Norm

While the tides are turning against male circumcision, doctors still remain pretty darn trigger-happy when it comes to modifying infant genitalia. Did you know that in America, about two thousand babies a year undergo some form of clitoridectomy?[5] No, we're not talking about the female genital mutilation perpetrated on young girls in some African countries; we're talking about surgically removing some or all of the clitoris of a newborn infant, a practice that takes place in modern American hospitals.

There's a considerable range in the possible size and length of the clitoral glans and shaft, and you can expect that if your baby girl is born with a clitoris that visibly protrudes past her vulva, your doctor may recommend a surgical "adjustment" just to minimize the perceived risk of future emotional scarring from the trauma of having a big clit! Needless to say, the results of this kind of surgery are totally unpredictable, and your daughter's sexual responsiveness could be irreparably harmed by the resulting nerve damage. Do *not* let this happen!

An estimated one in every two thousand babies is born intersexed, meaning that their sex organs don't fall in the neat categories of male or female.[6] Given our society's high anxiety around any gender ambiguities, the modern medical response has been to "assign" gender to these infants. Since removing an organ is easier than building one, most intersex babies are assigned female gender, and their genitals are surgically whittled down regardless of the effect on nerve endings and blood vessels. There's a growing activism among adults who suffered such surgery as children to put laws in place that would require doctors to postpone surgery until intersex babies are old enough to give informed consent. Until such laws are in place, consent remains in parents' hands. If your child is born with ambiguous gender, we'd strongly encourage you to contact organizations such as the Intersex Society of North America before agreeing to any surgical procedures.

When Your Child Has Disabilities

If your child is disabled, we urge you to take a stand in asserting his or her right to sexual self-expression from an early age. People with physical disabilities are in a far better position to advocate for themselves than people with developmental disabilities, and if your child is physically disabled, he or she will have access to an empowered and empowering activist community. However, if your child is developmentally disabled, you'll need to be prepared to take an advocacy role. You may find that one of the hardest first steps is being willing to acknowledge and validate your child's identity as a sexual being.

All people are sexual people, but the innate sexuality of the developmentally disabled is rendered invisible in a society where only the young, skinny, and good-looking are considered sexually viable. Despite, or perhaps because of, this denial, developmentally disabled individuals are particularly vulnerable to sexual abuse, with an estimated 30 to 90 percent of those who live in group homes or residential facilities being abused, usually by staff.[7]

Parents of children with developmental disabilities are understandably protective, and may default to a head-in-the-sand mentality around trying to convey sex education, but denying these children access to basic information and communication skills does them a terrible disservice. In recent years, advocates for the sexual rights of the developmentally disabled have been working to create training and education tools, such as classes on sexual anatomy and abuse prevention, or instructional videos on masturbation.[8]

If you're the parent of a child with developmental disabilities, you may initially find it difficult to envision a future for your child that includes sexual and romantic relationships. Take the time to prioritize research in this arena; the resources are out there to help support your child in enjoying intimate adult relationships of his or her own.

OTHER SOURCES OF INFORMATION

You'll notice that throughout this book we refer you to the wealth of sex information available on the Web. On-line resources are a boon to the sexually curious and can be a lifesaver to members of marginalized communities (transgendered folks, gay teens, folks with disabilities, practitioners of responsible nonmonogamy). Many of our survey respondents sing the praises of on-line forums, where they can find support and encouragement from other moms. The accessibility of the Web enables grassroots information sharing, while the anonymity inspires candid confidences about sex.

We encourage you to take advantage of the Web, but keep a salt shaker at hand while you're surfing; you'll need to apply the proverbial grain of salt from time to time. Make sure any sites you visit for sex or medical information clearly indicate their affiliation (such as whether they're sponsored by a university, government organization, nonprofit, or drug company). Check out a site's mission statement or its author's qualifications to get a sense of the underlying philosophy and to determine how much of the content is opinion and how much is verifiable. Keep in mind that even verifiable data doesn't translate into gospel truth; research articles, studies, or surveys are fascinating reads, but you needn't feel compelled to swallow their conclusions whole. Check to see how the research was conducted. When it comes to sex research, people tend to be more forthcoming and honest in phone interviews than face-to-face interviews, and in filling out anonymous on-line surveys than anonymous paper surveys. See if you can ascertain who funded the research. Organizations tend to seek out researchers who can support their political slant.

When you're swapping advice with pals in an on-line forum, retain the same healthy skepticism you might have when chatting with moms at a playground. Chat rooms and bulletin boards can be like a fast-moving kids' game of "telephone," with information becoming a bit more garbled with every transmission. Medical information is particularly susceptible to miscommunication, since even with the best intentions, folks on-line can confuse facts or extrapolate from their own experience.

Keep your skeptic's cap on while you're sorting out fact from fiction, but don't forget to remove it when the time comes to swap personal details with other moms. We've all endured so many judgments about the right way to be a parent or to be sexual that we have a tendency to turn around and pass judgment on one another. Yet every woman's experiences of sex and parenting are utterly valid. You can gain a lot of comfort and perspective from another mom's experience even when it bears no relation to your own. As the following quotes attest, one of your best sources of inspiration and support as a mother may come from interactions with trusted friends, family, and peers.

My Woman's Circle is an environment of complete sanctity and respect, and, because of this, I feel free to ask about anything I'm curious about. It is amazing the wealth of information contained amongst twelve women.

Our couples' therapist is a great support. We spend so much time laughing in our therapy sessions. Laughter heals. Also we belong to a lesbian moms' support group. We don't talk about sex there, but it helps with our sex life, because if you feel bad about being a lesbian family, you won't enjoy lesbian sex.

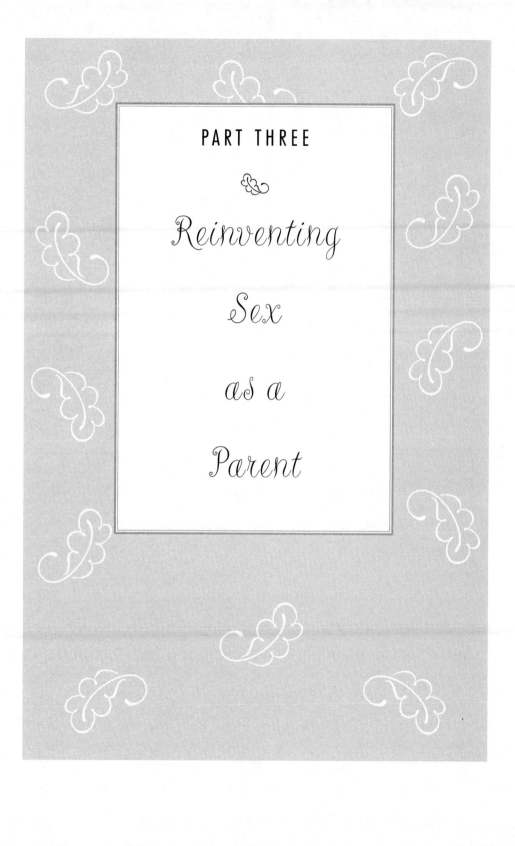

PART THREE

Reinventing

Sex

as a

Parent

SURVIVING SCARCITY

HERE'S nothing like a child in your life to make you realize what an abundance of everything you had when you were without one. Sleep, time, energy, even friends seemed more plentiful in those long-ago lazy days. Being in love, enjoying sex alone or with partners — it all flowed so naturally and effortlessly because you had to think and act only for yourself. But kids enter your life with all the impact of a hurricane, blowing out the routines and self-indulgences, leaving you to weather a new regime of scarcity and self-sacrifice.

There will never again be enough time, energy, privacy, etc., once you become a mom. You must claw and scratch for every last moment.

Bleak as it sounds, calmer winds will prevail, particularly if you hone a few survival skills. Navigating the sea of scarcity depends entirely on your ability to take care of yourself. Without this, you can't function effectively as a parent or a loving partner. If you have a hard time reconciling your maternal identity with the perceived "selfishness" of prioritizing your own pleasure, keep in mind that being a wiped-out, bedraggled, resentful mom won't benefit your loved ones. Do your family and yourself a favor, and look out for number one.

To that end, this chapter is geared toward helping you survive some of the most common scarcity issues: lack of time, spontaneity, privacy, and energy. Typically, when these things fall by the wayside, so do your chances of a satisfying sex life. And while we recognize that sex may be the last thing on your mind (especially if you're a new mom), continuing to view yourself as a sexual being is an important part of your emotional and physical health. The last thing we want is for sex to become one more pressure-filled goal, but we can help you create space in your hectic life so that basking in a little sensual pleasure is both desirable and easily within reach. And besides, scarcity has its upside, as these moms found.

> The quantity of sex has suffered, but the quality is better. It's more special when we do find the time. We're more adventurous and creative in our lovemaking. It's lowered my inhibitions and made me more daring.

> "Lack of spontaneity" is not always bad; I get lots of pleasure in my (very few) spare moments looking forward to Saturday night.

This chapter has a particular focus on negotiating the life changes that result when your children are young, but much of the advice will be useful even as your children grow older. For tips specific to single moms, see the Sex and the Single Mom chapter (page 244).

TIME: IT'S NO LONGER ON YOUR SIDE

Your experience of time changes in three ways once you have a child: You no longer have enough of it, you start to experience it differently, and you feel like it doesn't really belong to you anymore. Sure, you still have the same number of hours in a day, but the demands on your time increase drastically. When you tally up the number of hours spent changing diapers, watching Disney movies, picking up toys, driving kids around, or attending school events, cloning starts to sound like an attractive option. When you're constantly squeezed for time, hobbies, exercise, and sex come to seem "indulgent" and often get sacrificed unless you make a conscious effort to include them in your routine.

You will find that your day can no longer be divided into neat little compartments—work at nine A.M., lunch at noon, cocktails at six P.M., dinner at eight P.M., nookie at ten P.M.—because babies could care less about clocks or schedules. As a result, the relationship between the quality and quantity of time you spend doing any one thing changes dramatically. A morning stroll through the park may appear restful to others, but you'd trade it in a heartbeat for just five minutes alone with the newspaper. There is a silver lining: You learn to stop and smell the roses, your patience threshold goes way up, and you really, really relish what once were simple pleasures.

Money-saving Ideas

If you're reading this chapter, thinking, "Well, that sounds nice, but I can't afford it," let us gently remind you that you can't afford not to. Economics certainly plays an important part in child-rearing, but there are plenty of ways to generate a little extra cash without having to take a second job. Just remember to earmark this money for the things that will help you cope—whether it's baby-sitters, massages, or a new washing machine.

- Find lower interest rates on credit cards and loans.
- Get a roommate to share expenses.
- Host a foreign student—organizations pay stipends to place visitors in homes.
- Share a house with another parent; this can save on baby-sitters.
- Buy secondhand clothes, appliances, furniture.
- Bring bag lunches to work.
- Sell your car and start taking public transportation.
- Give up luxury expenses that you don't really use: cell phones, cable TV, gym memberships.
- House-swap for your vacation and save on rental fees.
- Use e-mail to communicate and save money on postage and phone bills.
- Comparison-shop on-line for lowest prices, special offers, reduced rates, free shipping, etc.
- Sell your old books, CDs, and clothes, and spend the cash you earn on sex toys!

The attitude adjustment you're forced to make translates well into the sexual realm. For example, you learn to take advantage of the sensual moments you find throughout the day; patience will make you a more skillful lover; and something as simple as a passionate kiss can be as erotically thrilling as any midnight rendezvous.

It makes sense that time no longer feels like your own, considering that the bulk of what you're doing is being done for another person. Many people who cope well with demands on their time in professional life find it much more difficult to get their marching orders from children. Not only do the demands come without warning or structure, there's no overtime pay, and no one's going to promote you for doing a great job. Putting another person first—usually without any acknowledgment or reward—is a great sacrifice, and it will suck the life out of you if you don't build in some time to call your own. You don't necessarily need to spend this time alone, but you must spend it the way you want to, and spend it on yourself. Don't free up an hour just so you can go grocery shopping. Use it for sleep, cuddling, masturbation, or sex, but use it for something that will relax and rejuvenate you.

Freeing Up Time

You can squeeze extra minutes, even hours, out of your day simply by reviewing your routine with an eye to more efficiency. In some cases, a monetary investment will buy you time (in the form of labor-saving devices or hired help), so if you're short on funds, please consult the sidebar for money-saving tips. Even if you employ only one or two of the following suggestions, you'll be surprised at the difference they can make in your quality of life. If you're a brand-new parent, you may be so overwhelmed by your total loss of control over the day that efficiency tips are difficult to contemplate. After all, there are days when simply taking a shower is a major achievement. If you can incorporate some of these suggestions before your baby arrives, they'll stand you in good stead. But it's never too late to put any of them into effect.

Get a computer and go on-line

If you live in an urban area and can afford a personal computer you're just a "point and click" away from convenient shopping, bill-paying, and banking. No more running around town doing errands; they can all be done from the convenience of your home, with the items delivered to your doorstep. And competition is still brisk enough to keep prices in line with those at retail stores.

> On-line grocery delivery has changed my life. I can do the shopping at night and my order is delivered *to my kitchen* the next day. I don't miss lugging all that apple juice and laundry detergent up my stairs!

Hire help

Bring someone in for housecleaning, or pay a neighbor kid to do errands, chores, and gardening. If you're a stay-at-home mom, hire someone to baby-sit one day a week so you can have a day off.

Order takeout

You can always count on pizza and Chinese takeout, or have your partner pick something up on the way home. Let your friends know that one of the best gifts they could give a new parent is to send over casseroles, groceries, or dessert. And thanks to the expanding world of on-line commerce, home-delivery cuisine options may soon know no bounds.

> I was so tired one day I said to hell with dinner. I went on-line and found a vendor who delivered a pint of ice cream, gourmet sandwiches, and a CD that I'd been meaning to buy.

Shop and cook in bulk

Instead of going to the supermarket every day, plan your menus in advance and shop once during the week. Similarly, when you cook a meal, make a double batch and freeze some for the future.

Invest in labor-saving appliances

If your apartment or home has the hookups, do whatever it takes to get a dishwasher and washing machine. You don't have to spend much more on reconditioned appliances than you'd spend in a year at the laundromat. Kids generate a mind-boggling number of dirty clothes and cups—you don't need to spend your time dragging it all to the Tidy Wash or washing baby bottles to the tune of "One Hundred Bottles of Beer on the Wall." And by all means, if you're determined to use cloth diapers, get a diaper service—you'll save a huge amount of time. If you have the money and space, buy an extra freezer so you can fill it with meals made ahead of time or with frozen entrees. A microwave will defrost in a jiffy (but don't use it for breast milk).

Throw out the white gloves

It's time to lower your standards—get used to a little clutter and let the dust bunnies breed. Probably the number-one tip from our survey respondents is to get comfortable with a little dirt.

> An immaculate house will not matter in the end. It's the time invested in your relationships—with family, with your kids, with your friends, and above all your partner—that matters.

Managing Time

These suggestions are specifically geared toward creating time for you and your partner to be together, but some also allow you to create more time alone:

Overlap shifts

If you work different shifts so you're rarely home at the same time, try overlapping by an extra half hour, just so you can check in with each other about your day.

Extend day care

Consider leaving your child in school or day care for an extra half hour, while both of you plan to arrive home at the usual time.

Job flexibility

If one or both of your jobs permit, schedule some regular time during the working week to be together, even if it's only during lunch.

NOONERS! They are the absolutely best thing that has happened to my sex life since my children were born.

Sometimes while the baby is engrossed in her favorite TV show, which thankfully comes on at my husband's lunch hour, we sneak into the bedroom for a quickie.

Cancel appointments

If one or both of you is heavily scheduled, agree to cancel one appointment each week and spend the time together.

Family nap

Institute a "family nap" during which everyone—including you—goes to their rooms for quiet time. You can explain to the children that you need your privacy or "grown-up" time and don't want to be disturbed.

Enforce bedtime

No matter how desperately they plead for one more drink of water, beg for one last TV show, or charmingly offer to help you get ready for bed—do not give in to your kids' stall tactics. Enforce regular bedtimes so you can count on adults-only time. Kids actually thrive on routine, so if you can train them to respect morning privacy too, you're that much better off.

Because of "grown-up" time, we are really uptight about bedtime schedules now with the second child. With the oldest, we were really lax about schedules and paid dearly by never ever being alone.

My husband fixed the old lock on the bedroom door and on Saturday mornings, we insist to the kids that they respect our time alone while we "have a cup of tea," and they simply have to wait and we'll see to all their needs when we get up. This is of course with older children (seven and five) who have something to do and can understand the request.

Use the media

Take advantage of cartoons, videos, or computer games to sneak in a little private time.

Saturday morning cartoons—there can be no other justification for the existence thereof. I say kids should be forced to watch as of age one.

Look for opportunities within your routine

You never know what interesting erotic rituals will be born out of necessity:

> My husband and I like to watch certain shows in the evening. If we like the shows that are on at eight o'clock and nine o'clock, but not the one at eight-thirty, we have sex at eight-thirty. It works out great.

> My husband came up with something we refer to as "the booty call" and it is great. We go to sleep (because we really need it) and he wakes up in the middle of the night and starts to fondle me and whisper to me, which leads to wonderful dreamlike sex.

> We took the television out of our bedroom and started just turning the lights off right when we went to bed, so that rather than watch TV or read, we'd be motivated to talk or be intimate.

Vacation at home

You don't need a special occasion to send the kids to a beloved relative's house. It creates a fun getaway for your kids and leaves you home alone together with a long stretch of free time.

> Our kids went out of town to stay with relatives (just for fun) and we spent the whole weekend together, just the two of us, enjoying our time and ourselves. It rocked because we almost never got out of bed!

Multitask

You'd be surprised what you can accomplish with a little imagination.

> Make the most of your time and energy. We do this by showering together regularly. We can have sex, get clean, and lock the doors all at the same time. Take long drives with sleeping children in the car and pull over—hand jobs can be great and discreet. We have yet to have a child wake up on us, and even if they did, they couldn't see anything anyway.

Use Baby-sitters

Find, use, and appreciate good baby-sitters—they quite simply are the key to your sanity.

> I know people who have never left their children alone overnight. EVER. And you know what? Their relationships suck! You have to get away. Even

for just one night. The best sex my husband and I have had the whole time we've been together is during romantic weekend getaways.

It's never too soon to overcome your reservations about leaving your precious bundle with someone else. If you learn to leave your infant with trusted adults, he or she will grow into a more social, engaging child, and you'll be able to retain some independence. Here are a few options for baby-sitters:

Relatives

If you like your relatives and are lucky enough to have some living nearby, they are an ideal source of (usually) free baby-sitting. Many grandparents, aunts, and uncles can be tapped for an evening, afternoon, or an overnight, and hopefully will thrill at the opportunity to develop a special bond with your child. Older siblings, nieces, and nephews might jump at the chance to be a "grown-up baby-sitter," especially if you throw in some money.

> God bless my mom and dad for those occasional days that they pick our daughter up on their way home from work and take her to their house for dinner.

Friends

Responsible friends and roommates are another source of cheap child care. Now is the time to take up any offer you ever received from a friend or a coworker to baby-sit. They want to help you out, so let them.

> Schedule in friends who can watch the kids at their house from the time they are little.

Friends without kids might need a little "cultivating" to overcome their anxieties about baby-sitting. Invite them along on a few outings with you and your child so they can observe your routine. Or simply have them over to baby-sit while you relax somewhere else in the house. Make every effort to talk openly about what their concerns are, and give heaps of positive reinforcement. And don't be shy about soliciting child care; you can get creative in your approach:

> I told my friends that I didn't want them to buy me presents at birthdays and holidays, but that I'd love coupons good for free baby-sitting or evenings out sans kid.

Other parents

Trade off baby-sitting with another parent—this costs nothing and gives your child a playmate. But be vigilant about reciprocating! Join a play group or a mothers' group to meet other parents, or network with the parents at your child's day care or school.

> Arrange with someone else to swap child care—alternate Saturday nights, or you get Fridays and the other parent(s) get Saturdays. Once a week is way better than hardly ever.

Baby-sitters for hire

Even if you have an active network of family and friends who baby-sit, the backup of a paid sitter is great to have. Get referrals from other parents, look for ads in parenting magazines, try finding or posting flyers at day-care centers, community centers, high schools, and kids' clothing stores. Look for agencies or listings on-line and in the Yellow Pages. When you're traveling out of town, see if your friends can find someone, or try the Internet.

With paid sitters, you should make every effort to be a conscientious employer. Be timely, pay promptly, and call when you are unavoidably detained. With gratis sitters, like relatives and friends, encourage regular visits and make it easy for them—bring the child to their house, or leave a cooked meal if they're coming to your place. And remember, if you're balking at the expense of a paid baby-sitter, keep these wise words in mind:

> It's cheaper to spend the money on a baby-sitter and go out, even for an overnight in a hotel, than to get a divorce, no matter how little you think you make. Don't quit dating each other.

SPONTANEITY: IS IT GONE FOR GOOD?

The answer is yes and no. Combustible spontaneous couplings can still be a key component in your sex life after the baby arrives, but now, instead of seizing the perfect moment, you need to be ready to seize any available moment. Kids' naps and other short-term distractions provide an opportunity to connect.

> When that baby goes down—GO INTO THE BEDROOM. Stop folding laundry, doing dishes, whatever. My husband and I take turns dragging each other kicking and screaming into the bedroom—inevitably one of us is "too grumpy or tired." One helps the other get into it and we are always glad that we did!

We have gotten into "quickies" when our child is preoccupied elsewhere. They are very short, explosive sessions where quite a bit of our clothing stays on.

It's true that you don't have the luxury of waiting around till the mood strikes, but you may find that the novelty of tackling each other in unconventional times and places can really turn up the heat. You can also discreetly equip your house so that it's quickie-friendly: Put condoms in several rooms, buy a quiet portable vibrator, and make sure there's lubricant stashed away. If baby sleeps in your room, and you live in anything bigger than a studio, you can designate a guest room or a corner of the living room for your trysts.

You will probably discover, however, that the demands of parenting greatly reduce the opportunities for spontaneous trysts. If you previously counted on having sex whenever the whim hit you, the constraints on your time and energy may short-circuit your libido.

Sometimes my partner doesn't even want to have sex because we can't be spontaneous. He doesn't think it's fun because we don't have the limitless time to do lots of fun things like we used to.

Once you're a parent, you can no longer enjoy sex that is both spontaneous and unrestricted. You are going to have to either cultivate your taste for quickies or plan for sex. Many couples find this one of the most daunting barriers to resuming a sex life and assume that scheduling sex is bound to feel artificial and antierotic. But if you cast your mind back to just about every hot date you've ever had, you'll have to admit that a certain amount of premeditation was involved — perhaps you made reservations at a nice restaurant, dressed provocatively, rented an erotic movie, or purchased some new toys to try, all in preparation for an amorous exchange. Sure, being more forthright about your intentions means you can't pretend to be swept off your feet, but you do get to enjoy the anticipation of a planned night of passion that can add an inspiring erotic tension to your day.

We have designated Saturday as "sex night" — when we hang out all night together with a bottle of wine or margaritas after the kids go to bed. That's when we have the opportunity to get into more relaxed sex or multiple "episodes" if we want. Almost nothing is allowed to get in the way of our Saturday nights. During the day we tease each other about what's going to go on — knowing it's going to happen adds to the excitement, so that we're practically ripping each other's clothes off by the time the kids go to bed.

If the idea of "planning for sex" strikes you as rather clinical, with sex reduced to a routine physical exchange accompanied by the ticking of a clock, it's time to think outside the box. Your goal here is intimacy; how you define sex is up to you. For some it's a kiss, for others it's a bag of tricks.

> We kiss a lot, say "I love you" a lot. I make an effort to kiss very consciously and deeply, and press my body hard against his. Usually it doesn't lead to anything, but once in a while, he'll kiss me a little harder, then I'll kiss him a little harder. We take it very slowly, step by step, so that if one of us isn't really into it, the other can easily back off with no hurt feelings.

> Just the intimacy of a little make-out session, a bit of oral sex, or a furtive hand job can help with the sense of "we've had some intimate time."

And just because your date is planned doesn't mean the sex has to be.

> My boyfriend and I have recently started using the book *101 Grrreat Quickies*, and we are having a blast! So far all the treats have been something that can be done after the kids are in bed, but they are sufficiently unusual and fun that there's always a sense of surprise and anticipation—I wonder if he'll give me the coupon tonight or later in the week?!

Spending regular time together where you won't be interrupted by a needy child and can engage in adult conversation (preferably not about your child!) and relax at the same time will go a long way toward establishing a comfortable environment where your sexuality can begin to flourish. By scheduling time with your partner, you ensure that the relationship does not get buried beneath all the other obligations, you affirm his or her importance in your life, and you keep a grasp on your own identity as an adult, sexual woman.

How do you go about planning? The same way you plan for dinner, doctors' appointments, and vacations—by scheduling it on your calendars, Filofaxes, or Palm Pilots. Pick the best time each week, or choose the same time every week. Remember to keep it manageable, especially at first. The idea is to relax and reconnect with each other. Be flexible and communicate honestly, so if one of you isn't feeling romantic, you can spend the time being intimate in other ways.

> We make a date for sex ahead of time, then because it has been planned for, neither of us will get sidetracked by a book or the dishes. That way it's a little more special, and if we find that later we're not really into it, we can at least have that time together to talk or watch a video.

Spending recreational time together without the kids helps build intimacy. You don't need to be gazing deep into each other's eyes and sharing all your hopes and dreams every week. Simply being alone with each other, doing things you like to do, will go a long way toward reaffirming your connection. If you get tired of planning, you can buy season tickets to favorite events, take turns picking movies or restaurants, play board games at home, or go on walks together after work.

PRIVACY: A LITTLE LOCK GOES A LONG WAY

The freedom to make love wherever the mood strikes has always been regulated by standards of public decency, and you've probably limited your lovemaking to the confines of your home. Now even that sanctuary is under assault from the curious eyes of your offspring. With kids around, you develop a keen appreciation for privacy, whether you're escaping a bed shared with a slumbering infant, minimizing the chances a jealous toddler will sabotage intimate moments, or sharing a house with a teen who's "grossed out" to think of parents "doing it."

> Kids seem to have an amazing sixth sense of when adults are about to do it—it can be frustrating. My teenage daughter complains bitterly every time I have sex. She bangs on the ceiling with a broom if she thinks we're making too much noise—and somehow she always knows!

Regardless of how much time you free up or whether you've moved mountains in order to spend the evening together, if you have no privacy, you won't be able to relax and enjoy the ride.

> My children know that our bedroom is off limits. It's our private space, and they respect that. We have a lock on the door, and we use it. This keeps me from worrying that they might walk in during sex, as I've found that anything at all that makes me inhibited is a bad thing for intimacy.

If you find that privacy is practically nonexistent in your house, we suggest checking to see if you can implement a few of these changes:

Assess Your Physical Space

Get a lock on your bedroom door

This simple, inexpensive solution holds the key—literally—to your peace of mind. Perhaps our biggest collective anxiety when it comes to having sex is the fear that our kids will barge in on us midorgasm. While this is hardly going to irreparably traumatize your children (certainly not as much as the prospect seems to traumatize parents!), why worry about something so easy to prevent? Installing a lock gives you a perfect opportunity to explain the concept of privacy to your children, a concept they will embrace with enthusiasm as they grow older (see the Teaching by Example chapter, page 321, for more on the subject of privacy and disclosure).

> A closed door must be respected. Privacy and Mom's needs need to be stressed.

Create privacy

If you live in a one-room apartment, you might want to hang a curtain or put up a screen to create a feeling of privacy. That way, when your child is absorbed in an activity alone, you can be quietly affectionate without being visible.

Alternatives to the bedroom

Cramped living quarters necessitate a creative approach to lovemaking. You'd be surprised at the variety of alternatives moms have come up with.

> Once or twice we jumped into the shower while our child was engrossed in something else on the other side of the house.

> I have almost all my sex outside on the balcony.

> Activities like mutual masturbation, dry-humping, things that can be done in a car, or the kitchen, under a blanket we do a good deal of, because it's quicker, and you don't have to explain why Mommy is on top of Daddy, or vice versa.

Several mothers reported that one of the benefits of practicing family bed (see below) was that it forced them to have sex outside the bedroom, which infused their sex lives with a greater sense of adventure.

> I found that having sex in the living room or office right after I nurse her to sleep for the night (that way I know she is sound asleep and won't wake for at least two hours) has the right touch of sneakiness, spontaneity, and feels a bit naughty.

> We set aside our guest room as our "playroom" for a while and would retreat there as our "getaway right at home." I mean just a candle, some body lotion, a "toy" or two stashed in there and we were in the mood.

Assess Your Habits

Tone it down

Lovemaking that involves screaming and moaning can be understandably confusing and frightening to a child. Lower the audio if you can do so without dampening your enthusiasm. Otherwise, consider soundproofing your room by putting carpeting on the floors or investing in some insulation. If your bedsprings are squeaky, put the mattress on the floor, get a new mattress, or try a futon. If your room is next to your child's, have sex somewhere else in the house. Use quiet sex toys like the handheld electric vibrators that resemble hairbrushes, or use them under the covers so the fabric muffles the sound.

Think twice about family bed

If your baby sleeps with you in a "family bed," you need to be realistic about the impact this will have on your sex life. Family bed, also known as "cosleeping," refers to the practice of letting a child (or children) sleep in the same bed as their parents. Advocates of family bed maintain that this practice strengthens the bond between parent and child. Many parents actively choose this practice, while others fall into it during their child's infancy either because nighttime breast-feeding is easier with the baby close by, or because baby falls asleep in the bed while nursing.

While we don't doubt that family bed benefits children, it does exact a price on adults. You are sharing your most intimate space with your child, and unless you make a conscious effort to create other opportunities to be alone together, the effect is to demote your adult relationship to second string. This situation can lead to a sense of neglect, resentment, and ultimately no sex. If you're single, family bed may be even harder to resist, since your child fills a need for closeness and physical contact. In either case, should you want to reclaim your bed for yourself and/or a partner, evicting the child will be no picnic. During infancy, family bed may be the only way to maximize your sleep, but we recommend teaching your child how to sleep alone as soon as you can.

Those who practice family bed have mixed reactions about its effect on their sex lives. Some find it rejuvenating, since it forces them out of a sex-in-the-bedroom rut.

> Our third child is cosleeping with us, and I have found that has revitalized our sex life and knocked us out of the nighttime, bedroom-sex routine we'd fallen into. We're challenged to find new places and new times.

Others, like this mom, find that the baby's proximity interferes with sex in practical as well as psychological ways.

> It's been hard to have a sex life for a lot of reasons. Part of it is that we have a family bed, and the baby wakes up any time we start to have sex. I'm not comfortable having intercourse when I've got the baby on one arm, nursing or whatever.

The most sensitive issue family bed raises is whether or not it's appropriate for parents to have sex with a baby in the bed. Culturally, we are schooled to keep our kids and our sex lives separate, so most people treat the prospect of children's being in the presence of any adult sexual activity as a violation of the most primal taboo. But a sleeping baby is oblivious to its environment, so if your hanky-panky won't disturb his or her slumbers, we say have at it.

> Sex and motherhood don't really mix well in the public imagination. For example, when I read in this really popular parenting book that sex with your infant in bed was disgusting and deplorable, I thought, Okay, the baby

in bed during sex is unacceptable and perverse. But the fact of the matter is, we don't have that many opportunities to make love. And if the baby is sleeping in bed with us, we are not going to risk waking him up by moving him to his room. It takes a bit of reckoning to be your own person, rather than a mother who toes the mainstream, conservative line.

Bear in mind that in other cultures where space and privacy are not options, kids of all ages sleep in the same room with parents (who presumably continue to have sex). In fact, the majority of parents around the world sleep with their children in the same room. But we products of American culture are distinctly inhibited by the prospect of our children seeing or hearing our lovemaking. Most parents practicing family bed will choose to have sex in other rooms once their kids pass infancy. In the end, as the following moms attest, it's all about exploring your own personal "comfort zone."

> Even sharing the hotel rooms on vacation never really stopped us. Our daughter just said we kissed loud.

> You have to explore your comfort zones regarding sexuality and your children. My partner and I felt comfortable making love in spoons position while our baby slept next to me. Now that our children are older, we simply tell them that we are having some alone time. They know EXACTLY what that means (they like to giggle when we say that), and have learned to knock before they burst through our closed bedroom door.

Level with Your Kid

Although the previous suggestions are geared toward minimizing kids' awareness of your activities, knowing what you're up to won't kill them. Which is to say, don't freak out if they catch you in the act. And don't obsess over keeping them in the dark. By being honest with your children, you send the message that sex is natural, healthy, and nothing to be ashamed of. You can teach your children to respect your private time; answer their questions in an age-appropriate way as they arise (see the Kids Are Sexual, Too chapter, page 267, for more on this subject).

> I think it's okay for children to see their parents being sexual. I mean, you want to be prudent and respectful, but if they see a healthy sex life in their home they will better be able to filter through all the hang-ups our society has about sexuality and hopefully recognize the unhealthy, belittling, exploitative, and controlling portrayals of sex out there in our media and society.

I grew up in a house where I could hear my parents having sex. I didn't know what they were doing, but I don't think most children jump to a conclusion that something bad is happening. I think it's a healthy household noise! Children should be accustomed to it and raised in an atmosphere where this kind of expression is understood as healthy. And, of course, they should be encouraged to ask questions . . . even the hard ones!

ENERGY: WHEN POWER BARS ARE NOT ENOUGH

Women are told that the physical exertion required for childbirth equals that of running a marathon. We'll take it one step further and contend that raising children is the physical equivalent of participating in a decathlon—one with no finish line! First event: childbirth. Second event: breast-feeding. Third event: sleep deprivation. Fourth event: day care. Fifth event: back to work. Sixth event: housekeeping . . . you get the picture. Nonbiological moms may skip the first two events, but they have to hit the ground running once their child arrives. It's no wonder so many women complain that they've lost their libidos—they're too busy running the race to look for them.

Since sex requires a certain amount of energy, overextended parents might find themselves preferring sleep or a quiet meal over a roll in the hay.

I find that the thought of sex can often make me even more tired. However, actually having sex can boost my energy level for weeks. So, as weird as it sounds, as an unpartnered single mom, I try to make sure that I have sex at somewhat regular intervals.

As this mom notes, the beauty of sex is that it actually rejuvenates you—replenishing mind, body, and spirit. So if you find that you're too tired for sex, too worn out to masturbate, or too stressed out to fantasize, we urge you to examine a few of the following ways to boost your energy. (See the Desire Revisited chapter, page 197, for tips on what to do when your sex drive takes an extended vacation.)

Exercise
Make exercise a part of your daily routine, and you will experience a noticeable change in your energy level. The endorphins released during exercise improve your mood and give your libido a lift. Your self-esteem surges because you're doing something just for yourself, and you're getting back into shape. Go on regular stroller walks, join an aerobics class, sign up for yoga.

Eat well

Whatever you do, don't skip meals. Unfortunately, some new mothers are so horrified that their bodies don't magically snap back into shape after childbirth that they diet compulsively. If you're breast-feeding, you need to eat regularly and nutritiously both for your sake and the baby's. If you're not breast-feeding and you want to diet, just make sure you're eating well-balanced meals. A Power Bar might be great for a mid-day energy boost, but subsisting on them will leave you run-down.

Sleep

Who wants to have sex when you can SLEEP!?

When you've got to have it, nothing else will do. With infants, try to sleep when they do. Get your partner to take the night shift or have a friend or relative sleep over a few nights so you can rest. With older kids, try to go to bed earlier. Take catnaps during your lunch break. Skip chores, cancel appointments, call in sick, if it means you can catch up on some sleep.

Get out of the house

Escaping your routine can go a long way toward boosting your energy level. Whether you go for a walk, have coffee with a friend, or plan an overnight getaway, just removing yourself from an environment that revolves around children can help you feel less like a mom and more like a woman.

> An annual parents-only vacation has made a huge difference for us. Even after we come home, a bit of that romance lingers for us because we actively create it. We buy music on vacation or art or clothes that we can see and touch and hear to remind us of those intimate days alone.

Do things alone

As much as possible, try to arrange regular chunks of time to be by yourself. This practice allows you to step outside your role as mom and take a break from the demands on your time and attention. Trade breaks with your partner or hire a sitter, but make this a priority. Set aside time to read your favorite magazine or newspaper, visit a museum, go to the gym or the movies, but spend time on yourself.

Get help with household chores

Despite the fact that vast numbers of women now also work outside the home, they still do the bulk of the child care and housekeeping.[1] Needless to say, this arrangement can lead to resentment within relationships unless you figure out a way to split the duties or compensate for the inequity. Many women cited frustration with domestic issues as a cause of diminished desire—see the Chore Wars sidebar for some practical tips on combating the issue.

> We fuss more about household responsibilities, and that leads to anger that sometimes affects my desire for sex. I can't feel very sexy if I've spent all day cleaning up after a grown man who puts forth little or no effort to help, and that leads to resentment and decreased energy, which leaves him out of luck sometimes. After all these years, that's the biggest battleground for us.

Keep an open mind

With the overwhelm of motherhood, slipping into the "We're too tired/busy/tense to have sex" mode is hard to avoid. But sexual pleasure can be relaxing in and of itself, and often moms find that simply being receptive to the idea leads to encounters that replenish body and soul. For this mom, one of the benefits of planned sex is that it gives her an opportunity to get in the mood.

> I find I need some adjustment time between going from "mom" to "lover," and he gives me that time, even if it's just a half-hour soak in a bubble bath between putting the kids to bed and starting our evening together. That time helps me adjust, lets me relax, gives me a few minutes for a new headspace to kick in.

Others simply accept fatigue as part of parenthood and discover ways to balance their sexual needs with their bodies' demands.

> We make an assumption: Great sex means we're going to be tired the next day, no question about it. If the sex is good enough, it's worth it, so we don't bother having lackluster sex now. And it's not like we're not tired all the time, anyway! We have small children!

> Being tired is the main difference. I have learned to work with it. There is rarely a time when I'm not tired, so even though I may not want it right at the same moment my partner does, I always give him a chance to "convince" me. I have to say he is usually successful at convincing me. I have yet to regret his advances.

Chore Wars

Chores were bad enough before the kid, but now your little bundle of love makes twice as much work; you feel stuck in an endless cycle of picking up toys, doing laundry, and cleaning up food disasters. By their very nature, chores are unpleasant—they're time consuming, tiring, and monotonous. It's easy to resent the amount of time and energy you spend on them—who wouldn't prefer to be lying poolside with a cold drink in her hand rather than vacuuming up the day's cookie crumbs? This resentment can sour a relationship, but with a little planning, you can avoid waging World War III over the mashed carrots on the carpet.

Itemize the Chores

Make a list of the chores and include child care and parenting activities. Keep track of the duties performed by each of you during an average week (or month) and write down how long each task takes. Use this list as a starting point to discuss a redistribution of work. If your partner is relatively oblivious to his or her domestic comforts, it may help to see—quantifiably—how much time is involved in upkeep.

Assess Your Standards and Goals

How clean does your house really have to be? It's hard to give up a tidy house, but if you're the only one who really cares about a spotless toilet bowl and smudge-free mirrors, maybe it's time to lower your standards a teensy bit. Clean the house once a month instead of once a week. Pick up the toys on the weekend instead of every evening.

Agree on Your Split

Do you want to divide up the chores fifty/fifty or use a different ratio? Be attentive when assigning a higher share to stay-at-home moms. She may not be punching a clock, but the care, feeding, and teaching of children is definitely hard work. If you agree in principle that the chores should be split equally, but one of you doesn't have enough time, consider letting her or him pay for a housecleaner or baby-sitter.

Compromise

To minimize the drudgery, divide up the chores according to what suits each of you best. Choose chores which match your skills or interests, and they won't seem as much like work. If you both like the same things, take turns choosing a chore from the list, or you can alternate your duties from month to month.

Schedule Time to Do the Chores

Don't assume they'll take care of themselves, or Sunday nights will be hell in your house—the kids will be whining about going to school as you whine about the laundry. Make a schedule and keep to it, but give yourself the day off once in a while!

Negotiate

If you can't do your chores, negotiate some alternative solution rather than just blowing them off. Bribe a kid to do them (don't make a habit of it), or swap with your partner: "If you do the laundry today, I'll make dinner tomorrow."

Don't Criticize

Everyone has his or her own style, so don't disparage your partner's efforts by complaining about the work. If you don't like the artful design vacuumed into the rug, keep your mouth shut! At least the darn thing is clean, so why not just compliment your partner on his or her unique domestic aesthetic?

Be Flexible

If one of you misses a chore, don't panic. There are more important things in life than housework, so allow for higher priorities. And give yourselves the weekend off once in a while so you don't miss out on more enjoyable pursuits.

Get Help

You don't have to do it all yourselves. Teach your kids how to pick up their toys, make their beds, and help out around the house when they're old enough. Hire professionals if you can afford it, or avail yourself of some time-saving alternatives (on-line shopping, a dishwasher, diaper service, etc.).

Reward Yourselves

Make rewards part of your routine, whether it's treating yourselves to a night out, taking turns with massage, or playing hooky from your chores once in a while!

SAYING NO TO SUPERMOM

Inevitably, women take on a crushing sense of responsibility when they become moms. Because mothers are still considered the primary caretakers, they shoulder the blame for everything that is less than perfect in this new being's life. Of course, every mom we know is also holding down a job and managing day-to-day household responsibilities. Instead of addressing the inequities of what's been called a mother's "second shift" with societal solutions such as subsidized child care or mandatory flexible work schedules for both male and female parents, our society has come up with the ridiculous ideal of Supermom. You know Supermom. She doesn't see any reason to change society because she can juggle two or three shifts and never break a sweat. She's white, middle-class, well educated, and somehow manages to raise attractive and well-behaved children according to the latest received wisdom on parenting, all the while holding down a successful corporate job. Did we mention that she has retained her girlish figure and that you'll find her on many nights sharing a gourmet dinner with her husband over candlelight and cell phones, the kids tucked safely in bed?

Supermom is a complete nightmare of a role model, and we say wake up! The pressure to live up to the ideal is killing us. In our efforts to be good moms, good partners, and generally likable people, we make a lot of sacrifices. We shouldn't have to work so hard to get access to the simple things—time, privacy, sexual pleasure—that renew and replenish us. Child care should be subsidized, baby-sitters bountiful, partners understanding, and children cooperative. But this is usually not the case, so we tend to compensate by protecting our children's quality of life at the expense of our own. But don't you deserve to live the kind of pleasure-filled life you want your kids to grow up and have? After all, how are your sons and daughters going to avoid the trap of impossible ideals if you don't show them how to trust their own experience? We invite you NOT to be Supermom. Let something go. Do for yourself. Be selfish. So what if you can't leap tall buildings in a single bound? You will love yourself, and from there all good things will come.

DESIRE REVISITED

I get "upset" if I'm not getting turned on like I want to. I feel like something is wrong with me.

SOUND familiar? For many of us, sexual desire is the barometer by which we measure both our health and well-being and our compatibility with a partner. An absence of sexual desire, no matter how brief, tends to fill us with fear. When our libido takes a dive, we assume it will never resurface. When our sex life becomes bland, or our sexual encounters become fewer and farther between, we begin to wonder if our relationships are doomed.

In the Ebb and Flow of Desire chapter (page 43), we examined a variety of factors that affect a woman's sex drive and encouraged you to accept fluctuations over your lifetime as natural and inevitable. However, even a supremely self-accepting woman is bound to find this attitude hard to sustain once she's negotiating the ebb and flow of libido with a partner. Trying to harmonize your sexual desires with someone else's can quickly deteriorate into a game of cat and mouse, rife with frustration, missed opportunities, misunderstandings, and petty cruelties. But you can change the rules of the game, and the first rule to go should be the notion that diminished desire signifies a failed relationship. On the contrary, as psychotherapist Jack Morin points out in his book *The Erotic Mind,* "Experts blame waning passion on lack of communication, lack of intimacy, trust, etc. But good relationships don't automatically lead to good sex. Often in the best relationships passion becomes elusive."[1] In this chapter, we'll take a closer look at why passion disappears, suggest ways to get it back, and show you how to keep your perspective.

REALITIES

While much of the material in this chapter is applicable to both single and partnered moms, it's of particular relevance to couples in long-term relationships. For reasons we discuss below in the Nostalgia section, waning desire is seldom an issue in the early stages of a relationship. But if you've been with the same partner for more than two years, you probably already know how difficult it is to stay in tune sexually. If you've read any sex manuals or discussed this subject with a therapist, you may recognize several clinical terms. "Desire disorder" or "desire dysfunction" are the umbrella terms for ongoing difficulties achieving arousal or orgasm. When couples are dealing with libidos that aren't in sync, they're described as having a "desire discrepancy." And the colloquial term for a couple's mutual, ongoing disinterest in sex is "bed death." While all of these terms have an ominous or downright pathologizing ring to them, they actually describe perfectly healthy situations that are common to a large portion of the population. The fact that your sex drive has headed south, that your partner doesn't seem remotely interested in sex, or that neither of you seems in sync does not indicate that there's anything wrong with either one of you. Desire issues usually result from the fact that our realities don't match our expectations. If you cultivate more realistic expectations, you can learn to appreciate your own desires, wherever they may wander.

Good Sex Takes Work

As the entertainer Bette Midler once quipped, "If sex is such a natural phenomenon, how come there are so many how-to books?" Few enough people in our society receive accurate information about the biological basics of sex, and practically no one receives accurate information about the emotional complexities of sex. In an age touted for its scientific discoveries, technological advancements, and communications revolution, we still aren't providing accurate sex education in schools, homes, or medical settings. Instead, the media substitutes as our instructor. Disney teaches kids that one kiss will solve all life's problems; movies and glossy magazines dish up airbrushed, blissed-out celebrity unions; and the advertising industry assures us that only the young and beautiful deserve to get laid.

Nobody ever tells or shows us that a satisfying sex life requires work. Psychologist Lenore Tiefer points out that there's no bridge between our own experience (or lack of experience) and our cultural expectations:

Imagine how you would feel if playing gin rummy, and playing it well, were considered a major component of happiness and a major sign of maturity, but no one told you how to play, you never saw anyone else play, and everything you ever read implied that normal and healthy people just somehow "know" how to play and really enjoy playing the very first time they try! It is a very strange situation.[2]

When sexual relationships show any sign of faltering, we start by worrying, move on to pointing fingers, then we panic, and often we flee. But sexual fulfillment requires just as much information gathering, communication, and persistence as parenting does. A new sexual partner won't know how to please you for the first time without your explicit feedback, and a long-term partner won't know how to please you for the thousandth time without your explicit feedback (trust us, your feedback *will* have changed). Self-awareness is crucial, and it does take effort to get to know yourself: from your sexual anatomy and responses to your hormonal fluctuations to your deepest erotic desires and fantasies. Ultimately, only you can teach yourself how to have good sex, because only you know how you define good sex. And you're going to define your terms in different ways throughout your life.

Challenges for the New Mom

The logistical challenges of parenting (see the Surviving Scarcity chapter, page 175) are a piece of cake compared to the emotional and physical challenges that make you and your partners so susceptible to a decreased sex drive while your kids are young. Plenty of women gain a sense of power and accomplishment from becoming mothers that ultimately boosts their sexual energy. But you'll probably experience a decline in libido and a corresponding decline in sexual activity during the first year or two of your child's life. Or, as a typical survey respondent put it:

> Sex? What is this "sex" of which you speak? I've heard of it, but for the life of me I can't remember what it is.

This lowered libido may or may not trouble you and your partners. Some women are perfectly blithe about their shift in focus, and many parents are self-possessed enough to take the long view.

> I have absolutely zero libido. Just want to nibble on the baby's plump sweet body. Can't even feel aroused at the site of a handsome movie devil's triceps.

I just don't sweat it. I'm in my marriage for the long haul, so short-term lapses in romance (and I consider a year or two to be short-term) are no big deal. My husband agrees.

In the Fourth Trimester chapter (page 138), we discussed the impact of physical recovery, fatigue, changing self-image, changing priorities, and postpartum depression on a biological mother's libido. The following common sources of stress affect biological and nonbiological parents alike and offer ample reason to cultivate compassion for yourself and your partners.

Hormones

The impact of hormonal changes on a biological mother's libido can't be underestimated. Many of our survey respondents commented that they had no warning that a postpartum drop in estrogen and the rise in prolactin accompanying breast-feeding would have such a sexually depressive effect. As one mom put it:

> Let women know that desire does return. I thought my pussy had died after three births in three years, accompanied by seven years of nursing, but it has made quite a comeback.

But biological mothers aren't the only parents affected by hormonal shifts — which may explain why they aren't the only parents who can experience postpartum depression. Some evidence suggests that fathers of infants experience an increase in prolactin levels (probably as a result of bonding) and a decrease in testosterone levels (probably as a result of stress). Presumably nonbiological moms would have the same experience. Lowered testosterone levels can result in a lowered libido in both men and women.

Guilt

New parents, especially moms, often become completely wrapped up in caretaking and feel guilty if their focus wavers for an instant. If you perceive sexual pleasure as at best a frivolity and at worst a dangerous distraction from the more important task at hand, you won't be particularly motivated to be sexual.

> My sex life changed dramatically because I went from being self-focused to being child-focused. I spent much less time on my own pursuits.

> Initially I couldn't fathom having sex. It was a total cognitive dissonance for me. It took many months (and I'm still working on it!) before I didn't feel

guilty having sex. I believed I should be totally focused on my daughter, even when she was sleeping. Sex took me away from her, and at times I was anxious something awful would happen to her while we were having sex.

One of your greatest challenges as a mother will be walking the line between selflessness and selfishness. Part of a healthy selfishness is recognizing that kids can't—and shouldn't be expected to—fulfill your needs for emotional and sexual intimacy. You need to prioritize your adult relationships as much to be a better mother as to be a happier woman. Of course, as we'll discuss later in this chapter, adult relationships present challenges that the relatively straightforward relationship of mother and baby does not.

Parents should put themselves first, put their relationship on the front burner. That took a while to sink in—realizing that we can't be good parents if we are not a good couple and partnership. Sometimes it is harder to be a wife than a mom.

Loss of self

Becoming a mother can present a serious identity crisis, since in our culture it can result in what anthropologist Sheila Kitzinger refers to as a "virtual annihilation of self." While increased status has typically accompanied a woman's transition to motherhood at other times and in other cultures, here's how she describes the effects of this transition in the Western world:

When a woman turns into a mother she is treated suddenly as *less*, not more. She tends to be perceived by men, and by other women who are not themselves mothers, as having fewer skills, and reduced competence, intellectual capacity, and commitment to the things that matter. Her identity has become that of "a mother," and it is as if the rest of her—her working skills, her career goals, and all her other interests—has vanished.[3]

Maintaining your own identity is not only essential to your mental health, it's vital to the health of your relationships. Without a strong sense of self, you won't necessarily feel entitled to your own desires.

I think that I have in some ways become shy about addressing my own wants and needs and that sometimes I play the mother role as an unhealthy buffer to avoid dealing with the issues I do have about safety and trust. I hide out in my motherhood.

On a practical level, you may well feel like you don't have time or space for your own desires. Caring for children, especially infants, is both incredibly demanding and incredibly gratifying, so everything and everyone else in your life might recede into the background upon their arrival. You may resent this narrowing of your horizons, or you may delight in a sense of higher purpose.

> Having a baby and integrating her into my life has been emotionally and physically draining. It is like my brain cannot fit in any need other than the baby, so it is very difficult to find the energy even to give my partner a hug when he needs it.

> I'm fulfilled by my child, so sex isn't as important anymore.

Mothers are expected and encouraged to put all their energies into bonding with their babies. The current philosophy of "attachment parenting" is based on perfectly sound ideas about the importance of providing infants with consistent, attentive care, but in time-honored tradition it places the ultimate responsibility for this care on mothers.[4] (Parenting trends may come and go, but Mom is invariably left holding the bag.) If you spend your days in constant contact with an infant, you're more likely to spend your nights dreaming about getting a little personal space than getting a little action.

> Not only is my sex drive just about gone, but practicing attachment parenting makes having sex nearly impossible. My son sleeps in our bed and sleeps the exact hours we do, so there is literally no time for sex. Plus, I hold him so much during the day that I am touched out by the end of the day. I just want to be left alone at night.

The intimacy you have with an infant may feel so all-encompassing that it's difficult to make room for any other feelings.

> I felt almost a chemical change, where sex became completely secondary and my entire affection was directed toward my child. I wanted to give all my physical love to my child. It freaked me out a little at first, but I was so in love with my child it really didn't matter. And in the end, as your child grows, you regain your sense of your self and your sexual self.

As the survey respondent above suggests, the infatuation phase with your infant will wear off, and your old familiar yearnings and appetites will come back to you, in a flood or a trickle. We all know that motherhood has a lot to teach us about self-sacrifice and nurturing, but no one ever points out that spending time with an infant has a lot to teach us about the integrity of human desires. If you can learn to apply the same attention, respect, and acceptance to your own desires as you do to your child's, you'll be well equipped to enjoy being both a good mother and a satisfied lover.

> Becoming a mom has caused me to become MUCH more aware of myself as a sexual being. I feel much more in touch with my body, and I have no embarrassment anymore about masturbating, experiencing sexual pleasure, or trying new things.

Challenges for the Relationship

Becoming parents presents a huge challenge to even the strongest relationships. Statistics show that marital satisfaction plummets during the first two years of parenting, an occurrence that takes most parents by surprise.[5] As Harriet Lerner, psychotherapist and author of *The Mother Dance*, explains, "Nothing is more stressful than the addition or subtraction of family members. We understand the subtraction part, because loss is the most difficult adaptational task we deal with. But we underestimate the incredible stress of adding a new family member to the system." An appreciation for the magnitude of your adjustment can help you keep your perspective. "Don't expect to have a sex life during the first two years after the child's birth," advises Lerner. "If it happens, consider it to be an 'extra.' But reduce your expectations to zero because a new baby is a crisis of enormous proportions in the life of a couple, and especially the mother from whom more is expected."

> I'm happy having less sex right now. However, I'm unhappy with the perception that I must have some problem if my sex drive is low. It seems perfectly normal to me that people who have averaged three to four sleep interruptions per night over an eight-month period, plus hauling a heavy child around all day, have less need for sex than other creature comforts.

Whatever conflicts your relationship may have had prior to having children will only be amplified by their arrival. Most new parents consistently fight about the same things: money, child care, housework, careers, social life, and sex.[6] Although both partners are dealing with the demands of parenting, heterosexual women typically bear the greater burden because the division of labor tends to break down along traditional gender lines (studies do show that lesbian parents share child-care tasks more equally than heterosexual parents).[7] In other words, mothers with male partners end up doing more household chores, assuming primary responsibility for child care, sacrificing or postponing a career, etc. As one typical survey respondent describes this scenario:

> I all of a sudden became the mom of two instead of one. Once we decided that it was best if I was the one to stay home, I acquired a full-grown child who sees me as a mom, not as his wife anymore.

As a result, studies show wives often experience greater marital dissatisfaction than husbands, which researchers suggest has to do with the gap between their optimistic expectations and the harsh realities of domestic life.[8] You don't need to be a rocket scientist or a sex therapist to figure out how this frustrating state of affairs could negatively impact your sex life.

> Find a partner who contributes fully in terms of child care and household duties — it is impossible to feel sexual if you're the one getting up three times a night to take care of your newborn while the other snores away.

Preparation, communication, and compromise will be your biggest allies in achieving domestic harmony. Face it, both you and your partner are dealing with the same stressors, even if you each sometimes feel like the other is the primary source of your stress. You probably both face economic anxieties and guilt: guilt about how much or how little you work outside the home, about how much time you are or aren't spending with your children, and about how you are or aren't meeting each other's expectations. Domestic stress frequently decreases sexual desire, but if you work together to create coping mechanisms, you'll be laying the groundwork for rediscovering your erotic interest in each other. "Renegotiating the marital contract, which may mean he negotiates reduced hours at work, does a lot for a better time in bed," says Harriet Lerner. Once you make a decision regarding the division of labor, maintain an ongoing dialogue about the arrangement. Even if you consciously decide to make a certain sacrifice, your resentment about this decision can flare up when you least expect it, and you'll need to continually fine-tune your agreements. Keep partners apprised of how stress affects your sex drive and what they can do to help:

> I need nonsexual attention — help with the babies, the housework, time to relax by myself (Calgon, take me away!), because without it, sex becomes a chore — just one more thing I have to do before I can get some sleep.

The bottom line is that you have to communicate about difficult or highly charged topics in order to keep your relationship vital—or even remotely interesting! If you keep a mental list of all your partner's perceived failures but never articulate your distress, the resulting hostility will eat away at your sex drive. If you feel resentful about giving up your career but never share this with a partner, you'll never have the chance to explore possible alternatives. If you're the partner of a new mom and feel jealous of or excluded by the mother/child bond, you'll only distance yourself further by staying silent. Revealing your most petty emotions is risky, but risk is the very element you might need to reinvigorate your relationship. Certainly it is the very element that will bring sexual tension and erotic excitement back into the mix.

Defining Your Own Terms

I was never too tired for sex, but my ex had a very low sex drive, which was the problem. I think that people who are highly sexed will find the time and place. For others, having children is an excuse to give it up or reduce the frequency.

I don't like the assumption that you have to prioritize having sex. I think there are phases of life where sex is more and less important, and it's fine if I'm taking a bit of a break right now.

Not enough is written or said about total loss of libido, and I am sure it is a very common experience. So much of what we read is about how to find time to have sex as if we are all just chock-full of desire and the one problem is finding time. But I avoid contact with my husband because I am not interested in sex.

Few topics seem to elicit quite so many judgments or so much defensiveness as defining an appropriate level of sexual desire, particularly in relation to a partner's: How much is too much? How much is too little? Will the real sick ticket in this relationship please stand up? The truth is that we're all entitled to enjoy as much or as little desire as we please. Although the focus of this chapter is on keeping the sexual flame burning in your relationships, we don't mean to imply that a relationship is meaningful only if you're sexually active together. As the survey respondent below points out, just because you're not "doing it" doesn't mean you lack an erotic connection.

I actually had a consensually celibate relationship for about five months when my son was three. We did a lot of thinking about how sex would impact each of us, our differing beliefs about abortion, my need for true intimacy, his fears about "entrapment," and we decided we would stop having sex, after one time. One VERY hot time. It was difficult, but I learned more about my sexuality in that time than I learned in all the years before! I felt truly listened to, was tenderly touched, enjoyed great kissing, and we even slept together occasionally.

Plenty of parents are philosophical about the fact that it's difficult to keep sexual passion high on the agenda when there's a small child in the house.

We share love, compromise, friendship, and the realization that the sexual part of any relationship goes through ups and downs. It helps to know that we won't have a one-year-old forever, and that someday down the road, we can just let her go out and play while we go upstairs and play!

Recognize that your passions need not be continuously stoked to a white-heat intensity for you to qualify as a sexual being. You should toss out the calendar rather than fretting over how many times this month you have or haven't had some kind of erotic encounter. Your sexual self-worth does not hinge on how often you do or don't have orgasms. This said, we're suspicious of women who proclaim that sex no longer matters to them because they're busy with the more meaningful task of mothering, and we have *very* limited tolerance for partners who become unable to view mothers as sexual creatures. We all live in a culture where sexual expression is viewed as a frivolous luxury and where mothers are expected to thrive on self-sacrifice. It's not always easy to distinguish between the social pressures herding your libido onto the back burner and your own natural ebb and flow of desire. Rather than redefining yourself as a sexless, maternal being, you might find it helpful to redefine what being sexual means to you. As Susie Bright put it during a panel discussion on sex and parenting:

I don't have to be "doing it" every day, minute, or week to prove I have a sexual life. If you think of your sex life as something that's just tick, tick, ticking like a heartbeat and you pay attention and recognize what affects that — that you have fantasies and daydreams — then your life is filled with sex. You're sensually aware that sex is part of being alive, and if you're feeling alive, then you're having a sex life.

ROADBLOCKS

If your sex drive, or your partner's, appears to have vanished without a trace, you are not alone. Our collective yearning for sustained passion keeps the mental-health professionals in business and fuels a million-dollar industry of self-help books. Books such as *Hot Monogamy*, *The Erotic Mind*, and *I'm Not in the Mood* all attempt to unlock the mysteries of sexual desire, while instruction manuals such as *101 Nights of Grrreat Sex* promise instant gratification. We consumers eat them up in the hopes that we'll learn how to time-travel back to that magical honeymoon stage of our relationship.

In fact, there are no time machines, effective aphrodisiacs, or money-back guarantees. The only fundamental truth is that your sexuality is unique: Techniques that enhance desire for one person might leave you indifferent, and vice versa. Your emotions, sexual history, values, and physiology all influence what arouses you. Add your partner's own particular sexual profile, throw in a variety of external factors related to your relationship, and you've got a chemistry that's exclusive to the two of you.

This is not to say that many couples don't stumble over the same obstacles or pass through some of the same phases in their relationships — they do. But you're more likely to overcome a problem — sexual or nonsexual — if you understand all the contributing factors. To that end, we invite you to examine how the following common roadblocks to sexual satisfaction might apply to your own situation.

Expectations

Many of us suffer from the unrealistic expectation that sexual partners should be perfectly in tune and perfectly sufficient to satisfy each other's desires. We find it threatening to experience different degrees of desire, to experience desire at different times, or to experience desire for different things. While we are hardly likely to take it as a personal affront if our partner feels like going for a jog or eating some ice cream when we don't, we tend to feel anxious, guilty, or irritated if our partner has sexual desires we don't share.

Few differences feel quite as threatening to a relationship as a discrepancy in sex drive. Since we equate sexual desire with love and attraction, we tend to leap to the conclusion "If you don't want to have sex with me, you must not love me." The truth is that sex drives simply differ from individual to individual. Or as Pat Love, psychotherapist and author of *Hot Monogamy*, comments, "some degree of desire discrepancy seems to be the human condition."[9] As we discussed in the Ebb and Flow of Desire chapter (page 43), there does seem to be a hormonal component to this naturally occurring discrepancy. Studies suggest that testosterone levels influence libido, and that individuals with higher levels of naturally occurring testosterone, or so-called high-T individuals, will have higher sex drives. While men, by definition, have much higher levels of testosterone than women, some researchers speculate that women compensate for this discrepancy by having a higher sensitivity to testosterone, so a little goes a long way.

Couples experiencing desire discrepancies may find it helpful to learn that their differences could have a biochemical component. When libido is conceived as something that fluctuates innately, rather than as something that "should" be at a certain "normal" level in a "healthy, loving" relationship, the desire discrepancy loses much of its negative charge. The low-desire partner is released from feelings of inadequacy and guilt and the high-desire partner from feelings of failure or rejection.

Identifying a desire gap does you no good if you're not also willing to strategize ways to bridge it, and we'll discuss this further in Let's Make a Deal, below. Rather than focusing on which of you seems to be high-T or low-T, you and your partner may want to get to know your respective body rhythms in order to make the most of individual highs and lows. Some women notice a distinct increase in libido at different times of their menstrual cycle—such as midcycle, when estrogen levels are higher. Some individuals notice a distinct increase in libido at different times of day—such as in the morning, when testosterone levels are higher.

> My husband knows that my monthly cycle provides me with about a week of feeling romantic, a week of lust, a week of slowing down, and a week of no desire. We work around that.

Playing biology professor can be useful and fun when it comes to mapping out your sex drives, but needless to say, there's a lot more to desire than biology. Plenty of emotional and environmental factors also come into play. Sometimes simply feeling freed from the pressure of a partner's expectations is enough to rekindle libido.

> The partner CANNOT take it personally when the mother is too tired or freaked to be sexual. Sometimes my desire came back simply because my husband said I didn't have to have sex.

Another common discrepancy that can jeopardize a couple's sense of sexual compatibility is a simple difference in what sex means to each partner. We're motivated to have sex for a variety of reasons: physical release, sensual closeness, emotional connection, ego gratification, and more. Our differences become problematic only if we think our partner's motivation is somehow not as legitimate as our own.

> The emotional and spiritual element of sex has become more and more important to me since having children, and my husband hasn't understood

that at all. Sex is still a completely physical experience for him, and I wish it could deepen.

My husband has always equated love with sex, and it took him some time to see that I could love him without always making love to him.

If you can let go of the expectation that sex should mean the same thing to both of you, and communicate honestly about your own motivation, you'll be more likely to get what you want out of your sexual encounters.

Nostalgia

Part of the reason so many couples in long-term relationships struggle with the gap between expectations and reality is that early in their relationship, expectations and reality seemed in perfect harmony. You probably have fond memories of the heady early days of your love affair: You couldn't keep your hands off each other; the simple touch of your lover's hand was enough to make your entire body tingle with arousal; you were willing to be more sexually adventurous; and you could stay up half the night making love and wake up raring to get right back down to action. Remember how intoxicating it all felt? That's because you *were* intoxicated — considerable evidence proposes that, during the initial euphoria of a love affair, we're under the influence of an amphetaminelike brain chemical known as PEA. What is sometimes referred to as "limerance" — the initial intensity of romantic love — is temporary and usually peters out between eighteen months and three years after your first date, as you settle down to sober reality.

One particularly sneaky aspect of this PEA infatuation is that it effectively camouflages any sexual incompatibility, which doesn't become apparent until the honeymoon phase is over. As Pat Love says, "In the infatuation stage, even a low-T person has a significant libido, a significant desire to be sexual. We start to believe that this is the way it always will be, we equate this physical desire with love, and we believe that this infatuation high is true love." During infatuation, both of you assume that your true passionate nature has either finally been uncovered or has finally met its match. If there is a noticeable desire discrepancy, bumping back down to reality once the limerance phase is over can be particularly disillusioning. But don't despair — as we'll discuss in the Silver Lining chapter (page 227), there are distinct erotic benefits to sticking it out and learning to work with each other's authentic patterns of desire.

Even if you're able to overcome the nostalgia for the good old days of limerance, you may find it hard to overcome nostalgia for the good old days without kids. The reality is that there are now three (or more) of you, and to a certain extent it's irresistible to reminisce longingly about all that loud, spontaneous sex you enjoyed prebaby. But you can't go home again, Mama—at least not until the kids leave home—so you might as well concentrate on creating some equally thrilling memories of the whispered, clandestine sex that's waiting for you to enjoy right here and now.

Attraction

When desire disappears, we sometimes assume that we no longer find our partner attractive. But attraction, like sexual desire, needs to be cultivated. When you first met your partner and were still intoxicated by PEA, all you could register was his or her fine points. Well, Cinderella, the spell wears off eventually, and then you and your sweetie see each other for who you really are, torn dress, thin hair, and all.

Bearing that in mind, try stirring the embers by remembering what you initially found attractive in your partner. Recalling an early sexual escapade can not only be arousing in itself, but it also helps you identify what it was that turned you on about your beloved—a movement, an attitude, a way of talking, a personality trait, or a particular physical characteristic. Share your memories, and be explicit about what it was that had such an arousing effect on you; your partner may be inspired to flex his or her charms again. But don't stay stuck in the past. Pay attention to what still gives you visceral pleasure about your partner.

Often our desire fades away because we no longer feel desirable. Biological moms confront a whole host of physical changes, while all moms have to deal with a certain disconnect between the roles of nurturer and hot babe. You may be uncertain about your own attractiveness, and you may project your uncertainty onto a partner. Both of you should discuss your anxieties in as nonconfrontational a way as possible.

> I felt really bad about my looks, but was relieved to find out my husband was still very attracted to me. I found that he was being so careful not to make me feel pressured or obligated to have sex that I felt like he wasn't sexually attracted to me. So now we are more open about exactly what is going on.

> My husband has talked about his fear that I'll "let myself go" the way he's seen other moms do, and this makes me furious. I have to remind myself that it took him courage to bring it up, but it really feels like an implicit threat that if I become fat and unattractive, he won't love me or want me anymore. I exercise and take care of my body, and I justify it by reminding myself that it's for me, and not about keeping my husband interested.

If your partner suggests that you've been "letting yourself go," the statement probably did take some courage, and it deserves your attention. The cultural bias that women are expected to prioritize being attractive to men is galling, particularly if you're a biological mom who's expected to snap back into shape overnight. But attraction is a two-way street, and you should feel just as entitled to request that your partner make efforts to keep up his or her appearance for your sake. We're fond of team efforts here — if you plan to diet or join a gym, do it together. If your partner gets the haircut you requested, repay him or her with lavish compliments. If he or she gives you a compliment in return, accept it without making self-deprecating comments. As this biological mom makes abundantly clear, confidence and validation can make all the difference:

> I think that having confidence in your body makes such a wonderful difference with postbaby sex. You just have to think of how hard you worked for those stretch marks, or that extra little lump on your tummy and hips. With positive sexual support from your partner, you can take your sex life and push it back up to where it was before.

Routine

The boredom, the utter boredom, of monogamy.

At the beginning of a love affair, you don't really have much to lose, so you might feel free to take more sexual risks. You enjoy flexing your seductive powers, experimenting with new sexual activities, or sharing fantasies you once thought you'd never tell another soul. But if the love affair evolves into a committed relationship, the dramatic tension of limerance is bound to dissipate, and you soon settle down into a comfortable pattern of familiar routines. Routine inevitably leads to boredom, and boredom leads to a loss of desire.

The trouble is, once you're in a committed relationship, you have a serious emotional investment at stake, which makes it a lot harder to disrupt your routines. You may be afraid you'll hurt your partner's feelings or cause him or her to see you in a less favorable light, so you choose not to rock the boat. The longer you wait to unburden yourself, the harder it becomes. In time, however, you run the risk of getting so bored with your sex life that you no longer desire sex, you resent your partner for not being in tune with your needs, or you assume you're simply no longer attracted to each other. When both partners grow disillusioned with the sex, the resulting "bed death" can be frustrating at best and damaging to the relationship at worst.

If you're not enjoying as much sexual excitement as you'd like — or simply as much sex as you'd like — take the time to question some of your sexual preconceptions. Make a list of the things you'd like to change about your sex life. Be specific! Don't write "I'd like to be more adventurous" if what you're really fantasizing about is renting a motel room for an hour and tying your girlfriend down to the vibrating bed. Don't write "I need more romance in my life" if what you really want is to listen to your husband read erotic poetry while you soak in a bath filled with rose petals. Then make another list—a list of all the reasons you're unwilling to share these proposals with your partner. You'll probably discover that you have a fair amount of shame about your desires and a lot of assumptions about how he or she will react to them. For example, perhaps you assume that your partner will feel rejected by your desire to introduce a vibrator to your sex play. But maybe deep down you're also afraid that your desire for a "marital aid" indicates that you're somehow defective or abnormal. You may think of yourself as a savvy modern woman, but sexual shame has many disguises and can creep up when least expected. If you acknowledge the fears you have about your own desires, you'll have a basis for empathy with your partner if he or she is resistant to some of your suggestions.

The prospect of raising the topic of sexual boredom with your partner is bound to make you anxious, but keep in mind that his or her reaction is most likely to be relief. The very fact that you're doing something uncomfortable, that you feel vulnerable, and that you're challenging each other's assumptions can create the erotic tension that may have been missing between you for some time. Either way, you will have taken a crucial first step, because there is absolutely no way to vary your sexual routine unless you talk about it. Communication is the key to ongoing sexual discoveries with a long-term partner, and its rewards are manifold: deepened intimacy, increased sexual self-awareness, and renewed sexual enthusiasm.

> I think what I love most about my sex life is that although it is monogamous, I feel a lot of freedom within my relationship to explore sexuality. I feel like the more I'm with my partner, the greater the depth of desire I feel.

REKINDLING PASSION

Every one of us will take sabbaticals from partner sex at different points throughout our lives. If you're single, you may be on a break right now. If you're in a long-term relationship, you may have already weathered your share of sexual dry spells—or you may be praying for rain this very moment. Parenting presents specific challenges to sustaining your sexual identity, but our suggestions for meeting these challenges will help see you through all the ups and downs of your erotic life.

We encourage you to make an effort to keep your partnered sex life alive for one simple reason: It's all too easy to lose momentum. While you might think of resuming partner sex after a hiatus as "just like riding a bicycle," it actually feels more like riding a bicycle on a high wire without a net. Fear, awkwardness, and performance anxiety can step in to short-circuit the exchange of erotic energy that used to seem so easy.

It has now been too long and we are both unsure of where to begin. It seems like once you get out of the habit of regular lovemaking, it's hard to get back into it. There is a gap we have to cross to reach one another again, even to think of ourselves as people who have sex. We need to find some kind of continuity.

Physical intimacy isn't necessarily the same as sexual intimacy. Many couples who haven't been sexual for months or years are exceptionally loving and warm with each other. But spooning through the night or holding hands wherever you go doesn't demand the same self-disclosure and risk as an erotic encounter. When you're distracted by your daily obligations and experiencing reduced desire, you can lose sight

Inspiring Words from Other Moms

"I find that with sex, the more I have it, the sexier I feel, and therefore the more comfortable I am with going after it, getting what I want during it, and giving my husband what he wants."

"I feel really good about myself sexually during lovemaking. For that length of time I forget that I weigh more than I'd like or that I have responsibilities to the babies. It's like a trip back to my 'me' self."

"I have to have physical contact with my partner at least once a week, even if it's only for an hour during nap time. Intercourse isn't the point. We just need an intimacy that reminds us that we're people independent of the little one."

"Sex allows me to feel like an adult and a woman, which is important after spending a day conversing with a three-year-old."

"We understand that sex has different roles in our lives. It can be fun, it can be romantic, it can just help deal with stress. It helps for getting a good night's sleep. It can take hours or minutes. I think the best is that we respect and trust each other. Sex is not used to prove anything, it's just a great way to show our love and affection."

of each other as sexual beings, and maintaining what Jack Morin calls "an erotic play-ground" takes an effort.[10]

> We are dissatisfied with our sex life. The biggest issue for us to overcome is shyness. We are really careful to work on intimacy in small ways, we talk dirty to one another, and we're trying to make actual genital contact a more regular occurrence in our life.

The good news is that, once you get over the hump, sexual activity can be its own best reward.

> Sometimes I've gone so long without it that I think my body forgets how great it is, and it needs some coaxing. It's like eating when you aren't hungry but know you haven't eaten all day and need it. Afterwards, I tend to go on a bit of a sex binge, as if I've just discovered sex, and I crave it often.

This is not to suggest that having partner sex after a hiatus automatically results in fireworks. Take advantage of the fact that you won't necessarily be connecting in as effortless or unconscious a way as you once did, and embrace change. Now could be a golden opportunity for you and your partner to expand your expectations to include a wider range of sensual activities than ever before. If shared pleasure, rather than intercourse or orgasm, is your goal, you'll have a reason to feel desire. And if you cultivate self-awareness in the ways described below, your eroticism will ultimately flourish.

Enjoy Yourself

> Everything I read about lack of desire just says "Oh, it's normal" and doesn't mention what you can possibly DO about it. I miss my sex drive.

If your libido has taken a hike, you don't have to sit and wait for it to come back into view over the horizon. You can get out your sexual compass and track it down. The first step to rediscovering a lost libido is to take the focus off the feelings you could or should be having for a partner and pay attention to how your own body feels and what your own imagination is telling you.

Masturbation
You've probably got a running list of all the self-improvements you're convinced would boost your energy and make you a more productive mom—eating well, join-

ing a gym, tucking yourself into bed by ten P.M. Well, we want you to add "masturbate" to your list (and we dare you to post it on the fridge). Masturbation is the single best way to stay connected with your sexuality. It allows you to explore your body and mind with ease. Not to mention the fact that it feels good.

> Even though I am currently in a sexual relationship, I never stopped "flying solo" whenever I wanted, which seems to have increased my sex drive, rather than using up my sexual energy.

Whether you're single or partnered, if your libido is ebbing, masturbation provides a low-pressure way to boost your sexual self-esteem, cultivate your fantasy life, and enjoy physical release. Masturbation can serve as positive reinforcement for investing time and energy in your own eroticism, and you may discover that a thriving solo sex life boosts your desire for partner sex.

> I think what helped me find my sex drive was starting to masturbate again. They say the more you are sexual the more you want to be sexual, and this has proven true for me. I needed to get back in touch with my sexual side by myself and then begin again with my husband.

Masturbation can also be a helpful tool for couples with desire discrepancies, since it provides an outlet for high-desire partners and a way for low-desire partners to recharge their sexual batteries. Furthermore, mutual masturbation can be a highly satisfying alternative to intercourse.

> Sometimes we masturbate together. Sometimes I just watch and vice versa. It's good just to come sometimes. It releases pent-up anxiety and frustration.

Fantasies

Sometimes all the libido needs is a little nudge. The reason the brain is called the biggest sex organ is that your imagination plays the biggest role in triggering your arousal. Fantasies can range from fleeting mental images to elaborate mental scenarios. Whether your fantasy is titillating (a flirtatious neighbor) or explicit (a sex fest at the construction site across the street), the bottom line is that it turns you on. If you think you don't fantasize, think again. All of us use our imaginations to enhance our sexual experiences. Pay attention to what thoughts and images pass through your mind while you're masturbating, or when you stand next to an attractive stranger on an elevator. If your fantasy pump needs priming, pick up a book of erotica, rent an X-rated movie, or explore the wealth of explicit materials on-line. Mentally reliving a particularly hot sexual encounter in vivid detail not only makes for great fantasy material but also gives you useful information about what turns you on and why.

Like masturbation, fantasizing can be a nonthreatening way to express your sexual self when you don't feel willing or able to be sexual with a partner. And it allows you to keep a sexual spark alive even when you're not partnered.

> I had a little crush on my gay male neighbor. It felt safe and easy. It made me feel sexual again, without having to worry about actually having sex.

> Since my husband left and I haven't had a sexual partner, my erotic dream life has flourished! I've had exquisite sex with a host of friends and famous people, and I inevitably wake up feeling quite satisfied.

Once you build up a repertoire of favorite fantasies, you can call on them to help you get in the mood for sex. During your breaks at work or at home, indulge in your fantasies. You may find that weaving a subtle thread of eroticism throughout your day sharpens your sexual appetite.

> It would have been really easy for me to just go and go and never think of sex at all after the birth of the baby. I made it a point to spend at least one day a week thinking of being romantic or sexual with my partner. That way, even if we didn't end up having sex, I didn't get into a rut of forgetting all about it.

Satisfy Your Senses

Sensual exploration is a bridge that allows you and your partner to reconnect and often to learn something new about each other. If you're trying to rekindle your sex drive, you may find that awakening your senses to their erotic potential is a valuable pick-me-up. If you and your partner are dealing with a desire discrepancy, sensual play can provide you both with pleasurable gratification, while getting you to expand your definition of physical intimacy. Letting go of intercourse or orgasm as the ultimate goal of a sexual encounter has several benefits: It encourages you to experience your entire body as an erogenous zone; adapts well to a variety of situations; is conducive to good communication; relieves performance anxiety; and can relax as well as energize you.

> We've become a lot more focused on sensation and mutual enjoyment than hard-core sex. Intimacy feels more critical than orgasm right now.

Touch

Many a tired mom looks at sex as just another "chore," but massage is a luxurious indulgence. Hands are capable of communicating much tenderness and affection, so let your fingers do the talking. Massages, foot rubs, back rubs, scalp rubs, and butt rubs can relax a tense mom, who may just discover a new pathway to pleasure along the way:

> Prebaby we had been doing some power-play experimentation, but now we're back to square one and gentle-gentle is what we need. Of course, after having our hair pulled and moles picked at all day, a gentle hand is greatly appreciated.

> Now I find that massages can lead to intimacy even if we had thought we were too tired. Generally a careful, caring massage can pull me out of even my most exhausted moments.

Similarly, moms should recognize that their partners might be feeling deprived of tactile stimulation. According to Pat Love, despite our cultural stereotype that men value genital sex over cuddling, "Far more men than women, by and large, will tell you that they don't get enough touching, both sexual and nonsexual." Offer to give your partner a bath after she or he gives the baby one!

> I try to make sure we spend time together touching each other. It feels good and it makes us feel more connected. I think sleeping together naked helps. I think skin-to-skin bonding is just as important with partners as with kids.

Sight

Between nursing, cuddling, swaddling, and changing, you may be so overloaded that you recoil at the thought of either touching or being touched by your partner. That doesn't mean, however, that you wouldn't appreciate some visual stimulation. Now could be a great time to try out a little voyeurism and exhibitionism. You can play the role of adoring fan while your partner strips, masturbates, or works out in the buff. Try looking at an erotic art book or a racy film together. Whether you decide to get physical, or you're content just to watch, you get to enjoy a potent new source of arousal.

Sound

Do you know what kind of music turns your partner on? If so, make a tape of his or her favorite erotic tunes and spend a candlelit evening dancing or kissing to the music. If you don't know, it's time you found out! You could make a game out of it one night: "Name the sexiest song from your teen years" or "What artist best captures sex in his/her music," etc. Use your newfound knowledge to set the scene for a later encounter.

Also, try to expand how you verbally express affection. Go beyond the generic "I love you" and get specific: Describe which of his or her traits particularly appeal to you, or reminisce about the first time you met. Whispering dirty secrets may incite your partner's lust; if you need practice, pick up a copy of *Talk Sexy to the One You Love*, by Barbara Keesling, or *Exhibitionism for the Shy*, by Carol Queen.

Smell

Ever notice your partner getting a little randy while baking pumpkin pie? Have your eyes ever glazed over at the smell of black licorice? Did you know that the aroma of these two ingredients, combined with cucumber, baby powder, and lavender, can increase female sexual arousal? That, at least, is according to the hardworking researchers at the Smell and Taste Treatment and Research Foundation in Chicago (and you thought ice cream tasters had the best jobs).[11]

For decades, scientists, chemists, and perfume manufacturers have been trying to identify and synthesize pheromones—odorless molecules emitted by animals and humans, which supposedly are detected by an organ in our nose and trigger sexual attraction. The degree to which researchers have been able to re-create these chemical secretions is debatable (some studies have found that men's cologne actually decreases women's arousal), but there's no denying that the nose plays a role in sexual arousal.

Sadly, our sense of smell tends to get assaulted more than appreciated these days. But if an aversion to heavy perfumes, pollution, car exhaust, or baby poop can do anything for you, it can serve to remind you to seek out pleasurable alternatives. Make a point of discovering what scents please your partner, and incorporate these into your routine. If he loves the smell of fresh air after a rain, go for a walk after a storm. If she loves gardenias, put some by her bed, or put scented oil into her bath. By reintegrating these subtle but profound pleasure triggers into your lives, you can experience sensuality as an everyday delight.

Taste

We ourselves are so fond of food that it's no stretch to equate the euphoria that accompanies eating a delicious meal with the euphoria that accompanies sex. In both cases, we enjoy exquisite anticipation, a consummation that stimulates all the senses, and pleasurable satiation. There's a reason lavish feasts have often been depicted as sexual foreplay. Unfortunately, with small kids around, mealtime usually feels more like a three-ring circus than a Roman orgy or the lobster scene from *Tom Jones*. Take our advice: Leave the macaroni and cheese to the kids and set your sights higher. Call the baby-sitter and treat yourself to a night out. Put the kids to bed early and order up your favorite takeout (with Web access, options abound for urban moms). If you can't afford to go out, take turns preparing a gourmet meal for each other. If you don't already know what foods tantalize your lover's taste buds, find out and get cooking! If you tend to do most of the cooking, you may find that having someone else cook for you is just as pleasurable as eating the meal.

As for foods that are reputed to be infused with aphrodisiac powers, we're here to tell you not to break the bank seeking out rhino horn and oysters. While there's no scientific proof that certain delicacies are sexual stimulants, there's certainly something to be said for the placebo effect, so if you've convinced yourself that crème caramel is the culinary Viagra, feast away. If you'd like to know more about the cultural and historical roots of a variety of reputed aphrodisiacs, check out our Resources section for the Web site Johan's Guide to Aphrodisiacs.

Make Your Mood

Sexual excitement is often made, not born. Sure, desire can wash over you when you least expect it, but more often, you have to take some initiative to get yourself in the mood. This can be as simple as enjoying a fantasy daydream on the way to work, or as elaborate as planning a romantic weekend out of town. In the past, you may not always have been aware of the ways you were priming yourself to experience desire. Now that you're a mom, you're going to have to put some serious energy into creating the mood, or desire will get so tangled up in that pile of sippy-cups, birthday party invitations, and dirty laundry that it will never penetrate your consciousness. But don't worry, cultivating desire is fun (much more fun than washing sippy-cups, mailing party invitations, or sorting laundry). All you need is self-awareness, respect for your own feelings, receptivity to your partner's feelings, and the occasional leap of faith.

You've got to be self-aware in order to be realistic about when and under what conditions you'd be interested in sex. For example, these women realize that there's no chance they'll feel desire unless they can achieve some distance from their children:

> When my stepdaughter arrived to stay with us for a while, I was so nervous that we would wake her that I found it difficult to relax and enjoy myself.

> Unless I feel secure that they are 100 percent asleep, out of the house being watched by someone else, or otherwise not in my "mom radar," I cannot focus entirely on physical pleasure.

You've got to respect your own feelings so you won't be pressured into a sexual encounter that doesn't meet your needs; this might mean that you have to take primary responsibility for initiating sex.

I find that since the birth of the children, my husband is much less likely to initiate sex. When we discussed it, he said this was because he knows how hard it is for me to be home with three children all day long, so if I've had a long day, he doesn't want to push me into sex that I might not be up for. So I initiate sex much more often than he does, but it's okay with both of us.

But you also need to be receptive to your partner's feelings, or both of you run the risk of getting bogged down in the dreaded initiation wars. The worst-case scenario is that you get stuck in a classic initiation standoff, with one of you assuming the role of "insensitive horndog" and the other assuming the role of "frigid wet blanket." Some couples can get so polarized that they have a hard time experiencing any physical contact without diving for their respective bunkers.

When the baby goes to sleep, I just want to be alone, but my husband sees this as an opportunity to have sex. It's hard, because sometimes he's just being sweet and affectionate, but I assume he always wants it to end in sex, so I get cold and unresponsive.

The key to breaking this self-defeating cycle is to meet each other halfway. Put the emphasis on identifying what you want out of sex and when you want it. As Pat Love suggests, "When you say no, say when. When you say no, say what. What really hurts relationships is a flat-out rejection or refusal." In other words, instead of snapping, "Quit poking at me," you could say, "I really just want to go to sleep in your arms right now, but Saturday morning, when the kids are watching cartoons, you're all mine."

You may be thinking, But what if I don't want to be poked at now *or* on Saturday morning? That's where the leap of faith comes in. To a certain extent, where sexual desire is concerned, you need only be willing and optimistic. You may be initially ambivalent about a sexual encounter, but if you allow yourself to be receptive to your partner's advances, you invite the possibility that a flicker of interest can be fanned into a flame of desire:

I have found that no matter how tired or overworked or underappreciated I may feel at times, I must remind myself that this person who wants to have sex with me is the love of my life, my partner, my daughter's father, and my best friend. I sometimes have to remind myself how much I really enjoy sex, how I have always liked a good fuck.

Although we appreciate the spirit behind the "just do it" approach to partner sex, this attitude works only if you feel that you can negotiate your terms or back out of an encounter if desire simply doesn't develop. Having sex out of obligation or fear is just about the most negative reinforcement around:

> I would have sex when I didn't want to, and that would make me feel like never having sex again.

The bottom line is that you need to take responsibility for requesting what would or wouldn't give you genuine pleasure. Sex should never be a service you provide for a partner or one more task to cross off your to-do list. Sometimes you'll be compromising with a partner, but by definition, a compromise means there's something in it for you! Once you learn what stimulates your desires, you can make your own mood instead of passively waiting to fall into it.

> I think of sex as a way of pampering myself. I take advantage of any impromptu blocks of time when my children are out of the picture. My partner is usually ready to go anytime, so I tend to initiate the unexpected sessions. If it's been a while, sometimes we rent a porno to really rev things up. I'm definitely of a lower libido, but am happy that our sex life has gotten to a middle frequency that satisfies us both. This has taken a good three years.

LET'S MAKE A DEAL: THE FINE ART OF NEGOTIATING DESIRE

That's right, a deal. The fine art of negotiation. If you and your partner face a desire discrepancy, your chance of improving the situation depends on your ability to communicate and to compromise. While blaming each other for your mismatched libidos is certainly easier, working together toward a mutually satisfying solution is ultimately more productive. Doing so requires a generous amount of give and take, a willingness to look at the big picture, and a recognition that compromise is crucial in any relationship.

> I'm dissatisfied with our sex life. We just never have sex, and it bothers me a lot. My husband is much more comfortable getting a proper night's sleep than giving it up for sexual time. It causes a lot of conflict and frustration in our relationship.

> Sex has become a major source of tension in our relationship. He requires sexual attention daily, while I would prefer some tenderness and quiet time together. The result is often frustration and resentment for both of us, and the attempt to talk about the problem never goes anywhere.

Keep Talking

You may be frustrated by your past failures to resolve this issue, but that doesn't mean you can stop talking about it. Restrict your discussions to times equally convenient for both of you to share your thoughts. Do not discuss the situation right after one of you has tried to initiate sex and been turned down by the other—hurt feelings and defensiveness will only muddle your ability to communicate effectively.

Give Yourselves a Break

Remember that what you're experiencing is perfectly normal. It's rare for any two people's sexual appetites to be perfectly matched and unrealistic to expect them to be. Start by giving yourselves permission simply to be yourselves, without apology.

Don't Label Yourselves

Common wisdom holds that men have stronger libidos than women. Actually, Pat Love comments that sex therapists see as many women as men who report higher desire than their partners. This gender stereotype can cause unnecessary shame for low-desire men, who may feel somehow less "manly" for not meeting their partner's level of desire. A corollary of the stereotype that men innately crave sex more than women do is the notion that lesbians suffer from bed death more often than heterosexual or gay male couples. This idea gained currency in the early 1980s due to research on the frequency of sexual activity in long-term relationships.

In fact, the researchers found that married heterosexual couples reported the highest frequency of sexual activity over the long haul, while frequency dropped for *both* gay and lesbian couples (while gay men had the highest levels of sexual activity overall, this was only because their activity shifted to sex outside their primary relationship).[12] Apparently, even when two testosterone-filled guys get together, their libidos can't always survive the challenges presented by a long-term relationship. Maybe a socially sanctioned sexual relationship creates a sense of entitlement that leads to greater sexual frequency—we can't know. One thing we do know is that all too many lesbians buy into the notion that they're somehow predestined to have less sex than anybody else. The truth is, it's pointless to categorize yourself or your patterns of desire based on gender or sexual orientation.

Practice Empathy

Just as you have every right to your sexual feelings, so does your partner. If one of you is feeling guilty and resentful, chances are the other is feeling rejected and unloved. When you're each able to see the situation from the other's viewpoint, you can approach the discussion with more understanding and less finger-pointing.

Define Your Terms

It's not enough for one partner to say "I want more tenderness" or the other to say "I want more action"—you both need to be specific. When you compare notes about what each of you craves—regular displays of affection throughout the day, more foreplay, verbal expressions of love, sexual encounters that aren't always expected to lead to intercourse, or sensual encounters that include genital stimulation at least some of the time—you may find that your definitions of "sexual attention" overlap more than you realized.

Examine Your Assumptions

The mom quoted above who assumes that her partner needs daily sexual attention may be correct, but she might be surprised to learn that she doesn't have to provide it every time. Her husband could be just as happy jerking off to her Victoria's Secret catalog, provided he was assured this wouldn't make her jealous. The husband who'd rather sleep than have sex may have developed a habit of refusing his wife's advances because he assumes that any sexual encounter has to result in intercourse, which he's not necessarily sure he can get up or stay up for. He might be surprised to learn that his wife would appreciate any kind of sexual expression on his part and would be perfectly content with letting him set the terms of their encounters.

Dig Deeper

Pick up a rock and you'll discover all sorts of hidden life teeming beneath it. Scratch the surface of your sexual dynamic and you'll uncover the complexities of your larger relationship. Which is to say, whatever problems are affecting your relationship will eventually show up in your bedroom. By probing a little deeper, you sometimes discover that you're each expecting your sex life to satisfy competing needs. One of you may need quiet time and tenderness because it provides a break from the demands of child care, you're depressed about quitting your job, or you can't relax enough to communicate without it. One of you may need nonstop sex because it relieves stress, you crave the ego boost, or it's your preferred way to show affection. By being completely honest with each other, you can explore other ways to meet these needs so that your sex life becomes more of a level playing field.

Share Information

Tell your partner what you know or have learned about your sexuality. Let her know that you've discovered your libido fluctuates with your hormones throughout the month, or let him know that a motel-room rendezvous far away from that pile of smelly socks on the floor might go a long way toward boosting your desire.

Explore Options

By now you're getting the idea that we want you to clear up any areas of ambiguity in order to accurately assess your situation. Once you've identified problem areas, you can strategize solutions. If one partner's voracious sexual appetite is a way of fending off stress, discuss other ways of reducing that stress (changing jobs, cutting back hours) or finding other outlets (sports, masturbation, yoga). If one partner is having a hard time feeling desire, discuss ways of getting in the mood (reading erotica, fantasizing during the day). Pat Love offers a practical suggestion: "The high-desire person might determine how often to have sex, but the low-desire person might determine how. It might be a quickie, it might be a romantic interlude, it might just be ordinary sex in your favorite position, or it might be a date where you go out and come home and get in the tub together. But you come to an agreement about what is best for the two of you and then you get creative about how you make it happen."

Compromise

Based on the amount of communication you've now done, you may emerge with a new awareness and appreciation of your sexual differences that allow you to accept your sexual dynamic for what it is. Or you may feel the need to change this dynamic, in which case compromises are in order. You might find that a compromise suggests itself when you compare what motivates you to be sexual; most people are motivated by the desire for physical pleasure and intimacy but crave each to different degrees and achieve each in different ways. Maybe you'd be satisfied by a combination of solo sexual pursuits, periodic sexual encounters with your partner, and more explicit reassurances of your partner's desire for you. Or maybe you'd be satisfied by regular non-sexual massage, periodic sexual encounters with your partner, and a half hour each night for intimate talk or relaxation together. If you practice self-awareness and mutual respect, creative compromise can be surprisingly easy.

Keep Working

As with any plan that involves behavioral change, you will need to evaluate your progress at regular intervals. You'll both always be likely to default to your more polarized positions in times of stress or conflict. Keep the lines of communication open, and don't hesitate to seek professional help if you find the task becomes too big for you to handle alone.

PULLING THE RABBIT OUT OF THE HAT

Sexual desire can seem like a magician's rabbit — one minute it disappears into thin air, the next it reemerges with the flourish of a top hat. But you have the ability to master a trick or two yourself; all it takes is a little strategically applied compassion, humor, reflection, and perseverance. Devote respect and attention to cultivating your sexual desires not only because you deserve a rich and rewarding sex life, but because your kids deserve to have one. Your children are watching you to determine what it means to be an adult, and if all they see is your daily grind of working and caretaking, they'll never want to grow up and leave home (and you'll never get to explore the erotic possibilities of the empty nest!). Whether you're single and dating, or coparenting with a spouse, take advantage of every opportunity to enjoy — and let your kids witness — the pleasures of adult relationships.

You know what having a child has taught us that I think is most important? To try to treat each other as well as we treat him. We realized that we'd fuck everything up if we treated him well but treated each other terribly. He won't learn how to expect a relationship, or how to make a relationship good, if he doesn't see it around him.

THE SILVER LINING: EXPANDING YOUR DEFINITION OF SEX

ANY of us, regardless of our chronological age, don't think of ourselves as being truly grown-up until we become parents. You're probably well aware that parenting has enhanced your emotional maturity, but you may not have thought much about the ways in which it can enhance your *sexual* maturity. After all, our culture perpetuates a model of arrested development with regard to sexual expression, and we get precious little encouragement to evolve past the stage of cootie alerts and adolescent peer pressure to a self-assured adult eroticism. But, in fact, if you want your sex life not only to survive but to thrive postparenthood, you're going to have to grow up about sex. The good news is that becoming a sexual grown-up is fun: You get to take responsibility for your own pleasure, show some initiative, develop your creativity, and be as "wanton" as you wanna be.

It isn't abnormal to be wanton and yet be a great mom.

YOU GET TO TAKE RESPONSIBILITY

Women are susceptible to a certain passivity when it comes to sex. We're socialized to put our sexual energies into being appealing and enticing, into being the fetching flowers that draw the attention of swarms of buzzing suitors. All too often, our eroticism is defined by our efforts to inspire desire in someone else: "What do I want? I want him/her to want me!" Enjoy the ego gratification of being a seductive siren, but if this is your default mode of sexual expression, you are missing out on a world of uncensored pleasure. It's human to want to be a desirable sex object, but it's divine to be a sexual subject. By "sexual subject" we mean someone who feels pure lust for her partner, who wants to get her hands on her lover's body and express her desire so actively that any concerns about whether she herself is good enough, pretty enough, or has her gut sucked in far enough fly right out the window.

> After my son was born, I felt very unsexy for about a year, but then I had an affair with a woman and I felt free as a bird and could care less. I still sometimes feel fat and very unsexy when I'm trying on clothes at stores, but then I read *Hip Mama* or call up my girlfriend and I feel sexy all over again.

Sexual subjectivity is a declaration of independence — independence from passivity, insecurity, and self-censorship. Once you cease defining your sexuality in reactive terms, you're no longer solely dependent on your lovers for ego or sexual gratification.

> I enjoy sex more often than my husband, so a vibrator has helped me not feel neglected. I realize my husband cannot please me every night, so my new vibrator has become a great friend.

Becoming a mother can be a valuable catalyst for transforming your erotic approach from reactive to proactive. In an adult relationship, love is inevitably colored by anxiety about reciprocation: Who loves the other more? It's empowering to discover your own capacity to love your children unconditionally, to enjoy feelings that aren't contingent on the responses they elicit. Parenting is positive reinforcement to break out of the reactive mode of relating; once you do, you're less likely to base your self-worth on other people's opinions. The ability to identify and value your personal experience is fundamental to a satisfying sexuality.

> The big issue was, hey, I'm getting older, isn't it about time we had a fabulous sex life? Having children made me realize I've got to get on with living my life — it's going by so fast! I can't settle for so-so sex anymore, so I let it be known if I'm not enjoying myself, and I no longer have "mercy" sex. When one of us wants sex, the other doesn't "just oblige."

We told each other what we really like in bed, not just ooh-aah, baby, but stuff that was almost embarrassing and very hard to reveal. We did it a little at a time and kinda played it out as we went along. Now sex is amazing.

Motherhood often brings a healthy pragmatism into the bedroom. For one thing, when your time and energy are limited, you're motivated to cut to the chase and assert what you want when you want it. And the realities of parenting can be a good antidote to a variety of romantic illusions. Women who discover how difficult it is to figure out what a crying baby wants, who struggle to soothe an upset toddler, or who come to realize that so-called maternal instinct boils down to repeated trial and error are less likely to get hung up on old saws like "If you loved me, you'd know how to please me without my saying a word."

I feel that my gratification is my priority, because I don't have time to mess around and not be fully satisfied! I think my partner and I are both more communicative now about what we want, when we want it, and when we need to go to sleep. We were both a little shy on these things BB (before baby).

We've learned that we both have needs and that neither one of us can read minds. We need to let our needs be known, in a nice way, of course. If we don't know what to do, we can't do it.

The Silver Latex Lining: Safer Sex

Must we really point out that you can't take responsibility for your sexuality without taking responsibility for your sexual health? Do you really need one more reminder of the myriad reasons to practice safer sex? Alas, perhaps we must and you do — certainly plenty of sexually active adults have their heads permanently stuck in the sand when it comes to the topic of sexually transmitted diseases (STDs). Yet the fact of the matter is that sexual contact — specifically the contact between precome, semen, vaginal secretions, and blood, and the mucous membranes of mouth, vagina, and anus — is a highly efficient way of transmitting viruses and bacteria from one person to another. This doesn't mean that sex is inherently dirty and dangerous, any more than your toddler's repeated bouts with head lice and the flu mean that a child-care center is inherently dirty and dangerous. It just means that any sexual grown-up owes it to herself to get a handle on some basic hygiene and to get her hands on some safer-sex supplies. The good news about safer sex is that following these simple precautions displays respect for you and your partners, inspires peace of mind, and enhances the creativity of your sex play.

Safer Sex 101

- Use condoms for vaginal or anal intercourse.
- Consider using condoms for oral sex (condoms are thinner and easier to procure than dental dams, and they can be cut open for cunnilingus or oral/anal sex); while unprotected oral sex hasn't been definitively linked to HIV transmission, herpes, hepatitis B, and bacterial infections can all be transmitted orally.
- Use condoms on shared sex toys or when you're moving a toy from anus to vagina.
- Use only water-based lubes with latex condoms or gloves; any oil or petroleum-based product will destroy latex.
- If you have latex allergies, use polyurethane condoms and gloves; polyurethane isn't as stretchy and supple as latex, but it is stronger and thinner.
- Don't use lambskin condoms; they are permeable to viruses.

If you're single and sexually active, practicing safer sex should be a given. Even if you're comfortable both asking and telling about your sexual histories, neither you nor your date can guarantee having all the facts about all past partners. If you're in a monogamous relationship and you and your partner have tested negative for HIV, hepatitis B, hepatitis C, syphilis, gonorrhea, chlamydia, and you've never had an out-break of genital warts or herpes, you may feel comfortable forgoing safer-sex precautions. But if you haven't been screened for all of the above, you should be—certain STDs are symptomless and can cause serious health problems if left undetected: For instance, chlamydia can result in pelvic inflammatory disease, and genital warts are a risk factor for cervical cancer. Given the six-month window period for HIV infection (it can take up until six months after infection before our bodies produce the antibodies that would be detected in an HIV test), you would need to practice safer sex for six months after the first HIV test and then repeat the test in order to confirm a negative result.

Unlike bacterial infections, viral infections can't be treated with a simple course of antibiotics, and you and your partner(s) will have to deal with these on an ongoing basis if you're positive for a viral STD, such as herpes, HIV, or hepatitis B. Develop a safer sex repertoire in order to enjoy the sex life you deserve. Too often, information about safer sex is presented in terms of preventing "the clean folks" from crossing over and becoming "the diseased." Anyone who's ever had an STD knows how painful and damaging this attitude can be. Furthermore, it's nonsense—the whole point of safer-sex techniques is that they allow sexual activity for one and all.

Whether you're with a long-term partner or a hot new date, whether you're STD-positive or STD-negative, safer sex is an erotic playground well worth exploring.

Condoms are available in a wide range of colors, sizes, shapes, textures, and flavors. Gloves cover dry skin and rough cuticles, transforming hands into smooth, slippery organs of pleasure. Many men report that condoms help prolong their erection, and applying lubricant to both the inside and the outside of the condom enhances sensation. You may feel more willing to explore the pleasures of anal eroticism — from rimming to fingering to penetration — with a barrier in place. Safer-sex supplies encourage communication, introduce humor, and expand creative possibilities. Plus, if your partners are men, condoms are highly effective contraceptives.

Basically, it's up to you to learn the facts, consider your options, and create your own risk-management plan. You might follow different safer-sex guidelines for different encounters. Practicing safer sex is a way of taking responsibility, showing initiative, and prioritizing your sex life — just the ticket for sexual adults like you.

YOU GET TO MAKE TIME

Many parents can testify that the key to maintaining an active sex life is planning. As discussed in the Surviving Scarcity chapter (page 175), kids generate more than their fair share of distractions, and if you don't make an effort, "forgetting" to have sex is just too darn easy.

> Weeks may go by and we don't connect sexually. This is often misunderstood as "Where have you gone? Don't you want me?" but the truth is, we just get caught up with the kids and all that they involve.

You might initially find that one of the biggest challenges to maintaining an active sex life is letting go of the idea that sex should be spontaneous. As we emphasize, the cult of spontaneity — the belief that unplanned sexual encounters are somehow more authentic or pleasurable than premeditated encounters — has quite a hold on our collective erotic imagination. For decades, popular movies, novels, and love songs have promoted the romantic notion that sex entails being swept off our feet and overwhelmed by passion. Some pretty obvious sexual shame lurks beneath all that bodice-ripping — we're reluctant to put any forethought into having sex because we're reluctant to acknowledge that we want to have sex! Sexual desire is supposed to sneak up on us and override our inhibitions.

You wouldn't have much patience with a teenager telling you, "Oops, I didn't know I was going to have sex until it just happened!" Surely you can marshal at least as much responsibility and self-awareness as you'd want your kids to exhibit. And you probably don't feel sandbagged by desire all that often. Couples who have been in long-term relationships soon learn that they need to be proactive in strategizing ways to stay sexually motivated, and this goes doubly for parents. As it turns out, there are myriad benefits to planning sexual encounters. Haven't you ever noticed that the planning stage is one of the most exciting aspects of a trip? As the moms quoted in the Anticipation sidebar prove, looking forward to a premeditated encounter is not only a powerful aphrodisiac but enjoyably arousing in and of itself.

Planning sex allows you to create the mood that best sparks your desire, to shift gears from mom mode to lover mode, and to guarantee you'll be prepared with birth control, safer-sex accoutrements, lubricant, or sex toys. Best of all, if you schedule a shopping spree at the thrift store, you can enjoy the best of both worlds by staging that bodice-ripping scene in your very own bedroom.

Anticipation

Planning for Sex Can Be Its Own Reward:

"Another time I take advantage of is while I'm at work. My partner and I often take a few minutes to call each other and talk about what we plan to do to each other later, or just say I love you. No kids around and it makes us both feel loved and appreciated."

"We talk or phone or leave notes or e-mail each other every day to discuss how to cope with the child, or how hot we are for each other."

"With a toddler sharing our bed, it's hard; we do a lot more sexy e-mails, suggestive ICQ, etc. We talk about sex a lot, only manage it a few times a month. There is a bit more self-satisfying going on."

"Since the quantity is so much less, the quality has to be better. It's more special when you do find the time. You're more adventurous and creative in your lovemaking. It has made me more inhibitionless and daring in my sex."

"We exchange glances, subtle touches, when no one is looking. We can play all day with each other, and then when we finally have a chance to get to the bedroom it is like having had hours and hours of foreplay. Even when we just play, the satisfaction of sharing an intimate glance with my husband is wonderful."

I visit the Salvation Army regularly to buy my daughter dress-up clothes, and I've discovered that costumes are fun for grown-ups too! When she was off on a sleepover last Saturday, I lounged around the house in a strapless evening dress and feather boa—quite inspiring to my boyfriend.

You may be resistant to the idea of planned sex due to performance anxiety—it's common to assume that planned encounters will feel uncomfortably awkward and staged. In fact, the prospect of sex in which both partners are fully awake and fully present can be a little unnerving. Feeling a little off balance won't ruin your mood, but the expectation that sex should be a silent, efficiently scripted event just might.

There's such a gap between the media portrayal of sex and sex as it really is: We don't have orgasms every time, it can be clumsy, there are good times and bad times. Some people's expectations of sex just don't seem real.

You'll be much more likely to enjoy the time you and your partner have set aside to be together if you approach it with an "anything goes" spirit of playfulness. Maybe you'll swap some erotic massage; maybe you'll describe your current favorite fantasy while you both masturbate side by side; maybe you'll put on an X-rated video with the sound muted and invent your own dialogue. You get to decide together what you'd like to do or what not to do. The beauty of regularly scheduled sexual encounters is that there will always be a next time to try something else.

We eventually worked out a standing play date for our kidlet on Sunday afternoons. Every two weeks he goes to his little friend's house, and we have three glorious hours to tear a piece off each other—whatever we want. This time is sacred, and is never to be squandered on repainting the dining room. We fill in the holes with night and morning sex, but he is not a night boy and I am NOT a morning girl, so those Sundays are the cement that holds us together sexually.

YOU GET TO HAVE FUN

You've no doubt watched the expression on a child's face as she jumps in a mud puddle or he comes barreling down a playground slide—sheer delight. Our own children have a valuable lesson to teach us when it comes to sex: playfulness. Somewhere along the path to adulthood we trade in bruised knees for bruised egos, an appetite for adventure for a comfortable routine, and unbridled enthusiasm for sensible

Give the Gift of Pleasure

You don't have to wait around for "the mood" to strike, you can make it happen with a bit of advance planning. These are the types of gifts that are as much fun to give as they are to receive.

- Give your partner a child-free day. Leave it open-ended so the recipient can claim the gift when he or she most needs it. This nonsexual gift allows your partner valuable privacy and an opportunity to relax and refuel—which could be all he or she needs to feel renewed enthusiasm for sexual intimacy.
- Plan a romantic evening and give your partner a handwritten invitation. Arrange everything yourself—baby-sitting, dinner, ambiance—don't let him or her lift a finger. You can do this at your own house or you can combine it with a night at a bed-and-breakfast.
- Give your partner an erotic bath. Pull out all the stops—set the mood with candles, scented oils, and heated towels. Throw in a slow, luxurious hand-and-foot massage.
- Give your partner a coupon good for a trip to a sex-toy store where he or she can pick out any item desired. Or buy a gift certificate and tuck it inside a toy catalog.
- Plan an erotic-video-viewing night. You can do this after the kids are asleep if you're not too tired. Rent several. Let your partner have complete control of the remote!
- Write your partner a sexy letter. You can retell the story of how you met, describe his or her most attractive features, relive one of your favorite sexual encounters, or detail what naughty things you'd like to do in the future.

restraint. With sex, we take ourselves far too seriously, inhibiting ourselves out of fear that we'll do or say something wrong, fail our partner, get messy, or embarrass ourselves. But the risk-taking, adventure, and down-and-dirtiness are precisely what keep sex from getting boring. Without that spark, sex starts to feel like a chore, and our desire diminishes significantly. In other words, being a satisfied sexual adult just might involve behaving more like a kid.

A Toy Chest of Your Own

Did you know that sex toys have a long and illustrious history? Dildos, for example, have been found among Paleolithic stone sculptures dating back over thirty thousand years. Leather and wooden dildos feature prominently in ancient Greek religious rituals, comedies, and vase paintings, and there are references to dildos in the *Kama Sutra* and Asian pillow books. More recently, electric vibrators were invented by American doctors in the late nineteenth century as an aid in the treatment of women's "hysteria."

As historian Rachel Maines reveals, medical experts of the day believed that women suffered from a variety of physical and nervous disorders that could be soothed via genital massage and orgasm — since vibrations were applied to the clitoris, not inside the vagina, "pelvic massage" was considered a perfectly respectable clinical remedy. Vibrators quickly became popular consumer appliances, marketed directly to the public in "ladies'" magazines and the Sears and Roebuck catalog, where they were promoted as palliatives for a whole host of ailments from asthma to tuberculosis. In fact, vibrators were the fifth home appliance to be electrified (following the sewing machine, fan, teakettle, and toaster, but preceding the vacuum cleaner or steam iron).[1] Once vibrators began appearing in the stag films of the twenties, their respectability tarnished considerably, and they dropped off the pages of needlepoint magazines!

While dildos no longer have ritual significance and vibrators are no longer medically prescribed, sex toys continue to delight playful adults to this day. A 1997 survey found that 10 percent of sexually active adults use sex toys in partner sex,[2] which means that literally millions of women and men around the country are slipping between the sheets with erotic accessories. But that doesn't mean they're talking about it — even those of us who are comfortable browsing the adult shelves of our local video and bookstores aren't likely to swap vibrator recommendations with our pals. After all, the topic of sex toys inevitably inspires snickers and jokes about trips to the emergency room. It's hard to shake popular stereotypes of sex toys as unnatural devices used by folks who are compensating for their own deficiencies: They're often viewed as "marital aids" designed to "fix" a sexual problem, devices to console the lonely, or equipment for the kinky.

The truth is that an adult's desire to bring sex toys into bed isn't any kinkier than a child's desire to bring bath toys into the tub. Toys offer expanded sensation and stimulate imaginative play. A silk scarf, an ostrich feather, and a clitoral vibrator all afford tactile stimulation. A partner's fingers, penis, and a dildo all provide pleasurable pressure and fullness. When you wrap a cock ring around his penis or slip a blindfold over her eyes, you get to explore the erotic territory where mind and body converge. Despite a common fear that toys (especially vibrators) will get you "addicted" to a specific form of stimulation, they're much more likely to help you break out of a rut in your sex life. If anything, experimenting with toys can expand your awareness of the myriad erotic possibilities of the world around you, suffusing your visits to the hardware store or the produce stand with a new sense of pleasurable purpose. After over a decade of selling vibrators, we ourselves remain unabashed boosters of the joys of toys and refer you to the Resources section (page 340) for some reliable sources.

> As a new mom, I discovered that sex toys helped me adjust to my changed body. It's a positive spin on thinking of your body in a new way — new toys create new and different responses.

Enjoying Erotica

Since becoming a parent, you've surely honed your skills at reading aloud. Why limit your bedtime reading to Dr. Seuss and Madeline? Recent years have seen an explosion in erotica and sexual self-help books. You can read to your lover from erotic anthologies encompassing a stunning range of styles and subject matters, or study up on every conceivable sexual wrinkle, including how to get in touch with your inner dominatrix, stimulate your chakras through tantric breathing techniques, enjoy your girlfriend's G-spot, talk dirty, massage your boyfriend's prostate with a strap-on dildo, or give better head. The Web is also an outstanding resource both for sex information and erotica.

> My husband and I both surf the Internet and send each other links from sites that have "how-to" ideas.

Adult videos offer their own special blend of home entertainment and sexual inspiration. While you may feel like this survey respondent who's frustrated by the low production values of many mainstream porn films, plenty of women and couples are flocking to video rental stores and have learned to identify specific directors, producers, or performers who reliably float their boats.

> Would you please donate a portion of your income from this book to an arts endowment fund created for improving the quality of erotic films?

Realistic expectations do help when you rent or purchase an erotic video. Production values are low, the sound track may be hokey, and plots, acting, and script are usually minimal. That's because most adult videos are made on a low budget; they aren't designed to inspire your aesthetic sensibilities, they're designed to inspire sexual arousal. If you can let go of your judgments and zero in on your visceral responses, you'll probably find that viewing porn is an entertaining way to create a mood, stimulate your imagination, expand your fantasies, or learn new tricks to try at home. Check our Resources section (page 340) for recommendations of retail and mailorder companies that offer more discriminating selections of both erotic and educational sex videos. And if you don't like the erotica you find, make some of your own!

> Writing erotic poetry and photographing myself have helped me in my sexual discovery and given me an outlet for my sexual energy.

A Word About Lube

> My sex life was saved by fantasies, humor, and lubricant in a tube.

Allow us to propose a toast to one of the most humble, yet most versatile, erotic accessories ever invented: water-based lubricant. Lube is the simple ingredient that can help transform a humdrum sexual encounter into the slippery, messy, glorious affair it deserves to be. Genital tissue is sensitive and deserves tender, loving care. Without moisture, the friction of genital stimulation can be distinctly countererotic. With moisture, penetration is more pleasurable, clitoral stimulation is more enticing, and gliding against your partner's body feels downright luxurious.

Both women and men often subscribe to the false notion that women "should" provide sufficient vaginal lubrication to handle any erotic occasion, and that a loss of natural lube reflects a lack of arousal. The truth is that a vast array of hormonal and environmental factors affect vaginal lubrication. The hormonal shifts of your menstrual cycle, and decreased estrogen—either postpartum, while breast-feeding, after a hysterectomy, or after menopause—can all reduce lubrication. Reduced estrogen levels also result in the thinning of vaginal tissues, which is one more reason to pour on the lube. Stress, allergy medications, alcohol, smoking, and jet lag are among the many environmental factors that can dry up your mucous membranes.

Essentially, there's no excuse not to use lube! It's a valuable safer-sex accessory, since well-lubricated latex creates less friction, is less likely to tear, and feels vastly more pleasurable for both parties. Lubricant allows you to enjoy much longer sessions of lovemaking and is crucial for any anal penetration (since the tissues of the rectum produce no natural lubrication and are much more delicate than the tissues of the vagina). Water-based lubricants are now available in a truly staggering array of formulas, ranging from thick and gel-like to smooth and silky, so there is bound to be one out there that has your name on it.

Fantasies and Role-playing

Kids everywhere relish role-playing, dress-up, fantasy adventures, and storytelling, and all these elements of play are valuable mood enhancers for amorous adults. Let your own imagination run wild, and you may find that playacting is just what's needed to refresh your erotic perspective. Whether you're dressing up as "cowboy and schoolmarm" or simply rejecting the societal roles that don't conform to your own erotic reality, the sense of unlimited possibilities can be hugely liberating—and arousing.

> Don't think you have to have parent sex, whatever that is. Sometimes people think they have to have nice, mellow sex after children, when what they really need is the back-against-the-wall, foot-in-the-windowsill kind.

Most folks have fantasies that fall into two categories: the impossible dream or the unforgettable reality. In other words, you can be aroused by fantasies of adventures that you would never, or could never, enjoy in real life (seducing your favorite movie star, having weightless sex in a spaceship). And you can be aroused by reality-based fantasies, those that draw on memories of past encounters or visions of future encounters. You probably enjoy your own "impossible dreams" without too much shame or anxiety, and you're probably comfortable with your partner's. However, you may be a little more ashamed or threatened by each other's reality-based fantasies. One of the challenges—and rewards—of becoming a sexual grown-up is learning to accept and enjoy the richness of the erotic imagination. In order to do so, you need to overcome the following common inhibitors:

Feeling left out

You'd doubtless be pleased and flattered to learn that your sweetie boosts his or her arousal during sex by reminiscing about particularly hot encounters you've shared in the past. But if some of his or her most powerful fantasies revolve around other past lovers or the cute babe who just moved in next door, you might feel a little threatened. Given our scarcity issues around erotic expression, we often fall into the trap of viewing lust as an either/or proposition: "If my husband desires her, he doesn't really desire me" or "If my girlfriend is turned on by attributes I don't have, she's not turned on by me anymore."

> My husband fantasizes about younger women who are not mothers, and that hurts me a lot.

The truth is, we're all capable of being aroused by many different people and many different attributes. Enjoying a fantasy about a past lover one day and a fantasy about a current lover the next is a natural way of keeping your erotic appetite stimulated. If you're so inclined, and feel secure enough to explore each other's fantasies with an open mind, you might notice that certain recurring themes are more responsible for your arousal than the actual cast of characters. And these themes—for instance, anticipation, teasing, virgin experiences, emotional closeness, being overpowered—can give you valuable information on how to turn up the heat in your sex lives (see Jack Morin's *The Erotic Mind* for more on this subject).

Feeling abnormal

Many people are comfortable with fantasies that they identify as "politically incorrect"—such as those that involve dominance and submission, exhibitionism, voyeurism, or inappropriate partners—because they're confident they won't enact them. After all, fantasies around taboo behavior are understandably common, since forbidden fruit has a powerful erotic charge. A certain amount of shame or ambivalence about your fantasies can make them more potent and pleasurable. However, if you would like to incorporate elements from your fantasies into your sexual reality, this ambivalence becomes problematic. People who share their fantasies with a partner are especially vulnerable to anxieties about whether their own or their partner's fantasies are "normal."

Whether your fantasies are normal is not the point. The point is to determine what aspects from your fantasy life you and your partner might like to explore together. All too often, when couples raise the topic of expanding their sexual repertoire, their shame and embarrassment polarizes them. The shame can be "Gosh, I must be a pervert if I want to be tied to the bed during oral sex" or "Gosh, I must be a prude if I don't want to tie her to the bed during oral sex." We easily default to a sense of insecurity and deficiency around both the sexual desires we have and those we lack, which can lead to a cycle in which each blames the other for being either too demanding or too much of a wet blanket: very negative reinforcement for further confidences. As the survey respondent quoted below suggests, a sense of trust and acceptance is often a prerequisite to sexual adventurousness.

> I'm open to things now that I would have recoiled in horror at ten years ago. It's nice to be really settled with the same partner for a decade and to have worked through untold amounts of relationship junk so we can really be friends and not worry about: "Is he happy with me? Is he going to find someone else better?" Knowing that this is it, that yes we are committed and in love, enables me to be open to his suggestions of things that I'm not totally comfortable with at first, often to discover that they're great. In the end, Settling Down has created the balance we need for very relaxed and intense sex.

It's perfectly all right if one of you fantasizes about activities the other doesn't wish to try. The whole point of being entitled to your desires is that neither of you is more or less entitled than the other.

> Since experiencing a return of my libido, I would like to try swinging, but my husband does not. But he is willing to try almost anything I want to in the bedroom. I desired anal sex, and since we started playing with that, I have discovered a whole new realm of pleasure. I would love to try a double penetration with two men, but doubt he would agree to it. Even so, we communicate more about sex now than we ever have, kids or no kids.

Fantasy is a powerful tool for self-awareness, and we encourage you to embrace, explore, and elaborate on your own, wherever they may lead you. Whether they manifest as random thoughts, mental images, or scenarios you role-play with a partner, your fantasies transform tactile stimulation into full-blown erotic arousal. They deserve your curiosity and respect.

YOU GET TO REDEFINE SEX

If you've been a parent for more than a month or two, you've probably figured out that when it comes to raising children: a) everybody's an expert, and b) nobody's expertise is worth squat except for your own. You can devour parenting books for tips and guidelines, but ultimately, you're the one who knows the individual quirks and personalities of your family members best, and you're in the best position to decide how to interact with your child. As Sheila Kitzinger puts it:

> It is not just a matter of a mother performing an action, such as breast-feeding a baby, but of how she *feels* about what she does—and whether or not she behaves in an easy, spontaneous, and above all self-assured way may be a good deal more important than the system of child-rearing she adopts.[3]

By now you can tell where we're going with this. Your self-assurance about the kind of sex you want to have is a good deal more important than what kind of sex that is. The best part of becoming a sexual adult is that you no longer have to restrict how you choose to define sex. We're all raised to envision sex in such painfully limited terms: "It's sex only if it involves mutual genital stimulation" or "It's sex only if it's penis-vagina intercourse; everything else is foreplay." If motherhood has taught you nothing else, it has most likely taught you that the boundaries between sensual and sexual, emotional and physical, self and other are simply too fluid to contain your eroticism in such rigid compartments. From now on, you get to define sex however you please. Here are just a few of the possibilities:

Sex Isn't the Be-all and End-all

Sex isn't the only way to express love, be intimate, or enjoy your body. On the other hand, every time you experience love, intimacy, or the pleasures of the body, you're in touch with your erotic nature.

> Sex is not the "be-all, end-all" in our relationship, and we know that we appreciate each other in many ways and can show that appreciation in many ways.

My husband would probably like to have sex more often (we're averaging once a month), but taking the focus off intercourse has also created a nice opportunity for doing other things, just for us, that aren't so sexual.

Sex Is Always Changing

Once you let go of the idea that sex should follow a certain predictable script, you'll be free to appreciate how your experience changes throughout your life and from encounter to encounter.

> I have fantasies of being middle-aged and alone with my husband again. Life has its cycles. Sometimes there's more room for sex, sometimes there's not. My husband and I can feel connected, emotionally and physically, with a lot or a little sex.

> Sometimes sex just feels comfortable, not mind-blowing. Other times, the fact that we've been together so long makes the sex way more meaningful.

Sex Is More Than Genital Contact

Sex involves your entire body. Try keeping your genitals off limits for a week and explore the myriad other ways there are to express yourself physically. Kiss the back of her neck; massage his calves; hump each other in the car with all your clothes on. Do you have fond memories of high school make-out sessions? Re-create them.

> Every once in a while we have a candlelit bubble bath when the kids are sleeping. We don't talk, just hold each other in the silence. It is needed.

> We've learned how to be sexual with our clothes on, our genitals out of reach. In other words, we've redefined sex. We cuddle a lot and hold hands on walks. We also tell each other what we would do to each other if we had the time (like when my husband calls on his lunch hour).

Sex Is More Than Intercourse

Kiss the tyranny of intercourse goodbye, and say hello to the anarchy of a full-bodied, imaginative sexuality. It can be challenging for heterosexual couples to replace intercourse with what's often referred to as "outercourse," because doing so forces us to throw out the rule book. After all, intercourse supplies the defining narrative thrust to so many couples' sexual encounters—a clear beginning, middle, and end that defines the all-American, indisputable act of "doing it." Once that framework is gone, how do we know if we're at the beginning, middle, or end of an encounter? Ah, we have to decide for ourselves and then talk about it, that's how! Maybe a sexual encounter will involve genital touch, maybe not; maybe it will involve an orgasm for one or both of you, maybe not; maybe it will involve five minutes of mutual masturbation on the sofa; maybe it will involve a full day of erotic phone calls. The only prerequisite becomes pleasure.

> Do long time lapses between bouts of penis-in-vagina sex mean you are no longer in love? For us, big NO. We were/are still in love, even more so, just have found other ways to be sexual together.

Sex Thrives on Intimacy

To sustain a sexual relationship over the long term, you need to feel a physical and emotional connection. Intimacy creates the context for the trust and acceptance that make erotic self-disclosure safe and appealing.

> Sometimes couples get in the habit of spending the evening separately. You know, like one's watching TV and the other is on the computer until bedtime, and suddenly you're trying to have sex and because you haven't seen each other, much less touched each other, all day, it's not working. So, I try to make sure we spend time together, that we touch each other.

> I also touch my husband daily, as in hugging or kissing, or pats, etc. just to feel connected to him. If I can't touch him a few times, I feel lost. And he says what helps is more affection both outside and inside the bedroom — more kisses, more spontaneous affection.

Sex Thrives on Independence

For your eroticism to flourish, you must feel entitled to your own desires, curiosities, and preferences. Intimacy with a partner will fuel passion only if you maintain your individual identities and honor each other's differences. Sexual compatibility isn't the ability to submerge your desires in your partner, but the ability to enjoy and balance competing desires. The balancing act you pull off as a lover and mother has the potential to enrich all your relationships.

> With children, everything is a balance. So without children, you're more free to have fun and work on just the individual relationship, but with kids, you wind up working on several relationships all at the same time. It is a

challenge, but in some ways feels more mature and, if done well, more bonding.

Sex Is Worth Prioritizing

Your feelings about your body will evolve, attitudes will shift, fantasies will reconfigure themselves, partners will change, kids will grow up and leave home. Your experience of sexual pleasure is in a continuous state of flux throughout your life, but your right to pleasure stays constant. And nobody can assert that right quite as well as you can.

> We've done erotic photo shoots, and we're nude models for life drawing classes at local galleries and colleges. We play at the local nude beach in the summer (our kids go with us), and our lives, in general, include our sexual natures as part of the picture. We don't compartmentalize ourselves. Does it sound like all we think, breathe, and do is sex? Nope. He's a lawyer, and I'm a workers' comp manager for a large company. Our kids are in the third and fourth grades. My son and I play on baseball and softball teams. That's my whole point—if you don't make your erotic nature a part of your life, it won't happen, and you'll be one of those couples that says the spark ended when the kids were born. And it won't be the kids that did it. It will be your failure to keep the spark alive.

SEX AND THE SINGLE MOM

F you're a single mom without a steady partner, sometimes the self-love sessions just aren't enough. You know what we're talking about: Even though you work double shifts taking care of the kids, there are nights when your head hits that pillow with one all-consuming thought: "I've got to get laid." A warm body, a comforting touch, a rollicking round of sweaty sex—these are the things that rouse us out of our maternal slumbers and rejuvenate our bodies and self-esteem.

But as you well know, wanting it and getting it are two very different things. Learning how to date again, trying to meet people, and navigating the logistical challenges around time and privacy are just a few of the obstacles littering your path to sexual communion. In this chapter, we take a look at some of the more common reasons single moms wind up sleeping alone, help you navigate the byways of dating, and offer suggestions for dealing with your kids.

By focusing on finding partners, we don't mean to imply that a single woman's solitary sexual pursuits are inadequate or inferior. On the contrary, solo erotic adventures such as masturbation and fantasy can satisfy one's carnal appetites quite nicely, and they often lead to a greater understanding of and comfort with one's sexuality. But despite the appealing fact that a vibrator won't cheat on you or hog the bed, it also can't say "I love you" or conform to the spoon position. So although we believe you can remain sexually vital without a partner, we think intimate sexual contact makes a unique contribution to your sexual well-being and is definitely worth pursuing!

WHY WE WIND UP SLEEPING ALONE

Figuring out the who, what, why, and how of a sexual relationship can get so complicated that many single moms adopt a "why bother" attitude. As logistical challenges, legitimate fears, and seemingly insurmountable odds pile up, throwing in the towel is tempting. Here are some of the more formidable forces which conspire against us, along with some suggestions for restoring a little optimism to your outlook.

My Child Comes First

When your days are jam-packed with work, chores, and child rearing, the last thing you need is another person demanding time and attention. After all, you have only so much to give, and by squandering it on another adult, you may feel you're depriving your kids.

> I plan on not dating until my son is two, at least. I feel that it is more important for me to be there for him than for me to be searching for some father figure that I'm sure won't show up. It's hard, but the most important thing is my child, sex or no sex.

> To me it's all about my daughter. As long as she's happy, I don't need a relationship at the moment.

Impossible as it sounds, you can be emotionally and physically present for your kids and have a sex life too. It takes a little work, but you wouldn't hesitate to put that energy into finding a new job or a place to live, so why not muster some for your love life? And as for the fear that your kids will suffer — on the contrary, they'll see a happy and fulfilled mom modeling good adult relationships.

> All I can say is, don't deny yourself and your sexuality and convince yourself that it's best to sacrifice your sex life for your children. It will always backfire on you. Plus, it gives your children a warped view of what it means to be a grown-up. If they see you making time to be with a man (or woman, as the case may be), yet not ignoring their feelings, they'll see adult relationships as a very normal part of life.

> It's sometimes easier to sacrifice your needs in the name of the child's best interests rather than look at what's really preventing you from getting back on that horse.

It's fine to take a break from sexual relationships, but by routinely avoiding intimacy, you actually end up doing yourself and your children a disservice.

> My advice is to get out there and get a life again ASAP. I waited so long I was almost dead by the time I got back out! I didn't really get to date until my son turned eleven and I started going out for a few hours and leaving him alone . . . it opened a door to a new life for me! Keep a social life at all costs. Pamper yourself to keep your sexuality!

Rather than postponing your needs for some indefinite time period, take another look at how a healthy sexual self-esteem can improve the quality of your life.

> Making time for yourself as a sexual person with needs and drives and desires is the single most important thing you can do for your sexual health. Keeping it separate from your children is not hard if you realize you deserve the attention and love that dating and sex can provide.

The Relationship Hangover

This is the "once bitten, twice shy" excuse for avoiding relationships, and its tenacity should not be underestimated. Many moms got to be "single" by breaking up with their child's other parent, and they carry the baggage from that breakup for a while. Whether you've been burned by a deadbeat dad or your lesbian coparent packed her bags, it's hard not to feel disillusioned as a result. You end up questioning your own judgment—how could the person you once loved unconditionally now be treating you or the child so badly? What's to stop you from falling for another loser?

The only cure for a hangover is time. If you've been through a nasty breakup, give yourself plenty of time to heal, and don't put too much pressure on yourself to make things perfect with your ex or to replace him or her immediately. Getting enough distance will give you a healthier perspective on that relationship and alleviate some of your guilt and anger—a perspective you'll need if you plan to continue parenting together.

> My best tip for other single moms is avoiding bitterness. It spills over into every relationship you have, including with the kids and other men, and does the actual husband no harm at all since by that time he couldn't give a toss. Staying tranquil inside (thanks to psychotherapy, in my case) was the only thing that really made a difference to me.

I think it's important, if possible, to try and have some sort of positive relationship with the father so that your child can know their other half. The father of my child, if we had not had a baby, probably would've been kicked to the curb immediately. But we both have the responsibility to raise our daughter, and it's been worth the effort.

If possible, try to approach new relationships with a clean slate — it's not fair to hold one person accountable for another's shortcomings. If you need help letting go of the past, consider therapy. Above all, learn from your past relationships and be clear with future partners about just what you need and expect from them. Your self-confidence will blossom, and so will your prospects for finding a partner.

Loss of a Partner

The way they play it in the movies, a wife gives her soon-to-be-widowed husband her heartfelt permission to remarry after she's gone. Ever notice that the dying husband rarely concerns himself with such sentiment? A woman who loses a partner is often relegated to the status of sexless widow, implying that to date again would amount to "cheating" on the dead spouse. Bucking that stereotype requires courage, a thick skin, and determination.

The death of a spouse is tragic for your entire family, but when your mourning subsides, you may entertain the question of whether or not to date. Don't be surprised if you experience feelings of guilt, fear, or betrayal — these emotions are normal, given the fact that you pledged your love and loyalty to someone who may be gone physically but whose memories remain with you and your children. Take some time to reflect on what would make you happy, and if that includes companionship, pleasure, and sexual intimacy, then these goals are worth pursuing. You can seek professional help to work through any residual guilt or anxiety, join a support group, or enlist the aid and understanding of more sex-positive friends and family.

Fear and Loathing

These emotions eat away at your self-image and your self-confidence, leaving you incapacitated when it comes to seeking companionship. Fear comes in many forms: fear that you'll be rejected, that your next partner won't be good enough, or that your kids won't like him or her. Loathing can manifest as general bitterness about relationships, guilt over a breakup, or negative self-image.

I'm satisfied now, but I could never reach orgasm before because of my extreme guilt about my daughter. I felt I was a terrible mother to be having sex in the next room with someone who wasn't her father. I realize now that that's absurd, but at the time it was a very real issue for me. Once I was reassured by my partner, and I felt okay about it, I was ready to try again. And it was wonderful! I just needed to know for myself that I wasn't doing anything wrong.

Harboring insecurities is absolutely normal, but if they become paralyzing, you need to confront them head-on: What are you most afraid of? What is the worst possible scenario? What is the best? If you don't ask someone out for fear of rejection, you also miss the opportunity to experience the thrill of acceptance. Whether you fail or succeed, you can improve your self-confidence simply by taking action.

I spent a lot of time and energy on personal ads and didn't end up finding anyone. But I'm so proud of myself for trying and feel good enough to do it again sometime in the future.

The Wet Blankets

My greatest difficulty was in finding peer support with regard to my need for companionship and sex. It was unbelievable how many people felt that I should forgo my feelings to "save" my kid.

As if you don't have enough naysaying going on inside your own head, you're probably surrounded by well-meaning, finger-wagging folk who have an opinion about every aspect of your mothering—neighbors, relatives, other parents, church members, even some of your friends. You can expect their eyebrows will arch clear to their hairlines when they learn you want to have—or are having—sex again. As a mother, your sex life becomes public property. Out come the moral yardsticks in the form of endless nosy questions: Does he have a criminal record? Did you let her sleep over when the baby was there? Don't your teenagers think it's hypocritical? Are you talking marriage? Simply imagining this cacophony of questions is enough to scare anyone celibate. And coming home from a hot date to a grand inquisition from your baby-sitter is the verbal equivalent of a cold shower.

Depending on your own personal style and your relationship to the interrogator, you can lob any number of replies which should get the point across:

Firm politeness
"Thanks for your concern, but my personal life is private."

Feigned insult
"I can't believe you think I'd do anything that wasn't in my child's best interests!"

Sarcasm
"Yes, I'm dating a criminal, and I plan to run away with him and leave my kids on your doorstep."

Blunt and to the point
"Mind your own business."

Fear of Losing Custody

The fear that we will be judged unfit mothers because of our sexual activities deters many of us from pursuing a sex life. Single moms get blamed for so many of society's ills that adding "whoring" to our list of sins comes naturally to our accusers. The only thing worse than having the intimate details of your sex life dragged out for public scrutiny by the courts is the idea that your kids can be taken from you as a result. Sadly, the law has a checkered history of defending mothers' sexual freedoms — lesbian moms, promiscuous moms, and breast-feeding moms have all been denied custody.[1] Admittedly, there's no easy solution to this problem; depending on where you live, your actions might earn you the support or the disdain of your community.

Standing up for your sexual beliefs is never easy, but when you engage in respectful, healthy relationships (with partners and children), you actively defy the stigma associated with sexual moms. Yes, be aware of the legal precedents in your area, but don't give in to a fear-based regimen of self-denial. If you find yourself anxious about the possible ramifications of your sex life, get some support. Talk to friends, a therapist, a lawyer, or other moms (go on-line where you can be anonymous). They can help you gain some perspective and take any necessary steps to ensure that you retain custody.

The Logistical Limitations

It's pretty simple math: A single parent has more work to do than two parents (even assuming couples don't split child-rearing tasks evenly). Plenty of single moms will read this chapter thinking, *Yeah, how am I supposed to have a sex life when I've got meals to cook, laundry to do, work from nine to five, my kid's sports events to attend, etc?* The question is legitimate, and one we don't take lightly. We do our best in this book to give you some practical advice on how to free up time, get help, and manage your workload. But the simple fact is, until society prioritizes the needs of moms — including quality child care (subsidized and on-site), paid maternity and paternity leaves, job sharing, and family-friendly work environments, we're never going to have enough time. So our advice to you is grab the moments you can for personal pleasure, and seize every possible opportunity to agitate for social change.

The New You

If you haven't dated since becoming a mom, you may be surprised to find that you now hold a whole new set of priorities when searching for a mate. With kids to consider, you may be more cautious when entering relationships, since any threat to your safety (or sanity) is a threat to theirs. Many mothers describe themselves as "pickier" when screening partners, and dates who don't measure up immediately to their standards or those of their kids get no second chances.

I don't have time for games and BS, so I weed people out quickly.

I don't even consider sex unless my dates are comfortable around my boy.

Some moms up the ante by seeking parental figures for their children.

One of the guys I met said single moms have it harder because they're looking for a partner *and* a father for their kids. I recoiled at this notion, but soon realized this described my situation to a T.

The downside of exercising so much discrimination is you may end up alone. If your expectations are set too high, you miss out on some pleasurable, if less cosmically significant, adventures. Give yourself some room, expect to make some mistakes, and eventually you'll find a balance that works for you.

Don't try to make every relationship a "family" — not every person you date has to be a potential parent for your kids. That's way too much pressure to put on yourself, your partner, and your kids, and it's a lesson I found hard to master at first. Once I let go, and dated who I liked, I had more satisfying relationships.

DEALING WITH YOUR CHILDREN

Even before you start dating someone regularly, ponder how you want to handle your sex life with regard to your children. If you've already decided whether you want your kids to meet your partners, where you plan to have sex, and what you want your kids to know, then you won't stumble into an awkward situation unprepared or do something you may regret later.

When Should My Kids Meet My Lover?

Most people agree that it's best not to let your lovers spend too much time with your kids until you've become more serious about your relationship. Although you may enjoy playing the field, kids form attachments easily and can be traumatized by a parade of people coming and going in their lives. Breakups can be tougher on children than adults; this mom makes a simple case for keeping her partners separate from her kids:

> Why should you AND your kids have to break up with someone?

On the other hand, don't err in the other direction and rigidly compartmentalize the pieces of your life. Kids do form attachments, but it's not as if no one ever leaves them — beloved relatives die; friends or baby-sitters move away. Although loss can be hard on a child, it's also part of living and loving. As long as you reassure them that *you're* not leaving, you can help them learn that change is a very real aspect of relationships.

Your values and circumstances will determine what approach works best for you. Some moms have the resources to keep kids and partners separate.

> I only see the man in my life when the boys are with their father.

Others manage to strike a balance by treating their partner as they would any other "friend."

> I've always had lots of male friends, so when I meet someone new I just introduce him as "Mommy's new friend." If he stays over, I make sure he moves to the couch in the morning.

We appreciate the simple pragmatism of this mom's advice:

> Try not to keep your dating life too separate from your parenting life. Have enough space to enjoy, but it is important for anyone you get close to to love your children and be able to have a relationship with them.

What Should My Kids Know About My Private Life?

You can expend a great deal of energy trying to prevent kids from learning about sex: by eliminating all traces of it from your home, avoiding discussion, or telling your kids they arrived on this planet via the friendly stork. But don't expect them to learn to be sexually responsible adults if no one gives them the facts, models good sexual behavior, or reassures them that their sexuality is normal.

As a parent, you will have the most profound impact on your child's sexual development. You can choose to conduct your sex life and base your child's sex education on lies, evasiveness, and ignorance or on honesty, openness, and information. Wouldn't you rather show your children an example of a healthy intimate relationship than pretend that you have no sex life? Conducting your sex life on the sly will teach your kids that sexuality is something to hide and be ashamed of, while an honest approach will improve your relationship with your child and contribute to a healthy sexual development.

> One day I sat my kids down—they were ten and twelve—and said, "There is someone I like and he is going to stay here tonight. I don't want to pretend to you that I'm not sexual and that I don't have a life outside of raising you, and I want you both to feel okay about whatever choices you make." My younger daughter's response was "Remember that boy last year that I went to the dance with? Well, I kissed him." She told me that she felt so much better now that I knew!

> There have been many times when my boys have surprised us with a visit when we thought they were doing something with their dad. I don't throw my sexual activities in their faces, but I don't lie. As they get older, I ask that they try not to just drop in when they know he is there.

> I do have women stay the night, sometimes even if it's not a serious relationship. It's tough, because my son does compete for my attention, even if he likes my lover. I try to speak to him in advance, and let him know how I feel about this person, and give him some clue that she might be staying the night. If he's somewhat emotionally prepared, he reacts better. I also found the impact on both of our lives is minimized if I get up with him in the morning and do some of our routine things immediately.

Don't treat kids as your confidants, either—they are not the ones you should be sharing your relationship joys or sorrows with. And in order to avoid confusing your children, be clear about the nature of your relationship with a date or partner. Kids are fed so many stereotypes that they may harbor unrealistic expectations about your new partner. You can explain that many unmarried people sleep together without any intention of marrying. You can let your kids know that the woman in your life is not a long-lost aunt but a girlfriend who sleeps with mommy. Similarly, don't set your partner up to play Daddy or Mommy to your child unless this arrangement truly reflects the situation.

Never, ever have your child call your date Daddy/Mommy!

Where Should You Spend the Night/Have Sex?

At some point, most single moms will grapple with the question of whether to invite a lover to spend the night at her home. It's definitely more convenient for you, but you need to be certain that it's safe and that you're prepared for the impact on your kids. Don't bring anyone home at any time if you harbor even the slightest reservation about having them meet your kids. If you decide that you are ready for an overnight guest, we suggest you level with your kids rather than trying to hide your lover, which can backfire.

> I would try to get the person in the house after my daughter went to bed and out before she got up, which didn't always happen — not to mention kids show up in your room in the middle of the night quite unexpectedly at times. Partners also tire of being kept secret and would question my commitment.

Of course, discretion and age-appropriate information should play an important part in your approach. Obviously, you aren't going to let your kids watch you having sex, but you don't need to avoid having sex in your house for fear that they'll "catch you" one day either. Use the lock on the bedroom door, and prepare yourself for their questions or surprise visits (see the Teaching by Example chapter, page 321). If the size and layout of your house allows it, maximize the amount of space between your bedrooms.

Younger kids are usually content with the explanation that your friend is a sleep-over guest, just like the kind they have over sometimes. Older kids can be told that sexuality is an important part of life, requiring companionship and privacy. If your teen asks why you can have lovers sleep over and she can't, you can simply tell her that you make the rules in the house, or you can take the opportunity to talk about the maturity and responsibility necessary for sexual relationships.

> A single mom needs to make it very clear to her kids that she deserves privacy and happiness too.

You can expect a certain amount of jealousy from your kids when the sleepovers occur (see the discussion below), so make sure to reassure your kids of your love for them, as this mom does.

The first time you have that big overnight sleepover with your lover, you have to get up the next morning and really do something fun with the kids. Have a big breakfast, go to the park, do something special so they don't feel pushed to the side.

If you're trying to minimize the amount of contact your kids have with your dates, obviously it's best if everyone doesn't bunk under one roof. If your ex regularly takes your children, you've got a perfect scheduling opportunity for dalliances.

I was lucky enough to have a very involved father for the first two years so I could count on a few nights a week to enjoy myself. It is nice to have at least one night to go wild—whatever your version of wild is.

Short of that, you will be limited to brief sexual trysts unless you can hire overnight baby-sitters or arrange to have the house to yourself. When your kids are old enough, they can sleep over at their friends' houses. Likewise, you can trade overnights with another single parent. Kids can be farmed out to relatives and good friends for the occasional sleepover, or you may find a baby-sitter who will spend the night.

What works for me for casual dating and sex is to plan activities during which my daughter is spending the night with family or friends.

Enlist your friends! You know all those people who offer to baby-sit? Tell them point-blank to not offer unless they mean it, as you WILL take them up on it. Call in those chips when you need downtime or date time or sex-fling time.

Shared housing gives you live-in baby-sitters and comes with a few other perks.

Sharing a house makes things cheaper, gives more baby-sitting resources and more options housewide for getting privacy. It saved my life as a single parent.

HOW TO MEET PEOPLE

Once you've given yourself permission to have a sex life, the next hurdle is finding someone to have it with. How do you find that special someone to grace your bed? Take these suggestions from your fellow moms on what works for them:

Friends' Referrals

As you probably discovered when trying to find child care, legal assistance, or trades-people, your friends can provide the most helpful referrals. Dating is no different, as your friends, relatives, and coworkers are your most valuable resources for future partners. Don't be shy about asking — let everyone know that you're interested in dating, and ask them to set you up with single friends. Boldly send out a group e-mail or casually mention it during your conversations. Once you put your mind to it, you may get quite creative.

> My sister wants to throw herself a "Find me a date party" where all the invitees have to bring a single friend.

> After I exhausted my pool of friends, I started asking trusted business acquaintances if they had any single friends. People were most sympathetic and genuinely tried to help.

The friends' referral option has several advantages. First, your dates are pre-screened — you have less chance of ending up with a psycho — and they're actually people your friends find interesting. Second, your friends can provide a nice alternative to awkward blind dates by hosting a dinner party or planning a group outing to which you're both invited. Third, you give your friends an opportunity to unleash their inner matchmakers.

And there's no better time than when you're single to get back in touch with long-lost friends. They may no longer be single, but hopefully they've made new friends that they'll want you to meet. Thanks to the Internet, it's getting easier to find people you've lost track of — some schools allow alumni to post e-mail addresses, and there are plenty of search programs to help locate individual e-mail addresses.

Getting Out

This option requires a certain commitment of time, but we think you'll benefit from pursuing activities that please you and enjoy the time spent in the company of other adults. See the Surviving Scarcity chapter (page 175) for suggestions on freeing up time in your schedule.

Join a group, class, or club

Why not reap the double benefit of indulging a personal interest and exposing yourself to new people? If you've always wanted to learn French, take a class at the community college and find yourself a study partner. Book groups abound, courtesy of local bookshops, schools, and libraries. If you crave a more disciplined exercise regime, sign up for a gym or an aerobics class. Join a single-parenting support group.

Go places alone

Although going to parties with friends might be infinitely more enjoyable, most people who do this spend the entire time talking to people they already know. By going alone you're forced to mingle, an activity that will endear you to your hosts and earn you a few new friends. Bigger parties are often rife with somewhat intimidating circles of friends gabbing in corners, but most often you'll find that by smiling and introducing yourself, they will respect your courage and welcome you with interest.

Similarly, consider going alone to events like book readings, the theater, gallery openings, or shows, since you will stand out as a single person. Look around during intermission to find other people, and start a conversation by commenting on the event or performance.

Kids' Hangouts

If you want to meet other single parents, you usually don't need to look any farther than your local playground.

> On Sundays all the noncustodial dads are out with their kids at the park/Chuck E. Cheese/zoo/movies/etc. Letting your kids play together is a good way to meet someone.

Neighborhood community centers, schools, and day-care facilities crave parent involvement. By getting to know other parents, single or not, you are able to tap in to their network of single friends. Even though your kids may provide the perfect icebreaker for starting a conversation, don't spend the whole time talking about them; you're better off trying to discover common interests other than children.

Personals

To the uninitiated, personals have a bad reputation — mostly as a forum for lonely, desperate creeps who've never been able to get a date. But actually, most personals' fans are just regular folks who, for one reason or another, want to expand their pool of potential mates. Tons of subscribers are relationship refugees reentering the dating scene, others are shy and find it difficult to socialize in person, some just don't get to meet new people very often. The people you meet through the personals don't usually have unrealistic expectations about meeting Mr. or Ms. Right every time they place or answer an ad, but they do appreciate the opportunity to cast a wide net in the hopes of one day landing the big one. And whether or not you succeed in finding a date, the whole process can help you get in touch with what you're looking for in a partner. This mom found the personals a convenient way to dip her toe back into the dating pool, as well as an effective way to screen out folks uninterested in kids.

> When I first left my ex-husband, I was pretty certain I wouldn't meet anyone until the kids were grown. I pretty much assumed that any man who heard I came complete with a set of children all under five years old would run screaming in the other direction. Since I didn't have time to actually go out much where people are likely to meet, I placed a personal ad. I mentioned the children, that I had them, and that they were my priority in my personal ad. That made all the difference in the world in finding someone who was able to deal with it.

If you decide to give the personals a shot, your first step will be to decide whether you want to respond to an ad or write one of your own. Depending on what service you use, you'll be charged either to answer an ad or to place an ad; if you're making your decision from a purely financial standpoint, find out how the billing works. If you're being charged to respond to ads, be careful, as the dollars add up quickly. Unless you're swimming in money, you'll soon learn to be very selective before picking up the phone.

When you call up the personals' service to reply to an ad, you enter the box number of your candidate, then you get to hear a more extensive voice message. After this, you can decide whether to leave a message of your own. The beauty of responding to ads is you have the luxury of exploring variety — do you like the clever one, the sincere one, the naughty one?

When you place an ad, you simply send in your carefully worded message, and the service sets up an anonymous voice mailbox on which you record a more detailed message about yourself. Callers leave messages (with their phone numbers), which you call in to retrieve. You're not obligated to return calls. The advantage here is that people come to you. You're free to describe yourself or your ideal partner in any way you like, so if they listen to your laundry list of physical shortcomings or odd personality traits and still leave you a message, you've got a live one!

On-line Dating Services

Where do you turn when you're too old for one-night stands, too busy to join any classes, and too tired to stay up late cruising clubs? To an on-line dating service! These services, with names like Match.com and Swoon, generally operate under the same principle as the newspaper personals, but you get to advertise more detailed information, attach a photo, and communicate on-line. So if you're looking for a forty-year-

Looking for Love

With both personal ads and dating services, it pays to put some thought into how you express yourself. A good personal ad is one that generates a few select responses. If your wording is too vague, you might get a lot of calls from people who turn out to have nothing in common with you. Think about what sparks your curiosity or turns you off in others' ads or profiles. If you're annoyed with overly cute or self-consciously clever writing, go for honest and sincere. Be yourself! Don't lie about your looks or your interests—the truth will only catch up with you eventually. (Surely you've noticed that the personals world is populated by a very high proportion of "attractive" people!)

> I love the personals, but what I do find galling is the superficial emphasis on looks. I shed my own baby fat in my youth, but once I became a mom, I found it difficult to shed the baby fat bequeathed to me by my daughter. I exercise, feel fit and sexy, but geez, there's nothing to dampen the old self-image more than reading through a bunch of ads written by men who are looking for "petite," "slim," and "slender" women. Don't even get me started on the "busty" and "buxom" crowd.

How much emphasis you place on looks, interests, and activities is entirely your decision. You might not like football or body piercings, but that doesn't mean you wouldn't be compatible (sexually and otherwise) with someone who does. There's a reason that "opposites attract" is a time-honored mating sentiment. While labels are inadequate, you have to come up with some way of defining your tastes that readers can respond to. You can always take out more than one ad and try different approaches.

When arranging a meeting for the first time, follow the safety tips listed in this chapter. Once you're finally face-to-face with your new pal, try to relax. It might help just to acknowledge the awkwardness of the situation and then take it from there. If you're the shy or tongue-tied type, come prepared with some questions to get the conversation moving. And if you're trying to assess if there's any sexual chemistry, give it some time. Between the conversation you're both working on, and the running commentary going on in your head, your body may barely have room to breathe. It might take several dates, and some time to reflect, before you discover whether there's anything worth pursuing.

old Irish Buddhist who listens to rap music and lives four blocks away (good luck!), you can search for him on-line.

Most services charge a monthly fee (with a free trial period) and offer a host of additional features like horoscopes, dating advice, discussion boards, and chat rooms. The benefits of on-line dating are numerous: You can do it at night when the kids are asleep, remain anonymous for as long as you like, save money on baby-sitting, and minimize awkward meetings. The convenience, anonymity, and prescreening capabilities can be just the inducement for moms to reenter the dating scene.

> It was very difficult to make time to get out and meet people, and it was hard to find a place to get private without spending a lot of money on dinner or a hotel room or whatever (I didn't want to be bringing people home all the time). That's why I turned to the Internet—I think it's a great place to meet people. Yes, there are plenty of freaks on-line who aren't who they pretend to be. But there are plenty more people who *are* what they say they are. And it's easy to be forthright with people when you don't have the fear of immediate rejection and repercussion facing you—I can say what I think on the Internet, to anyone, without worrying that they're going to reject me out of hand.

As this mom reminds us, the Internet is having a hard time shaking its undeserved reputation as a place filled with "freaks," including rapists, stalkers, and child molesters. Yes, these people exist, and yes, they can and do use the Internet to ensnare potential victims, but the degree to which these incidents occur is vastly exaggerated by the media. We'd much rather see talk shows and newspapers take a more responsible approach to the benefits and dangers of the Internet—extolling its educational virtues and advising people on commonsense ways to protect their privacy—but we realize that wouldn't pull in the ratings during sweeps week. So we'll provide the public service announcement and give you a brief primer on protecting your privacy.

Whether dabbling in the personals or on-line dating services, your best strategy is to follow your instincts and err on the side of caution. Use common sense when giving out information about yourself. Until you trust someone, don't give out your last name, where you live, work, etc., either in your profile or in person. Use a pseudonym or a first name only. If you're worried about what personal information appears on-line, do a search on your name or inquire with your service provider and ask to have personal information deleted. Complain to the site operators if you're being harassed, or if someone's being creepy.

When you arrange to meet in person, follow the safety tips listed below. Until you're confident that this individual poses no threat to you, take initiative in order to guard your privacy: make the phone calls rather than giving out your number (although some recipients might have Caller I.D.); arrange to meet in public places to avoid being picked up at your house or at work; limit the identifying details you divulge in conversation. If you follow these precautions, you'll be just as—if not more—safe with your on-line acquaintances than with folks you meet at your local bookstore. And you'll have acquired valuable practice in being assertive to boot.

Safety

When you find someone who piques your interest and you decide to get together, you should take a few precautions, especially if it's the first time you'll be meeting:

- Meet in a public space. Consider meeting during your lunch break; that way you have a built-in excuse to leave (and you save on baby-sitting).
- Arrive separately.
- Tell a friend where you're going and when you'll be back. Make sure you call your friend to let her or him know you've returned from the date.
- Bring a cell phone, your phone card, or change for a phone call.
- Bring plenty of money in case you need a cab to get home.
- Bring safer-sex supplies in the event you are swept off your feet.
- If you're coming from out of town, don't plan to stay at your date's house; book yourself a hotel room.

DATING ADVICE

When to Tell Your Date About Your Kids

If you haven't told your prospective love interest about your kids *before* your first date, do it *on* your first date. There's no point in pretending that your children don't exist, and it's not fair to your date to omit this vital piece of information. Hard as it is for moms to imagine, not everyone is fond of kids.

> Accept that some men will immediately avoid you because of your child, and try not to take it personally.

Besides, most moms find that full disclosure helps them separate the wheat from the chaff when it comes to screening out unsuitable partners.

> Be blunt, be prepared! The third sentence I say to any potential mate is (as I hold up my pager) "I love my new baby-sitter—she only pages if there's a problem." Most guys look at their watch and find some lame excuse to leave.

At the same time, be careful of dates who are too interested in your kids. You may find that it's not you they really want but your instant family.

So far the challenge I have encountered is accurately reading people's motives. I find that people fall into three categories — those with a pregnancy/lactating-mother fetish, those who want an instafamily, and those who want to be able to say they have another notch on the belt.

I keep finding people who want to treat me like I should take care of them in addition to my children.

Kids as Barometers

No wonder some people run from single moms — not only do they have to pass muster with the mom, but they have to face the daunting prospect of trying to charm someone else's children. Many of the moms from our survey were quite clear that they wouldn't waste time on anyone who didn't meet little Joey or Janey's approval.

Make sure you date the kind of people you want your children around. If my kids don't like someone I'm dating — really don't like, I mean, not simply trying to get rid of them because I'm dating them — then that's the end of that guy. I trust my children's opinions.

Fortunately, this mom can distinguish between the natural jealousy kids have for anyone who's competing for Mommy's attention and a genuine dislike. Don't allow your kids to sabotage your relationships, but do take the time to find out what they don't like about your new partner. You may discover that they have anxieties you can alleviate; for instance, letting them know they're irreplaceable in your affections and aren't expected to embrace your lover as a substitute parent could ease the strain.

Don't judge partners too quickly based on their initial success (or lack of success) with your children. People who aren't accustomed to being around kids may be awkward or somewhat fearful at first, but with practice, time to relax, and the opportunity to gain confidence, they can blossom.

Jealousy

Be patient with yourself and be patient with your lovers. They WILL get jealous of your kid. And be patient with your kids . . . they don't like these people showing up in Mama's bed.

What's a mom to do when there's only so much of her to go around? With your partners, be clear about your availability. If getting together is dependent on your schedule, make sure they're okay with this and show appreciation for their flexibility. When you're together, don't rattle on about your children, but focus on your adult time together. It's fine for you to explain that your kids come first in your life, but this fact shouldn't stop you from making your partner feel that she or he comes first in your personal life.

As for your kids, bear in mind that it's normal for them to be jealous of your affections for another, particularly if they haven't had to share you in a while or if you've recently broken up with or lost their other parent. With younger kids, explain to them that you have a special friend with whom you like to spend time, just as they have favorite playmates. Older kids can be told about the importance of intimate adult relationships and the value they have in your life. Make sure you continue to spend time alone with your kids, and don't pressure them into group outings with you and your new flame until they express interest or willingness.

Your Sexual Health

As one of our survey respondents puts it, "A happy mom is a good mom," and there's nothing like good health to lift your spirits. So honor your sexual health by making family planning and safer sex a routine part of your sex life. Carry condoms or dental dams with you (practice in advance if you're a little rusty) and talk openly about birth control and safer sex with your partner before you have sex. For more on this subject, see the Silver Lining chapter (page 227).

A Dating Plan

Most single moms find that once they start dating again, they establish something of a "dating plan." This philosophy incorporates what they've decided is best for themselves and their children and is used to establish boundaries with potential partners. What follows are three different types of plans, which all reflect forethought and experience.

> I am very careful about whom I meet, and where I meet them. After six months of trial and error, and a few close emotional calls, I have finally evolved a dating plan. We meet several times for lunch, sometimes as many as a dozen, until a comfort level is established. Then I suggest a "family" outing. Only a couple of men have reached this level — it is an effective way to weed out those who are interested in the short term. My theory is, my daughter needs to see a friendship develop before there is romantic involvement. Additionally, I see no point in "dating," which seems to connote romance, if this new friend and my daughter do not click.

After the birth of my second baby (as a single mom), I became very hesitant to involve myself in sexual relationships. I even swore at one point that I would not have sex again unless I was with someone I could feasibly marry and raise children with. However, after the first sexual hurdle (which involved lots of crying and confusion), I discovered that sex was a need for me — to make up for the pleasure deficit and stress overload that is the burden of so many single mamas. I am not interested in relationships now, so have learned to seek protected, mutually understood one-night stands or sex with good friends at periodic intervals. I have found this to work out quite well, despite the little deep-seated southern Baptist moral voice in the back of my mind. It is safe, fulfilling, and no strings.

On my first date with the man I've been with for two and a half years, I told him that my son was my first priority no matter what, and that if he ever had me apologizing for that, it would be over. Kind of heavy to lay out in the first few hours of knowing someone, but I'm glad I did. You need to have a bottom line to look to, so you can say: "I said that, I meant that, I'm going to live with it and you are too."

After you read this chapter and give careful thought to the issues we've presented, hopefully you will feel confident enough to craft your own dating plan. You may find it evolves over time, so our advice is to be flexible, learn from your mistakes, and celebrate your successes!

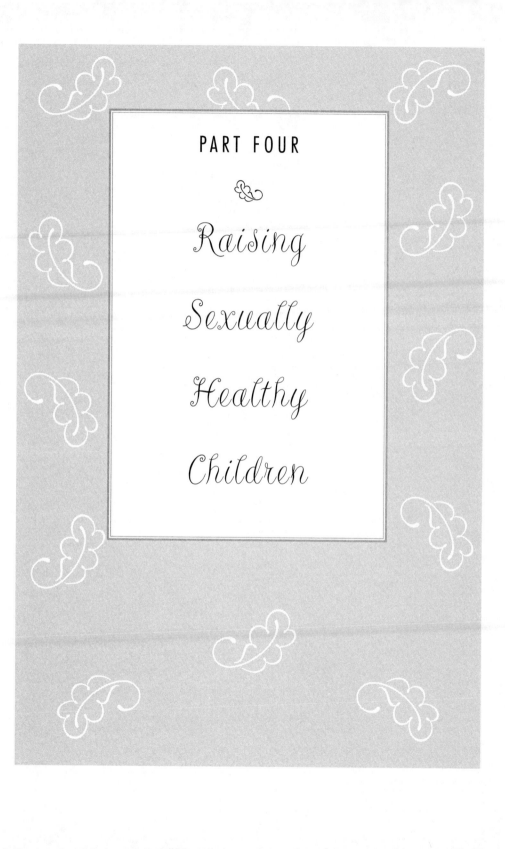

PART FOUR

Raising

Sexually

Healthy

Children

KIDS ARE SEXUAL, TOO

YOU might have noticed that most of this book focuses on how to have a good sex life *in spite of* your children. But we also want you to have a good sex life *because of* your children. When they see a happy, sexually fulfilled mom who conducts relationships consistent with her own values, they learn to embrace sexuality as natural and to form mature relationships of their own.

However, as much as we encourage you to be a good role model in deed, we urge you to be a good one in word as well. Talking to your kids about sex will go a long way toward counteracting the misinformation, stereotypes, discrimination, and sex negativity that can derail children's sex education. Unless you want your child's sexual journey to mirror Alice's trip through Wonderland—alternately nightmarish and thrilling—you need to cultivate an open and honest dialogue around sexuality.

In order to do so, recognize that your children are sexual beings and have every right to unfettered sexual development. We'll walk you through the primary stages of their sexual growth, and along the way we'll point out opportunities for fostering a sense of sexual well-being. To illustrate why the job of sex educator should fall squarely on a parent's shoulders, we'll briefly review what and where your kids learn about sex when left to their own devices. Armed with the knowledge and the determination to speak frankly with your children about sex, you'll be ready for practical tips, which appear in the next chapter, Talking to Your Children About Sex (page 301).

Since entire volumes have been written on this subject, we can give you only a quick tour and point you toward some valuable resources. But we felt strongly about including even a short discussion of sex education in a book about mothers' sexuality, since today's sexually informed children will be tomorrow's sexually satisfied parents. We all wish a better life for our children; freeing our daughters and sons from sexual guilt and anxiety and giving them the tools to cultivate a healthy sexual self-esteem is one of the greatest gifts we could possibly offer.

FREE YOUR MIND

Class, Your Dictionaries, Please!

We use the words "sex" and "sexuality" a lot, but what do they mean when we're talking about children's sex education? For most adults, sex represents an intimate activity involving genital stimulation. It's usually equated with intercourse and frequently with reproduction. When adults think about children's sex education, they often assume that any discussion should focus on sexual intercourse, which they consider either an entirely inappropriate topic for kids or one that can be addressed only as it relates to reproduction or disease transmission.

Sexuality, on the other hand, is much more fluid. How would you define it? You won't get any help from the dictionary; Webster's maddeningly defaults to "the state of being sexual." Start by examining your own sexuality and what factors affect it. We bet first on your list is your body and its capacity for pleasure. And you can't expect your body to process all those pleasurable sensations without your mind, right? Thanks to the mind, you get the thrill of erotic daydreams or fantasies. Your gender—where you identify on the continuum of male and female—is certainly a part of your sexuality, as is your sexual orientation. And in making decisions about your sexual behavior, you employ a unique set of values, right? You'll notice that all of these factors either exist at birth or evolve at various stages during childhood. A child's sexuality doesn't spring full-blown at puberty, it develops gradually over time, and as a parent, you are a primary influence.

We offer this clarification to provide some context for the following discussion of children's sexual development. You may equate sex education with high school "Family Life" courses, but your child's sex education encompasses so much more and requires active participation from you. We realize that some parents may have difficulty accepting the idea that children have innate sexual desires from the time that they're born. According to Joani Blank, the author of A Kid's First Book About Sex, our discomfort is due in part to our tendency to attribute adult sexual feelings to kids:

"If the child is masturbating, we assume that they're doing it with the same kind of emotions or fantasies as adults are." Too often, we opt to suppress children's natural sexual curiosity out of fear that it will lead them down some kind of slippery slope to premature adulthood.

Not only do we project our own sexual sophistication onto kids, we saddle them with our cultural baggage. Thanks to our sex-negative heritage, we've been taught to disavow our children's sexual feelings in the name of protecting their "innocence." But in denying this very real and natural aspect of their development, we consign them to a life of ignorance and insecurity.

Too Much Too Soon? Never!

During the decade we worked at a women's sex-toy- and bookstore, the comment we heard most often from parents looking for kids' sex-education books was "Oh, she's too young for that." Most of us graduated from the school of "too much too soon may be hazardous to your health." We either worry that we'll overwhelm our kids with indigestible information, or we fear that frank talk about sex might plant lascivious images in their innocent heads, encourage sexual precociousness, and somehow transform them into perverts or nymphomaniacs.

But making sex information available from the earliest age serves our kids well in several ways: We give them the opportunity to assimilate material at their own speed, we "normalize" sexuality by treating it as we would any other subject they might be curious about, we convey our respect for their ability to handle what they learn, and we communicate our own values and morals in the process. Letting children set the pace of their sex education can challenge your own assumptions.

> One of my toddler's favorite books is geared toward preteens. The text is way over her head, but she loves looking at the cartoon drawings of naked kids. This has given us a great opportunity to review her anatomy and talk about what makes boys and girls and men and women different.

As for how much information to impart, we believe it's better to err on the side of too much information than not enough. If children aren't old enough to comprehend what you're saying, they'll tune out and you can cut your narrative short. Ultimately, kids will process only what they can handle—just as your fine distinction between the proper and improper usage of the word "stupid" will go over a toddler's head, so too will some of your sexual pearls of wisdom.

With questions of timing, remember that teaching kids about sexuality is a process, not an event.

Don't try to explain the whole thing to them in one day. I spent my whole childhood learning how to cook from my mother, and I still learn new things. The same goes for sex. It's an evolving topic that will take a long time for a child to understand, so give it time.

Children are born sexual, and parents have countless opportunities to help them build self-esteem, teach them to love their bodies, encourage their curiosity, and answer their questions. Not only is it okay, it's a good idea to let Johnny play with himself during his diaper change, tell Suzie the names of her genitals during bathtime, and give a simple, straight answer about "where babies come from" instead of leaving her struggling to figure out what birds, bees, and flowers have to do with human reproduction.[1]

Bear in mind that it's *never too late* to teach your kids about sex. You may feel like you've missed so many opportunities that your kids will perceive any attempt you make now as too little too late. But even if your twelve-year-old gives you the I'm-so-bored-by-this glare during a heart-to-heart on sexual responsibility, don't despair! By being both proactive and approachable, you actively defuse awkwardness and mystery and send the message that you're always available to talk about sex.

If you're just getting started on sex education with older children, don't assume that they already know a great deal. Chances are they've acquired a garbage heap of misinformation on their own that has left them confused and cynical. Review the stages below, and begin by addressing some of the simplest topics. That way, you simultaneously lay the foundation for more complex subjects and practice your communication skills.

CHILDREN'S SEXUAL DEVELOPMENT

As with other developmental milestones, keep in mind that children will mature sexually at different speeds and in different ways. Not seeing signs of a specific behavior doesn't mean your child is developmentally delayed. For example, although many kids masturbate during childhood, many others — particularly girls — don't. As long as your daughter is not being discouraged from self-exploration, and she knows about her genital anatomy, she will develop naturally at her own pace.

Although we present the following topics according to the age at which they'll first arise, you shouldn't restrict your discussion of each topic to a onetime chat. Think of your conversations about sexual matters as building blocks — once you've laid the foundation, you can build upon it throughout your child's life. Besides, you can never be sure what information your child retains, so even though you may feel like a broken record, repeat your messages over the years. For example, we address the importance of explaining sexual anatomy in the toddler section, but we encourage you to make this topic an ongoing part of your sex education.

Infants and Toddlers

Sexual functioning

We're guessing your baby book doesn't come with fill-in-the-blanks for "baby's first erection" or "baby fondles herself." But why shouldn't it? Signs of fully functioning genitalia should give us just as much joy as our child's first smile, but we greet the former with quiet embarrassment and the latter with a news broadcast to the neighborhood. We realize that Aunt Betsy might be a little shocked at news of Timmy's erection, but there's no reason you should be. Ultrasounds reveal erect penises in the womb (can you imagine your health practitioner exclaiming, "It's a boy, I can tell by his hard-on!"), and although erect clitorises cannot yet be detected in utero (they're too small), girls do experience them from infancy on, along with accompanying vaginal lubrication. Kids are capable of sexual responses, including orgasm, at birth. Your adult sexual responses are more fully developed, but children have all the same equipment with none of the psychological baggage.

Masturbation

As infants begin to explore themselves and their surroundings, they soon discover that touching their genitals feels good. This early form of masturbation is somewhat akin to the pleasure you get from scratching a particularly persistent itch; it's largely a physical impulse. Your baby's drive to masturbate is no more innately harmful or evil than your drive to scratch your back, despite centuries of brainwashing to the contrary. In fact, masturbation helps develop bodily awareness and improves self-esteem. Parents who interfere with children's self-pleasuring by pushing their hands away or offering verbal chastisement teach them to associate their genitals and feelings of pleasure with "dirtiness" or "naughtiness." And since most kids (and adults) can't resist the urge to masturbate, disobeying a parent's directive will usually result in guilt, anxiety, and poor self-esteem.

During infancy, your job is simply to let your kids play and avoid sending any negative verbal or nonverbal messages. During the toddler years, however, don't just ignore or tolerate your child's masturbation, verbally acknowledge that what he or she is doing is normal. Try something as simple as "Does it feel good to touch your penis? That's because it's supposed to." You'll reinforce that your kids' behavior is okay and give them a solid foundation to counter any antimasturbation sentiment they will undoubtedly receive in the future. As your child becomes old enough to understand the concept of privacy, you can also incorporate statements such as "I know it feels good to touch your vulva, but I'd rather you did it in your own room where you can have some privacy."

Both of my kids have been enthusiastic masturbators. We have never discouraged it, nor told them it's wrong. We've said that it's a gift from God, and one they can enjoy their whole lives, even after they're married. We've also said that it should be a private pleasure, something like going to the bathroom. We've explained that our culture frowns on masturbating in public, just as it frowns on public urination. It took a while—a few phone calls from various preschools and camps—but eventually they got it.

If you're having any difficulty accepting masturbation as the natural and life-enhancing activity that it is, we encourage you to review the Self-Love chapter (page 36). Those in need of further reassurance might appreciate this insight from Heather Corinna, a former kindergarten teacher:

I got my best research on intuitive and natural sexuality not out of a book, in a brothel, or in a partnership, but in kindergarten classrooms during nap time. The lights go down, the covers get settled on gently, and near every kid I ever taught began to pleasure themselves in some way. Thumb or blanket sucking reigned supreme. Hair stroking was a biggie. Singing to oneself was another all-time favorite. Most of all, when everyone got quiet and restful, those little hands would almost inevitably and consistently wander to the nether regions of genital bliss.[2]

Sexual anatomy

A lot of parents don't know quite what to make of children's sexual anatomy. We're exposed to our kids' genitals daily during the diaper-changing and potty-training years, but our discomfort betrays itself through general avoidance and the use of cutesy euphemisms. Our culture reinforces this avoidance at every possible turn. For example, this mom was prepared to answer her daughter's question about why girls' sexual anatomy differs from boys', but not why Barbie's resembles neither.

My daughter wanted to know why the letter "B" was printed all over her Barbie's butt and genital area and whether this was going to happen to her. Not only does buxom Barbie have no genitals, now she has some mysterious alphabet disease.

How do we explain to kids why the clitoris is left out of most high school biology textbooks, why "N" never stands for "nipple" on Sesame Street, and why photographs of naked children never appear in sex-ed books? Our society is so uncomfortable with the notion of children's sexuality that it seeks to suppress it out of existence; as a result, kids learn to view their genitals differently than they do the rest of their anatomy—as something to avoid or to be ashamed of. If they never get accurate information about their sexual anatomy, they may experience problems with their sexual health and relationships later in life.

It's time for you to remove the black bar of censorship from your child's private parts. You'll have plenty of opportunities with infants and toddlers, given the amount of contact you have with their genitals in these early years. For example, during bathtime, make sure you wash the entire body—don't skip or skimp on the genitals; doing so only reinforces the notion that they are somehow different from the rest of the body. Rehearse the names of their genitals with your children, just as you would other body parts.

> Use real words. Teach what they have, especially girls, whose parts are less apparent. Be nonjudgmental, nongiggly, matter-of-fact about things. Be positive about the concept of touching and feeling good in their bodies. Answer questions honestly. Don't pass on your own hang-ups!

Avoid using euphemisms or slang, and make sure you've boned up on your anatomy. Many well-intentioned parents think their work is done once they've pointed to a little girl's genitals and said "vagina." You aren't doing your daughter any favors by defining her genitals in terms of something invisible, and you're actually mislabeling them. Her external genital area is called the vulva, and it contains her labia, clitoris, urethral opening, and vagina. Your son has a penis, urethral opening, scrotum, and testicles—let him know that some boys have a foreskin and others do not. Kids of both sexes have an anus, and they'll probably want to know all about it, because they're fascinated by their ability to poop.

> I find it my duty to constantly correct the kids who come to my house saying "Boys have penises, girls have vaginas." The anatomical equivalent of the penis is the clitoris!

Actually the penis and clitoris aren't precise anatomical equivalents any more than the penis and vagina are. There is no one single word sufficient to describe female genital anatomy (because it's so special!). You can most accurately refer to your children's external genitals as penis and vulva, but by all means let them know that both the penis and the clitoris are pleasurable to touch.

Once you put your mind to it, you can get quite creative and simultaneously take a stand for children's sexual emancipation. If you're tired of songs like "Head, shoulders, knees, and toes" that skip right over your daughter's middle section, add the verse

"Labia, clitoris, vagina, and anus" and sing it with her (no, we're not suggesting a playground sing-along). Write and illustrate a book for your son called "The ABCs of Sexuality" (we know, "Z" will be hard). Surprise your child with an anatomically correct doll—you can buy one on-line from a company called Corolle, a French company owned, ironically, by Mattel, the makers of Barbie (see Resources section, page 340, for information).

Diaper changes and potty training provide another opportunity to teach kids respect for their bodies. Remember that they find going to the bathroom a pleasurable experience and are naturally curious about the outcome, so try not to corrupt their learning process. No, we don't expect you to wax ecstatic over a foul-smelling diaper, but exclaiming "Oh, gross," "God help me," and "Yuck" will only teach your kids to view their genitals and their normal bodily functions as displeasing and disgusting. Similarly, potty training is all about children demonstrating control over their own bodies. Even though we empathize with parents' desperate longing to reach this milestone, too much pressure on children is counterproductive, since they will either rebel or be confused by your exertion of control over their bodies.

Sensual touch

One extremely important way to honor children's developing sexuality is to indulge their need for sensory stimulation, particularly touch, which helps them connect physical and sensual pleasure to an overall sense of well-being. By all means, touch, bathe, breast-feed, snuggle, kiss, and talk to your child. Let him or her run around naked. You may be able to identify some ways that your parents' sensual expressions of affection influenced your own sexuality—perhaps you have fond memories of your mom or dad gently stroking your hair, murmuring into your ear, or caressing your back. While the acts themselves are nonsexual, their ability to evoke a sense of peace and pleasure are what make them powerful forces in your sexual development.

What kids should know/feel by this stage

- Touching themselves is okay
- Their genitals are as natural as other body parts
- Pleasurable touching from family and friends

Preschoolers

Sexual curiosity

If you've ever been on the receiving end of a preschooler's firing line of questions, you inevitably start to fear the word "why." In an endless search for answers, he or she will follow each of your explanations with one more dreaded "Why?" During this stage of development, children's brains work at lightning speed to assimilate everything that crosses their paths. Imagine trying to acquire language, social behavior, and control of your body all at one time, and you start to appreciate the enormity of their task.

Children approach sexuality with the same voracious curiosity they do with every other aspect of their lives. One minute they're asking why the cat sheds and the next they want to know about penis size. Children will satisfy their curiosity not just by asking questions but by engaging in a variety of behaviors which, although perfectly normal, can trip up unprepared parents. Kids in this age group are constantly trying to reconcile what they know feels good with what they're learning from adults (namely parents) is acceptable behavior. For example, three-year-old Tammy loves watching her daddy undress because she's fascinated by how different his body is from hers. Dad catches Tammy gazing lovingly at him, finds it disconcerting, and yells at her to close the door. So Tammy gets two messages: It is wrong for her to watch him undress, and bodies are something to be embarrassed about. Dad could have explained that he prefers a little privacy when he's dressing (a concept she will be learning in other areas as well), then made a point later of asking Tammy if she had any questions about his body—a good opportunity to teach the differences in male and female anatomy.

We would guess many of you have memories of playing doctor with a friend, or of touching a sibling's genitals while bathing together. Unless you were caught, you probably just recall a sense of adventure and a tingling of excitement. Or maybe you remember that what seemed harmless and fun at the time erupted into a traumatic and humiliating episode because you were "caught" by an adult. Although these kinds of sex games among children are the norm, parents often overreact, causing needless amounts of grief. Remember that your child does not yet know the appropriate limits of sex play and needs to learn them from you in a supportive manner. Rather than yanking the children apart, giving the playmate marching orders, and telling your child he or she's been "bad," calmly explain to both kids that while curiosity about each other's bodies is normal, and it is always okay to touch your own genitals, it is not necessarily okay to touch someone else's. You may believe the incident is simply a good opportunity to reinforce the concepts of wanted versus unwanted touch. Or you may believe that it is never appropriate for children to touch each other's genitals, in which case you can communicate a message about respecting each other's privacy while reiterating that curiosity is perfectly natural.

Sex play among kids in many other countries is regarded as completely natural, and kids aren't reprimanded for their explorations unless one is harassing another. In the United States, however, most parents discourage this type of play. Our particular discomfort comes from both a Victorian ideal that childhood is a time of sexless innocence and an increased awareness of childhood sexual abuse. If we believe that children are not innately sexual, then any overt sexual behavior is taken to signify some sort of abuse, trauma, or dysfunction. Despite studies that conclude that sexual activity in children is not an indication of sex abuse,[3] and endless reassurance that sex play is a normal part of sexual development, parents still find it hard to overcome their panic when confronted by young children's sex games. In large part, we project our adult experience of sexual arousal onto our children.

The best way to proactively address your fears while respecting your children's sexuality is to make sure your children understand and can express the concept of unwanted touch. Sex educator Meg Hickling teaches parents and kids the phrase "The person who says 'no' rules," which empowers kids to extract themselves from any situation where they feel uncomfortable—whether it's bathing with a sibling, getting their cheeks pinched too hard by Auntie Bev, or playing doctor with a friend. Given that most child sexual abuse is perpetrated by an adult relative or friend, your child should learn that this type of relationship is not appropriate and that it should be reported to you or another adult.

> My daughter was being fondled by a relative. Teach your children proper terms for all of their body parts, and teach them to say no and say it loud and mean it. Teach them to have pride in the decisions that they make and to always think of what the alternative might be.

Bear in mind that the bulk of sex education your child receives in elementary school is focused on sex-abuse prevention, and that you will want to balance this fear-based curriculum with reminders that sexual pleasure is natural and good. As this survey respondent suggests, if you provide your kids with a healthy respect for their bodies, familiarity with their genitals, and a sense of appropriate behavior, they not only have the tools to protect themselves from unwanted touch but to appreciate their own capacity for pleasure:

> I am so proud of my daughter and her comfort with and knowledge of her body. When she was physically harassed by two of her peers, she came and told me that they were masturbating her. As we discussed it, I asked her if besides feeling violated, she also discovered that it felt good. She told me, "Yes, but I know it's something I should do for myself." The incident was reported and stopped happening and my daughter seems stronger than ever to me.

Gender differences

At this age, children are fascinated by the biological differences between men and women, along with the traditional gender roles that get assigned to each. Curiosity motivates much of their staring and prodding and questioning. "Why don't I have a penis?" "Can I grow up and marry Mommy?" "Why can't Daddy have a baby?" This age is also when kids are still flexible enough to enjoy exploring gender roles through dress-up and playacting. Parents, who live in a rigidly gendered world, find this kind of play both amusing and disconcerting. If you thought explaining Barbie's alphabet skin disease was hard, try telling your daughter why she'll (probably) never be able to grow a beard or your son why the kids at school will laugh at him if him if he shows up in a dress and nail polish.

Even if you want your kids to grow up "free to be you and me," you've probably thrown up your hands and abdicated responsibility for combating our deeply ingrained system of gender socialization. But a crucial aspect of ensuring a happy, healthy sexuality for your children involves taking a stand against attitudes that restrict acceptable behavior based on gender. Notions such as "Girls just naturally enjoy cooperative game playing" or "Boys just naturally enjoy competitive sports" are on the same continuum as "Women prefer to cuddle" and "Men prefer having their penis touched to anything else in the world." Every time you capitulate to the Blue versus Pink version of reality, you are letting your children down by limiting their sense of what's possible.

We're not saying that you should forbid your son to play competitive sports or try to discourage your daughter from being cooperative. And eliminating Barbies and guns from your children's toy chests would only fuel their obsession with forbidden fruit. The point is to *add*, not *subtract*, options — simply never to limit your child's sense of how he or she can move, talk, interact, and generally be in the world based on gender. Your kids may enjoy embracing gender stereotypes, but your job is to let them know what a stereotype is and to point out all the interesting people around you who are happily thumbing their noses at them. Perhaps you can convince the male teachers at your son's school to wear skirts one day, or maybe, like Ariel Gore, author of *The Hip Mama Survival Guide*, you'll stage impromptu minirevolts for the benefit of your daughter and her peers:

> Whenever I see one of those weird muffins that turn into a sexy little doll, I tell the children in the vicinity to repeat after Mama: "Women are not baked goods."[4]

For a provocative discussion of the distinctions among sex, gender, and sexuality — along with an inspiring call to embrace "gender independence" — we encourage you to check out Phyllis Burke's *Gender Shock: Exploding the Myths of Male and Female*.

How babies are made

Much to their credit, most preschoolers won't buy the old "You came from a stork" story (or its endless variations) and will relentlessly pursue the truth behind a process that involves some of their favorite things: bodies, parents, and babies. You'll need to gauge your explanation to your child's age and ability to understand the details of human reproduction. A three-year-old asking "Where did I come from?" might be satisfied with "A baby grows inside Mom and gets pushed out through her vagina." But an older or more developed child might understand "When Mom and Dad make love, he puts his penis in her vagina. Sperm from his penis joins an egg in Mom's uterus and forms a baby that grows for nine months and then comes out through her vagina." If you conceived by other means, or if your child is adopted, you can tailor your explanation accordingly; all children should learn about conception via donor insemination and in vitro fertilization, since they're very likely to have peers conceived through such methods. A good first step is to ask your children to tell you their understanding of "where babies come from," which gives you a chance to assess what information (and misinformation) they've already acquired. You may be surprised to learn that the details from the book you read out loud together aren't as crystal-clear in your child's mind as you had thought.

While preschoolers won't necessarily understand the connection between sexual intercourse and reproduction, let alone the fact that the two can be mutually exclusive, parents should make the point early on that sex is pleasurable even when the goal isn't baby-making. Most of what children are taught about sex focuses on reproduction, but discussing lovemaking, in whatever terms you find appropriate, gives you an opportunity to impart values, feelings, and expectations as well.

> When my son was five, he asked me where babies came from. I told him that mommies and daddies love each other in a special physical way that's called sex, and that sometimes they can make a baby. He was happy and content with that answer. Later on (around nine) we discussed the mechanics, with an emphasis on feelings and love.

> When kids ask about about the origin of babies, explain how the baby gets there. It is SO much easier when they are little. We explained that in order to make people want to make babies—so the species does not die out—the act of making babies had to be great fun. So much fun that most couples like doing it even when they don't actually want to make a baby. That's how we tackled it, and it has been no problem.

What kids should know by this stage

- Correct names for genitals
- Masturbation is okay

- Sexual curiosity is okay
- Exploring gender roles is okay
- Appropriate behaviors and how to say no to unwanted touch
- Where babies come from

Elementary school kids

Privacy

By this age, privacy looms large for kids, because the term is used so frequently as a way to bridge the gap between what's considered "normal" and "appropriate" behavior and what's not. Perhaps you have told your child that masturbation or lounging around nude is fine as long as it's done in private, or that going to the bathroom or picking one's nose is usually done in private. By now, children have internalized the various messages you've communicated, intentionally or not, about their bodies and their erotic behaviors. Since so much of what they've learned about sexuality involves privacy, children will continue their sexual explorations in private, away from the watchful eyes of parents.

Sigmund Freud referred to this stage as the "latency" period: Between the ages of about five and ten, children seem to show less sexual interest, particularly compared with the insatiable curiosity of toddlers and the obvious sexual blossoming of puberty and adolescence. Some physiological support exists for this theory, but since hormones never tell the whole story, most experts now agree that during so-called latency, children remain as curious and interested in matters related to sex as ever; parents just aren't privy to their activities. Especially if children have been taught that sex is somehow dirty, naughty, or taboo, they'll seek answers to their questions elsewhere and keep their activities a secret. Their natural curiosity may also give way to a sense of embarrassment over what they don't know. As parents, you'll probably have to work harder to integrate sex information.

> By about age eight, kids begin to be embarrassed about sex because of schools, so you have to create a real comfort level at home before this time.

Personal responsibility

Children are gaining a sense of personal responsibility during this time — a key sexual development that will enable them to make decisions relevant to their own and others' health. By learning how to care for and respect their bodies, they acquire confidence and self-esteem. An awareness and appreciation of their own bodies also helps them to understand how their actions can affect others, and they should be able to grasp why it's not okay to punch one kid at recess or beg another to pull down his pants.

Without a sense of personal responsibility, children are more likely to either perpetrate or be the victims of abuse and sexual exploitation, both in childhood and later in life. When you pass along your values, teach them the cause and effect of their actions, and promote a healthy relationship with their bodies, kids learn responsibility. Sadly, the only sexuality education young children usually receive in schools focuses on the prevention of child abuse, which, although necessary, will mark the beginning of a formal education that uniformly associates sex with danger, disease, and unwanted pregnancy. Parents can help provide a context for these lessons by supplementing them with examples of and information about the joy and beauty inherent in sexuality.

> My bottom-line message to my daughter has been for her to do the things which best promote her health and happiness. I've encouraged her to learn about her own body and desires and responses now so that when she is ready to enter into an intimate relationship with someone else, she will be a full participant, not just a passive recipient of whatever they give her.

Dirty words

Unless you keep your kids locked in your house with no TV, no radio, no VCR, and no visitors, they're going to pick up swear words and repeat them. Whether they use them because they sound fun, they know they're not supposed to, or they're copying your occasional lapse, hearing your six-year-old call his sister a bitch can be mighty disconcerting. When they're young, most kids don't know the meaning of these words, and it makes more sense to offer explanations than to run for a bar of soap.

Defining words like "cunt," "asshole," and "dickhead" gives you a great opportunity to review sexual anatomy and reinforce the notion that the body should be respected. You can also seize the moment to explain how words like "motherfucker," "bitch," and "whore" express disrespect and hatred for women, just as "faggot" and "queer" do for homosexuals. You're set up for a natural segue into a discussion of gender stereotypes or sexual orientation.

You don't necessarily have to wait till your kid throws one at you to bring up the subject of profanity. Why not periodically ask your child what slang is being used at school? This way, you can keep in touch with your child's environment, clarify your values, and reinforce your position as someone he or she can come to with questions. Your son may know better than to say "cocksucker" around you, but if the word is being uttered at school or on the playground, he's going to want to know what it means.

> My brother loved calling the neighbor boy a "dildo" when we were in grade school. It had such a great sound to it. I remember my mom chewed him out, but she never told us what it meant. I spent years trying to find out.

Fantasy and masturbation

When we asked survey respondents to our first book, *The New Good Vibrations Guide to Sex*, at what age they remembered masturbating for the first time, many mentioned five or six. Perhaps it's difficult to remember events earlier than this, or maybe our self-pleasuring really does take off as we become more conscious of our control over our bodies. Regardless of the reason, these early memories revealed an impressive resourcefulness: Girls remembered humping washing machines, rubbing dollhouse furniture against their clits, and perching on ottomans, while boys were busy poking their penises into knotholes and prodding couch cushions.

Contrary to the notion that a child's sexual interest declines during the grade school years, it's actually being pursued with studied determination. Typically, boys start masturbating sooner than girls, mostly because they handle their penises every day in order to urinate, whereas girls must dig deeper to discover the pleasurable clitoris. As we noted earlier, masturbation is a healthy and normal way for children to get to know their bodies and its attendant feelings. Children can learn from you that masturbation is an important aspect of their sexuality, and older children can be taught that it's a fine alternative to sexual intercourse.

Other people's genitals aren't half as important as learning to honor and pleasure and respect your own. No one should be allowed to touch you until you've touched yourself first!

During our talk about sex, my daughter asked me why would anyone DO THAT? I told her because they may want to conceive a baby or they are merely enjoying sex and how it makes them feel closer to the one they love. I asked her if she ever touched herself between her legs, and she said yes. I asked her why. And she said because it felt good. I told her that sex feels good like that. She asked me if I touch myself and I told her, "Of course!" I want her to understand that masturbating is the one great sexual experience that carries no risks.

Children also begin to fantasize or daydream during this stage, often of family members or close friends of the same sex. The nature of their fantasies may have no bearing on their sexual activities or orientation later in life, but it's another example of the ways in which feelings of security and comfort connect with feelings of sexual pleasure. If a child comes to you disturbed by his or her dreams, offer reassurance that dreams don't hurt anyone and don't mean that the dreamer wants to engage in the fantasy activity. This can be a good segue into a discussion of sexy feelings; your children will periodically find themselves being aroused by something they see or hear, and will need reassurance that this is normal.

Preparation for puberty

As children approach puberty, they will become more inquisitive about the changes that await them. Whether or not your children ask questions, you need to prepare them for the onset of puberty by explaining what will happen to their bodies and what to expect from menstruation and nocturnal emission. How many of us either experienced or heard horror stories of the girl who started her period and thought she was dying, or the boy who awoke from a wet dream, afraid he had a disease? Not only will you help smooth your child's transition into puberty, but you avoid being caught by surprise yourself. Once your daughters menstruate and your sons start ejaculating, they are capable of conceiving children, so now is the time to plan how you will approach the subjects of contraception and safer sex.

> Do not wait until the kids hit puberty. By then it's too late because they've already heard so much misinformation from peers that it would take years to undo it all.

The how and why of sex

Between the dirty words tossed around at school and the sexual imagery teasing him or her at every possible turn, your child will probably have a healthy inquisitiveness about the mechanics of and the motivation for sex. She or he may grasp the basics of reproduction but be mystified by references to things like oral and anal sex. Be prepared for a certain amount of "Ewww" and "Gross," but keep a straight face and impart the basics. Now is the perfect time to explain that there are a variety of ways that adults enjoy sex, including orally, anally, and manually, in addition to penis/vagina penetration. You also have an ideal opportunity to explain the difference between sex for procreation and sex for pleasure, and to illustrate the benefits of oral and manual sex as safer-sex activities.

AIDS and condoms

As you've undoubtedly discovered from children racing to your room after nightmares or panic attacks, they're scared of bad things happening to them. Because we think of AIDS and STDs as grown-up problems, we may consider discussing these with younger kids unnecessary. But kids are exposed to information about these subjects in the media, on the playground, and through adult conversations, and unless parents fill in the blanks, they can suffer unnecessary anxiety. They may not be old enough to articulate their concerns, which is why it helps if you simply address the issue matter-of-factly.

> Answer everything honestly. Try to relax and laugh with your child. Be up front about HIV, condom use, STDs, etc. when they are little. They won't

care, but it gives important knowledge to how casual sex can be dangerous. It empowers kids as they hear crap on the playground to know factual truths.

This preparation will help if your child encounters a classmate with HIV. You can avoid the hysterical parent stampede to traumatize *all* the children by teaching your own children facts about transmission, as well as instilling compassion.

Condoms are another subject parents usually avoid until their children are sexually mature. But condoms are discarded in public places where kids have been known to pick them up and blow them up like balloons. Far better to explain to your kids what they are and why couples use them. In explaining why used condoms shouldn't be touched, you can try educator Meg Hickling's approach: "I find it helps to compare condoms to Kleenex. When you buy a box of Kleenex in the store, they're clean and healthy, but you wouldn't pick up a used one in the street."

Diversity

Nuclear families are no longer the norm. Parents today come in all colors of the rainbow: straight, gay, unmarried, divorced, blended, and single, which means their children are playing hopscotch together at school. Children could care less about a playmate's skin color, family background, or religious affiliation; it's the parents who pass stereotypes down the line. We don't live in a perfect world, but you can help get closer to that ideal by teaching your child about diversity, tolerance, freedom of choice, and sexual expression.

> I want my children to learn that it is okay to fall in love with whoever makes them truly happy. Right now we have been teaching my oldest daughter about families and how there are many different kinds of families and that there is no one kind of perfect ideal family in the world. My oldest is six. When we got pregnant with our second child, we explained how babies were made. We gave her books and showed her videos about the process. And we explained you don't have to be the biological mother or father in order to be the parent of a child. So far she knows that a sexual act is something that people do when they love each other, or by themselves, and that it feels good.

When your children come home with questions about sperm banks or gay sex, you can topple a few stereotypes while providing honest answers. Like the survey respondent above, you can clarify that families are defined by love, not biology. You can tell a child curious about gay sex that gay men and lesbians have sex because they love each other, and that sex can involve any combination of oral, anal, vaginal, or manual sex, just as it does between men and women. Your child has probably heard that gay men have anal sex, and you can clarify that sexual identity isn't defined by specific sexual activities. Do your part to expose children to a variety of lifestyles and viewpoints early on. Several children's books address issues of diversity and can be a wonderful catalyst for ongoing discussions.

If yours *is* a "nontraditional" family, you'll need to be sensitive to and realistic about the societal pressures your child faces. Network with other families, and put your kids in touch with organizations such as COLAGE (Children of Lesbians and Gays Everywhere). Kids need to know that they're not alone in feeling conflicted about getting picked up from school in a van decked in lavender triangle bumper stickers, and that seesawing between pride and embarrassment about one's parents is part of every childhood.

What kids should know by this stage

- The concept of privacy
- Respect for their own and others' bodies
- A sense of personal responsibility
- The meaning of dirty words
- What to expect with the onset of puberty
- That masturbation and fantasy are okay
- How and why people have sex
- What AIDS is and what condoms are
- Differences in family types and sexual orientation

Puberty

Puberty is the child's rite of passage into adulthood. The journey is characterized by cracking voices, pimply faces, growth spurts, wet dreams, and periods, and biologically driven by newly manufactured sex hormones—testosterone for him and estrogen and progesterone for her. Technically, a child has reached puberty when he or she can reproduce (ejaculate, menstruate), but most people refer to the years of tremendous physiological change leading up to this event as "going through puberty." The path to puberty takes not just a month, or even a year, but several years. Puberty begins anywhere between the ages of nine and fifteen, and girls usually start a year or two earlier than boys. If you can remember when you hit puberty, you might have an idea as to when your child will. While increased health, weight, and body fat have caused the average age of a girl's first menstruation to decline steadily over the past hundred years, it seems to have leveled off at no younger than nine.

We will briefly review what changes to expect during puberty, but we urge you to have on hand some of the excellent books that have been written for this age group (see the Resources section, page 340). Kids will be alternately fascinated and mystified by these changes and will want, most of all, to be assured that they are normal. So do yourselves both a favor and get comfortable with the subject matter. You'll avoid horror stories like this:

> I had a friend that told her nine-year-old daughter that she got her period because there was POISON in her body!

Body changes

How do you know when puberty begins? Your child's changing sexual anatomy provides the first clue: A girl's breasts and a boy's testicles and penis will all start to grow. From then on, it's a roller-coaster ride of physical changes, with both sexes finding that their limbs, hands, feet, and facial bones will grow; they'll sweat more; their skin will be oily; and hair will appear under the arms and around the genitals. A girl's breasts and nipples will grow, the nipples may darken, her hips will expand and her body might appear more curvaceous, her ovaries will grow, she may see some vaginal discharge, and she'll start to menstruate. A boy's testicles will grow, his penis will lengthen, his scrotum will darken, hair will erupt on his face and chest, his voice will crack then drop, his Adam's apple may be more defined, he'll start producing sperm and eventually ejaculate. Boys worry about budding breasts (you can reassure them that these will disappear), penis size (explain that it takes eight to ten years from the onset of puberty for a boy's penis to grow to full size), and semen (let them know that the average ejaculate is about a tablespoonful, not a bucketful). Girls tend to worry about breast size (they may be sore and uneven for a while) and the intricacies of managing menstruation.

Emotional changes

Remember that, to the naked eye, puberty is a series of biological transformations, but to your child, it is also a time of tremendous emotional and psychological change. When a body you've known for a decade starts to sprout hair, leak, stretch out, and swell up, you can feel like a Transformer toy gone wildly astray. Your child will find it challenging to cope with the changes to his or her social system, regardless of the fact that other kids are going through the same thing. It's mortifying when your voice cracks while talking to someone you're trying to impress, or when a pimple sprouts up right between your eyes the night before the dance. Kids worry about the size of their growing body parts, maturing too early or too late, and whether their friends will still like them. The hormonal surges make them moody or absentminded, much to the chagrin of concerned parents.

In addition, children are coming to terms with new sexual feelings. Kids who've never masturbated before may start now, while others may be having their first orgasms. Some may worry that they're masturbating too much or that their erotic daydreams are naughty. Kids start grappling with the concepts of sexual attractiveness and sexual desire, both of which can be exciting and intimidating.

> Without the "family life" books my mom left on the shelf for us, I'd never have known what the real names for my genitalia were, how babies were made, or why I bled every month. But they were no help in figuring out why I yearned for someone to touch me, why I had painful crushes on movie stars, or why popular love songs moved me so much I burst into tears.

Children may be frightened by their body's new capacity and the transformations going on in their peer group. Because children are exposed to so much sexual activity in the media, they often need reassurance that it's okay not to want to have sex. They don't need another rundown of the mechanics, they want a point of reference for their feelings.

> Remember, little children ask about sex because they want the "anatomy lesson" — the penis goes into the vagina and the sperm meets the egg inside Mommy. Adolescents ask about sex because they want the "emotional lesson" — be sensitive to the other person's feelings, only do what you feel comfortable with no matter what your friends say, saying no is okay. . . .

Sexual relationships

We're amazed at how many parents feel okay about discussing puberty with their children but are unwilling to take the conversation to the logical next level: sexual relationships. Giving our sons and daughters a party or a pat on the back at puberty is all well and good, but what we're celebrating is the fact that they are physiologically able to reproduce. For many kids, puberty begs the question, Now that the motor's up and running, where do I go? Talking to your kids about puberty without giving them any sex information is like handing them the keys to your car without teaching them how to drive it — and then acting surprised when the car gets wrecked!

But while most advice books focus exclusively on the need to teach children the unfortunate consequences of sex (we'll do some of that later), we think the joys of sex should be given equal time. We're not suggesting that you give your daughter the *Kama Sutra* along with her first box of Kotex, but we do think it's an appropriate time to acknowledge her sexual feelings and discuss sex in a fuller context. Teach her or him the facts about safer sex, contraception, and family planning, but also acknowledge that sex between loving partners can be one of life's greatest pleasures.

Tell your children about sex for pleasure, not just sex for "making babies." It is more important for them to know about that side of sex in a healthy way, rather than being bombarded by unhealthy views of sex in the media.

Be honest about the fact that it can feel good to have sex, and it feels even better when it's the right time and done safely.

You have a perfect opportunity to empathize with what your child is going through by remembering your own sexual awakening.

Be realistic about kids these days—what they know and do—and try to remember how you felt as a teen. Try to fill the role for your kids that your own parents couldn't fill for you when you were young.

Now is also the right time to explain your values—perhaps that while sexual intercourse can be wonderful, it takes a level of emotional maturity, responsibility, and communication skills that most people don't have in their early teens. Finally, you can remind them of suitable outlets for their sexual energies, such as masturbation and fantasy.

You may think a discussion of sexual relationships is too sophisticated for your child, but given that teen birth rates in the United States are the highest of any industrialized nation, both of you should be prepared. Even if your child is not close to being sexually active, he or she is still about to enter the complicated world of dating and intimate relationships and will soon be grappling with issues like sexual assertiveness, building trust, self-control, and peer pressure. Try to clear up any misinformation your child may have about sex, reproduction, and contraception. A lot of kids are confused by euphemisms for sex; they might think "sleeping together" means you can get pregnant by lying next to someone, or that "making love" means you'll get pregnant from kissing. Other, more sophisticated kids might think that oral sex doesn't "count" as sex (heck, plenty of adults suffer from this misapprehension too!), or that STDs can't be transmitted through oral sex.

Sexual responsibility

Make sure your child understands the concept of sexual responsibility—*before* he or she becomes sexually active. Hopefully, you've laid this groundwork throughout childhood, so that he or she takes the idea of respecting one's body—and a partner's—seriously. Information about reproduction, contraception, STDs, AIDS, and safer sex is standard fare in many high school sex-education programs, but given that many kids are sexually active before they get to high school, parents need to review the information with their children during puberty.

Be honest and open, and don't make up stories to scare kids away from sex. Kids will have sex whether you want them to or not, and I think it is better to educate a child as to the pleasures and dangers from sex, rather than having them learn something the hard way and end up pregnant, or catching an STD.

Furthermore, school sex-ed curriculums are largely designed to frighten kids into abstinence. Kids don't necessarily take these one-dimensional scare tactics seriously enough to modify their behavior,[5] but they do learn to associate sex with fear, paranoia, and guilt. As a parent, you can balance this sex-negative message by communicating that sexual pleasure and sexual responsibility need not be mutually exclusive.

Discussing sexual responsibility provides an excellent opportunity to address the double standard governing sexual expectations of males versus females. In our society, a son's sexual experimentation may be tolerated, even encouraged, but a girl's earns her a reputation as a slut. Boys raised to be aggressors may feel fine pressuring a girl to have sex, while girls raised to be passive or submissive may have trouble resisting. Youth who have little experience with relationships run the risk of defaulting to these age-old dynamics, unless you've given them the tools of self-awareness, respect, and self-confidence. You can find plenty of examples of sexual *ir*responsibility in the news that allow you to drive your point home.

> When my son was seven, Mike Tyson was being put in jail for rape. It was difficult for my son to understand how a great athlete could be put in jail for anything. He didn't understand what rape was. It was our first technical discussion about intercourse. I explained the basics of intercourse and said, When both people want to have intercourse, it is a pleasurable experience. It should never be forced or used to hurt someone. I used enough details so he could understand. As usual, the conversation changed to something else. When he left the room, I thought, Great, my son's first real lesson about sex was brought about because a woman was raped by a man my son thought was a hero. Be straight with your kids. You both get a good view of the world.

Your biggest gift to your children during puberty is information. By remaining active and involved, attentive and receptive to questions, you can help them weather their journey to adulthood with humor, grace, and self-respect.

What kids should know by this stage

- That they're normal
- What changes puberty brings for both boys and girls

- Basic information about reproduction, birth control, teen pregnancy, abortion
- Basic information about STDs and safer sex
- Intricacies of social and sexual relationships
- That sexual feelings are valid
- The difference between sex for procreation and sex for pleasure

Teens

What teens want to know about sex

Teenagers want to know everything from the basic facts of reproduction to detailed explanations of sexual technique. Simple curiosity fuels your toddler's desire to know how babies are made, but your teenager's need for reproductive facts is all too urgent. Advice columnists report that most questions from kids in the ninth to twelfth grades are about how to avoid pregnancy. Because many are engaging in sexual intercourse, the depth of their ignorance comes flowing forth: "Can I get pregnant if we do it standing up?" "Does Coca-Cola kill sperm?" In classroom settings or on-line environments where teenagers are allowed to ask questions anonymously, queries run the gamut, covering basic sexual anatomy (Is my crooked penis normal? What's the clitoris for?) to technique (How long should thrusting last? How do I avoid gagging during fellatio?) to curiosity about sexual pleasure (What does an orgasm feel like? Will it hurt the first time?).

We recognize that despite your lifelong effort to remain an accessible parent, your teen may avoid you like the plague. As Meg Hickling says in her book *Speaking of Sex*, "Detached silence is a form of rebellion common to adolescents who fear disclosure of ignorance."[6] What's more, teenagers need to separate from their parents in order to become adults, and rejecting you may be part of this process. You can poke and prod into their private lives all you want, but don't be surprised if they're either oblivious to your existence or hostile. Don't take it personally, but don't use it as an excuse to stop your sex education. Teens need information more than ever, so bookmark useful Web pages, leave educational books or videos out for them, or ask a trusted friend or relative to step in.

Sexual activity

One third of all teenage girls in this country have sexual intercourse by the ninth grade, and two thirds will by the twelfth grade.[7] Although the federal government has sunk billions of dollars into abstinence-only educational programs, teens are becoming sexually active at increasingly younger ages. As this survey respondent points out, kids suffer from the lack of a well-rounded sex education.

> Don't sell yourself or your kids short. They know more than you think they know, so you might as well make sure they understand it all. The kids most likely to start having sex too young are the ones to whom it is still a mystery.

By now, you realize that we don't want you to deny your children's sexual feelings (which by this age are extremely powerful). Instead, we want you to provide them with the information, guidance, and support that will help them make responsible decisions regarding their sex lives. One responsible decision might be not to have sexual intercourse. Many of even the most sex-positive sex educators emphasize the fact that teenagers' physiological drives outpace their ability to realistically assess the consequences of their sexual behaviors. On the other hand, plenty of adults well past the age of consent lack the self-control, self-esteem, and communication skills required for responsible, safer sex — while some teenagers have enough of all three to safely negotiate consensual sexual activity. Certainly, teens in European countries, raised with comprehensive sex education and ensured access to family-planning services (Swedish schools even schedule field trips to family-planning clinics), manage to be sexually active without destroying the moral fiber of their nations.[8]

We believe your teenager should know that many forms of sexual expression carry no risk of pregnancy and minimal risk of disease transmission — oral sex with latex barriers, mutual masturbation, dry humping — and that being sexually active as a teen isn't incompatible with maintaining self-respect and behaving responsibly.

However, it's challenging enough for adults to behave with sexual maturity, and we would also acknowledge that there are many good reasons for your teen to postpone diving in over his or her head. For one thing, the riskiest form of sexual expression — vaginal intercourse — is still the activity by which our culture defines "having sex," and your teen could feel that delaying genital sex with a partner until young adulthood is safer and easier than trying to challenge this monolith. Either way, your job will be to provide understanding, practical advice, and unconditional acceptance. Equipped with these, your teen will have what it takes to develop into a thoughtful sexual adult.

Peer pressure and sex

Take a deep breath and admit to yourself that even though you've raised a "good girl" or a "nice boy," you cannot overestimate the intensity of their sexual feelings and the social pressure to engage in sex at this age. Most girls do not cite "love" as the number-one reason they have sex for the first time; it's either curiosity or "peer pressure,"[9] whether it's a partner saying "If you loved me, you'd show me" or the sense that "Everyone else is doing it, so I should too." Now is not the time to contradict or lecture your children. Give them information and point them toward tools that enable them to make their own decisions. Peer support is the best antidote to peer pressure — see the Resources section (page 340) for several peer-based books and Web sites which help walk teens through a variety of questions and issues to consider before engaging in sexual intercourse, including discussions of possible consequences, such as abortion, adoption, and becoming a teen parent. However, this kind of peer support should be in addition to, not a substitute for, your active and ongoing support.

Sexually active teens will be struggling with a different set of dilemmas, such as learning how to insist on (and use) safer sex or birth control. Your children may be clear on the importance of protecting their sexual health, but the logistics can be intimidating. Depending on your teen's willingness to discuss these matters, you might want to practice various scenarios to teach assertiveness, or provide a book or video that does the same. Whether or not your teen is sexually active, you should ensure that your daughter has regular gynecological appointments and discuss birth control, family planning, and abortion with both your son and daughter. Communicate your values, and the responsibilities of becoming a parent.

Sex, drugs, and alcohol

If you've ever had sex after a few drinks, you know firsthand how alcohol can unlock your inhibitions, so it should come as no surprise that alcohol and drugs are closely connected to teens' sexual activity. We don't advise being the party police, but you should be up front with your kids about the connection between intoxication and impaired judgment. Expecting your teenagers to make it all the way to high school graduation clean and sober may be unrealistic, but you can make it clear that you expect them to avoid getting into uncomfortable or dangerous situations. Give them practical tools to extricate themselves from a bad situation: Make sure they never go to a party without cab fare, a cell phone, or a friend you both trust.

Sexual orientation and gender identity

Teens often develop strong sexual feelings for friends of the same sex, whether they manifest as intense friendships or more overtly sexual relationships. Most advice books reassure parents to fear not, that this healthy, "normal" sexual exploration isn't any indication as to their child's ultimate sexual orientation. We resent the implicit suggestion that a homosexual son or daughter is a parent's worst fear. Sure, we live in a society where heterosexuality is the norm, but that doesn't mean we should treat bisexuality and homosexuality as less desirable possibilities for our children.

So stop worrying about your child's sexual orientation and focus instead on loving and accepting him or her during what may be a critical time. Whether your child is experimenting with same-sex play, or has identified as gay, lesbian, bisexual, or—in the current parlance—questioning, he or she will need your understanding, since getting it from anyone in high school is particularly unlikely. Gay teens often feel isolated, rejected, confused, and suffer at the hands of their peers. They're more likely to get beaten up, are relentlessly teased and disparaged, and have a much higher suicide rate. Anything you can do to create a safe, supportive environment could save your kid's life.

Teens who have gender-identity issues face even greater isolation and the potential for even greater abuse than other queer teens. You can help—not by trying to change or deny your child's experience—but by seeking information and a connection to a supportive community. Particularly good resources for transgendered people exist on-line (see the Resources section, page 340). Compassion and acceptance can be liberating for both of you.

> I suggest talking, talking, talking. I felt that I was the most open-minded person on the planet and was floored by my reaction to my son telling me he wanted to be a girl. Gay I thought I could handle. Kinky, of course. But he was unhappy with his gender!? After I panicked and freaked out, I took a step back, listened, encouraged, made him feel no shame, and in the process, opened my own mind even more.

What kids should know by this stage

- Your value system around sexual behavior
- The connection between sex and alcohol; coping mechanisms
- Your acceptance of their sexual orientation; support for gender identity
- The responsibilities of becoming a parent

IF NOT YOU, WHO?

Although most parents, sex educators, and children agree that parents should be the primary source of their children's sex education, we give ourselves a failing grade. According to a *Time* magazine poll,[10] adults believe teens get their sex information from the following sources: Friends: 45 percent; TV: 29 percent; Parents: 7 percent; School: 3 percent.

We parents see ourselves as painfully ineffective sex educators, yet our kids are clamoring for more participation from us. In one study, 70 percent of teens interviewed said they were ready to hear information their parents thought they weren't ready for.[11] So, parents, ditch the dunce cap and move to the head of the class. To illustrate why you are the best candidate for the job, take a look at what your kids are learning from these other sources.

Friends

About half of today's kids are getting the bulk of their sex information from other kids, who presumably are getting it from . . . other kids. While peer influence plays a major role in every child's physical and emotional development, most kids are more qualified to give advice about choosing Nikes than Trojans. Condoms are the tip of the iceberg when it comes to shared sex information, but the tidbits kids parcel out are often rife with errors. Because the misinformation is not filtered or supplemented by someone who can correct factual errors and offer context and perspective, kids make stupid decisions. When someone tells your daughter that girls can't play soccer as well as boys, you can counter this misinformation with a poster of the women's World Cup champs and a pair of cleats. When a friend tells your son he can't get a girl pregnant if he withdraws before ejaculation, you need to be able to tell him how conception occurs and what methods of contraception are effective.

> Remember, what you don't tell kids they learn from peers at school. Do you want your children's views and opinions shaped by a bunch of horny, misinformed, big-talking teenagers?

> As uncomfortable as it may make parents to talk about sex with their kids, it'd be better for the kids to hear it from them than from some asshole on the street.

TV and Other Media

Unfortunately, the second most popular source for children's sex information, TV, isn't any more likely to provide clear, thorough answers to your children's questions. They won't learn how to have safer sex, what an orgasm is (beyond moaning and puffing), or even what to do when a period starts during math class. They will learn that usually only beautiful heterosexuals have sex, that sex is a commodity, and that it's better to "do it" than to talk about it.

> Don't think that their seeing you snog will warp them . . . better to see their parents have loving sex than some skinny nighttime-drama babe and her latest fling! They have to know that it is a real and wonderful part of life.

> Some networks tip their hats to more responsible programming by delving into subjects like teen pregnancy or gay relationships, but these tend to focus on "lifestyle" choices rather than the realities of sex. Daytime talk shows present a particularly

Embracing the Internet

Although most parents view the Internet as a positive new force in their children's lives, you wouldn't know that from the media.[12] As the talk shows and news articles would have us believe, the Internet is one big land mine of corruption and vice, peopled by pedophiles and pornographers. But ask anyone who's watched a kid use the World Wide Web to play a computer game, research a homework assignment, or chat with a friend, and they'll tell you the Internet is not getting its props.

However, even folks who recognize the contribution this technology makes to their children's development get scared when sex is added to the mix, blindly following the latest "safe surfing" recommendations to use filtering software to limit their child's on-line access. They don't realize that when it comes to sex education, the Internet is a valuable resource for parents and children. Filtering software and rating systems often don't distinguish between porn and sex information and ultimately deprive families of these possible scenarios: An eleven-year-old girl consults with peers about pimples and pads on Kotex's Girls' Space; a sixteen-year-old boy learns about condoms from the Safer Sex Page; a parent picks up tips for talking to kids about sex from Planned Parenthood and SIECUS (see the Resources section, page 340).

Parents worry about the abundance of pornography on-line, but the truth is, young children are unlikely to wander into X-rated sites, and older children who want to seek them out will do so whether you've got the filters or not (we all know that once something becomes "forbidden," it holds a greater charge). In either case, we recommend addressing your child's on-line experiences rather than restricting them—they provide an excellent opportunity to convey your values and expectations around sex.

As for the pedophiles lurking around every virtual corner, we urge a hearty dose of levelheadedness. The media has blown this risk completely out of proportion, exploiting the fear that is every parent's worst nightmare—having a child abducted or harmed. Just as you empower your children to protect themselves by telling them not to get into cars with strangers, you can do so by teaching them to follow basic, commonsense precautions when surfing. Larry Magid, author of *Child Safety on the Information Highway*, offers these tips for kids, which you can print from his Web site (www.safekids.com) and post on your computer:

- I will not give out personal information such as my address, telephone number, parents' work address, telephone number, or the name and location of my school without my parents' permission.

skewed view of sex—by and large pandering to the lowest common denominator, focusing on sexual betrayal, and presenting most sexual desires as "deviant."

As for the rest of the media, the results are mixed. Sexy advertising featuring waif-like babes and ripple-chested studs sends kids the message that their bodies aren't good enough—consider that, by the fourth grade, 20 to 30 percent of girls are already trying to lose weight[14] and boys are taking steroids to bulk up. And when we're taught that sex can be used to sell cars, food, and clothing, we're also learning that sex can be used to acquire such things.

Your child has somewhat better odds of learning useful sex information from the news media, but it's often colored by the tone of the program, newspaper, or magazine. The daily newspapers and news broadcasts rarely report more than sex scandals, sex crimes, or the latest survey results. However, stories about teen pregnancy rates, condom distribution in schools, or the latest AIDS research can give teenagers useful facts to help them make decisions.

Women's magazines saturate their pages with sex instruction, usually with a retro man-pleasing focus: "We'll teach you how to give better head in order to keep your man from straying" or a competitive slant: "Seven steps to multiple orgasms." Mainstream men's magazines can provide a struggling adolescent with insights into men's and women's sexuality, but only if he can peel his eyes off the soft-core fashion spreads. And as for men's sex magazines, the average teen is destined to be extremely confused, disappointed, or surprised by his girlfriend's naked body after viewing page after page of silicone-injected models with no pubic hair!

When it comes to music, our parents might have been scandalized by our singing along to the Rolling Stones' "Let's Spend the Night Together," but now it's our turn to shriek with horror as the words "smack my bitch up" come blasting out of a child's boom box.

> Popular culture is very sexual. I personally have reacted against the misogyny of some gangsta-rap music (and the general bleakness of the rap worldview). I've mentioned this to my kids — not to condemn it, but rather to say that relationships don't have to be that way, that there's more to life and love than pimps and whores. I think they see my point because they know this is true from their own lives.

Like this father, we're not suggesting you jump on the censorship bandwagon, but be aware that music can be a powerful teaching tool, whether it's the misogynistic message in the aforementioned rap lyrics or a song about saying no to a guy's advances. If you're offended, instead of shouting "Shut that filth off," you might try taking a moment to talk to your child about the lyrics from the song and how they make both of you feel.

Believe it or not, the place your kids are most likely to get accurate sex information is from a place most parents wish would just go away: the Internet. Yes, the Web does have thousands of cheesy porn sites with enough T&A to make you go blind, and yes, chat rooms are visited by the occasional pervert trying to pick up kids. But there are also plenty of excellent age-appropriate sex information sites that can fill in the gaps in your kid's formal sex education. Often these sites seem like a beacon in the dark to kids who are too embarrassed or afraid to approach parents; they provide a supportive community of similar youths and some straight-shooting advice. Check out these sites yourself and bookmark the ones you want your kids to visit.

School Sex-Ed Programs

If anything suffers from the "too little, too late" syndrome, it's sexuality education in the schools. Parents, teachers, students, and politicians have been battling for decades over what, how much, and when to teach kids about sex. Chances are your child's formal education will cover abuse prevention, the physiology of puberty, reproduction,

HIV and STDs, and possibly some birth control and safer sex. But since abstinence-only programs prevail in most schools, contraception and safer-sex instruction are by no means guaranteed, and sexual pleasure or homosexuality are seldom addressed.

Our refusal to recognize our kids' sexuality and provide them with thorough information has landed us with one dinosaur of a sex-ed plan that doesn't seem to be working for anyone. Educators often feel unprepared to teach the subject, frustrated by lack of parental support, and tired of having the curriculum dictated by shifting political winds. Students consider the programs largely irrelevant to their lives. Parents who claim they want schools to teach sex education (so they don't have to) can't decide what they want the teachers to teach, yet they reserve the right to interfere with the school's curriculum.

Five percent of U.S. schools teach something known as comprehensive sexuality education, designed to promote a positive view of sexuality in children, and to provide information and skills that will help them make decisions regarding their sexual health. Pioneered by an organization called the Sexuality Information and Education Council of the United States (SIECUS), the program goes from K through 12 and covers "the totality of sexuality: human growth and development, personal skills, relationships, sexual health, sexual behavior, and sexuality in our culture."[15] The program recognizes the many stages of sexual development outlined in this chapter and provides consistent, accurate, and age-appropriate information so that by the time children reach adolescence, they're more capable of making responsible decisions around sex.

We heartily endorse comprehensive sexuality education and urge you to supplement your teachings at home with this effective school model. We refer you to SIECUS for more information—they have a plethora of handouts, bibliographies, fact sheets, and guidelines, so you can learn how to advocate for the implementation of comprehensive sexuality education in your local schools.

TEN REASONS WHY PARENTS SHOULD TALK TO THEIR KIDS ABOUT SEX

1. They want you to
Your child may not leave you a note on your pillow saying "Teach me about sex," but she or he is looking to you for information and guidance. Most children, when asked how their sex education could be improved, request more time and information from parents and more realistic sex education in the schools.[16]

2. Someone needs to set the record straight
Without your participation, most children will be fed the contradictory notions that "sex is dirty" and should be "saved for someone you love." We can't expect our children to emerge as sexually satisfied adults at some magical age if all they've heard

about sex is that it leads to abuse, disease, bad reputations, and unwanted pregnancies. Parents can raise children to honor and respect their sexuality throughout childhood, explaining the joys as well as the responsibilities of sex.

3. You help them build self-esteem

A girl who feels too fat or a boy embarrassed by penis size will be plagued by these same insecurities in their adult sex lives unless we help them to love and accept their bodies as normal. When teens are taught to understand and value sex rather than fear it, we nurture a self-esteem (versus a self-loathing) that will help them make responsible decisions about sex. Simply telling your kid not to do something—whether it's staying out late, having sex, or doing drugs—won't have much effect unless they've got the self-esteem to recognize what is right for them.

> Sex happens and it's better to arm your kids with information and the confidence to say no if they don't want to.

4. They learn your values

Babies are born amoral and from that moment on develop a set of values based largely on input from their parents. We instill concepts of goodness, compassion, respect, fairness, and integrity in our children through our words and actions. These values give children the foundation on which to make decisions regarding their sexual health and successful relationships throughout life.

5. Nobody does it better

We'll let you in on a big secret—talking to kids about sex doesn't come easily for anybody. So although you might find it awkward and embarrassing, don't expect that there's somebody out there who will do a better job than you. Maybe your teenager will develop a special bond with another relative or teacher who can answer their questions, but their sex education starts long before that, when you're the only one in the driver's seat.

6. Good communication prevents social problems

The most comprehensive study of adolescent behavior ever undertaken in the U.S. found that young people who feel close to their parents and are satisfied with family relationships are less likely to engage in risky behaviors like drug and alcohol use, violent behavior, suicide, and early sexual intercourse. The study's authors recommend that "Parents who wish to prevent risky behavior in their children should spend time with, talk to, be available to, and set high standards for them, and send clear messages about what they want them to do and not to do."[17]

7. Ignorance does not equal abstinence

Nor does it equal bliss, especially when the subject is sex. Parents who believe that the less their kids know about sex, the less likely they are to have it, underestimate teens' sexual impulses and the power of peer pressure. As we mentioned earlier, your children will gain a sex education from a variety of other sources, most notably their friends, who also happen to exert the most pressure to engage in sex. If you're a firm believer in the "Just say no" approach to sex education, consider that the bulk of research on abstinence-only sex education proves that it does not delay first intercourse.[18]

8. Sex education does not equal promiscuity

Some parents worry that sex information will breed promiscuity in their children. They worry that either their explanations or the school's teachings will be viewed by teens as tacit permission to engage in sex. But you can give your child information and resources while also reminding him or her of your values, whatever they may be: that you aren't condoning sex before marriage, that sex requires mature relationships, that protecting your sexual health is imperative, etc. In fact, no evidence exists that links comprehensive sex education to increased sexual activity—more often the result is delayed intercourse, reduced activity, or more responsible sexual behavior. It's also worth noting that the first study of condom distribution in schools found not an increase in sexual activity but an increase in condom use among those already sexually active.[19]

9. Sex-positive outlook breeds understanding and tolerance

By raising children who respect their own sexuality, you're teaching them to respect others' as well. When they are taught that sexuality is a lifelong process, they learn to respect the sex lives of people of all ages. When they learn that their own varied sexual preferences are normal, they learn to accept that others' preferences are normal as well.

10. You can teach by action as well as word

By approaching your child's sex education with openness and honesty, you do not risk living a double standard that would require you to be secretive about your own sex life. By recognizing that your sexual desires and healthy relationships have a positive influence on your children, you create an environment where both parent and child can celebrate sexual expression as a routine part of life.

KEEP LEARNING

We've tried to cover a lot of territory in this chapter, and we wouldn't be surprised if you're feeling a little overwhelmed. You doubtless have many more questions spe-

TALKING TO YOUR CHILDREN ABOUT SEX

E'VE given you the why, what, and when of talking about sex with your children, so now we need to spend a little time on the "how." Even when you sally forth with the best of intentions, you inevitably run into problems. Perhaps you seize a golden opportunity to raise a sex-related topic only to find yourself flushed, tongue-tied, and counting the minutes until your chat is over. Maybe your child bombards you with a wave of questions, some of which you don't know how to answer. Or maybe, despite your repeated attempts to talk about sex, your child stonewalls you with somber silence. The good news is that many parents and educators have traveled this road before and have plenty of wisdom to share.

EARN YOUR CREDENTIAL

You don't need a Ph.D. in human sexuality to talk to your kids about sex, but you could probably use a refresher course on some key issues. By reflecting in advance on some of the areas that influence your understanding and awareness of sexuality, you will be better prepared for questions or situations that you'll encounter.

Evaluate Your Own Sex Education

Fear and embarrassment contribute to our discomfort talking about sex. We're afraid we'll be asked something we don't know, we'll send our kids the wrong message, or we'll say something we might regret later. We're embarrassed because this whole practice is unfamiliar to most of us. It's not like our parents greeted us each afternoon with "Hi, honey, how was school? Anybody mention sex today?" When you consider that talking about sex is hard enough with a partner, who can at least empathize with our awkwardness, the challenge of speaking to a wide-eyed kid who expects the gospel truth from us begins to seem rather daunting. You can jump-start your courage by putting yourself in your child's shoes and making a point to get the information you need. If necessary, practice talking about sex with a partner, friend, or relative to help gain confidence.

> Don't let your child be the first person you've ever had a heart-to-heart talk with about sex. You need to be comfortable talking honestly and openly about sex before you talk to your children.

What do you wish you'd learned?

Look back at your own sex education as a way of figuring out what you'd like to avoid, emulate, or modify in your approach. Even if your parents never spoke about sex, or surprised you with one big talk at puberty, think about what you learned from their actions or their silence. How were you made to feel about masturbation? Fantasy? Your body? What questions did you have, and where did you get your information about sex? If you were lucky, your parents set an example you want to emulate.

> In high school, my mom was great and always told me to come to her if I started to be sexually active. She promised she wouldn't judge or ask questions, she just wanted to make sure I was educated about birth control, got an appointment with an OB/GYN, and knew that I could confide in her. It worked! I told her when I wanted to have sex, with my now-husband, and she got me to the doctor for birth control.

> I remember when I was in grade six, I asked my mom what a rubber was. And she told me exactly what it was. I remember asking my dad about what exactly a blow job was and he told me the truth. I respected that and, in turn, respected them, and the next time I had a question or needed to talk to them about sex, I knew I could.

But for many of us, our parents' approach to sex education serves as a lesson in what *not* to do with our own children.

> My mother told me squat about sex. Her explanation of getting your period was that sometimes, when a woman goes to the bathroom, a little blood

comes out in the toilet, but it's no big deal. No talk of body parts, ovulation, certainly nothing about (gasp) penises. So everything I learned was from fifth-grade health class, a movie entitled *Swedish Erotica*, and my husband.

When I was nine and asked about sex, my mother gave me a book to read. While it was useful, I didn't learn that sex was supposed to be pleasurable. It was presented to me as an obligation among married people. I don't plan on making the same mistake with my daughter.

What do you still need to know?

All of us can benefit from a little Sex-Ed 101 now and then. We hope you've learned a lot from this book, but if you still have questions about female or male sexuality, sexual anatomy, reproduction, technique, safer sex or contraception, by all means pick up a book, rent a video, or go on-line in search of the answers. You may not have used a condom in years, but if you expect your teen to do so, you should at least know how to get one out of the wrapper and unrolled. We also recommend investing in age-appropriate materials for your children, as these will help you focus on what are likely to be the most pressing emotional and physical issues for your child at each stage of development.

Face Your Past

Sometimes we hold our kids hostage to our own sexual histories. Maybe you don't want to talk about sex with your children because you don't remember sexual feelings being an important part of your own childhood. Perhaps you're afraid that if you teach abstinence as part of sex education, your kids will find out that you had pre-marital sex and expose you as a hypocrite. Or deep down, you might just not want your kids to make the mistakes you did, so you pretend you were never in their shoes. Realize that your past is *yours*, not theirs, and that your kids deserve honesty above all else. By keeping them in the dark, hiding your secrets, or pretending to be something you're not, you deny your kids the opportunity both to learn from your mistakes and to learn that we're all constantly evolving as sexual beings. You don't need to apologize for your past, nor do you need to wear it on your sleeve, just keep it in perspective.

Use nongraphic anecdotes from your past. It makes them see you not just as parents, but as people who once were just like them.

As far as sexuality goes, I want my kids to remember that just because Mom started having sex at fifteen, that wasn't necessarily cool. First, it was illegal.

And second, I didn't know what I wanted from relationships, and I made a lot of what I now see were stupid choices. I put myself into dangerous situations, I had sex with people I didn't want to just because they wanted me to, I equated sex with love. I want them to be able to find people they trust, people with whom they'll be safe.

Question Cultural Norms Around Sex

Every society develops a set of cultural norms about sex that are reflected in laws, teachings, beliefs, and everyday attitudes. While these norms are frequently held up as fundamental laws of nature, a little scrutiny reveals that they're far from absolute. Within a society, sexual norms are constantly evolving or being replaced to reflect generational shifts in attitudes and expectations.

Perhaps in reflecting on your childhood, you discovered some areas where you were—or are now—in disagreement with your parents' attitudes about sex. By periodically evaluating your stance on these issues, you can identify where a particular belief came from, examine its merit or relevance, and decide whether to dispose of, modify, or embrace it. This way, you'll be prepared for discussing these issues with your own child, since they usually provide the testing ground for individual moral convictions.

It helps to be up to date on the times. What was true for my parents just didn't hold for me.

Be honest, don't push double standards down your kid's throat. Women are just as sexual as men, and that should be OK.

Here are some examples of cultural norms that are continuously being challenged:

- Sex equals intercourse.
- Women are frigid and men oversexed (or men are a slave to sexual desires, women are above them).
- Girls should remain virgins till marriage, boys should have experience.
- Sex should be saved for marriage.
- Sex should be for procreation only.
- Children are not sexual.
- Old people are not sexual.
- Homosexuality is abnormal.
- Masturbation will lead to insanity, blindness, and moral degeneration.
- Anal sex is a practice exclusive to gay men.
- Oral sex is a perversion.

Stand By Your Values

At some point, your children will call on you to defend or justify your principles, which can be a good opportunity to reevaluate your attachment to a position or to strengthen your resolve. For example, you know that your son and his lover share a bed in their home, but it makes you more comfortable if they sleep in separate rooms in yours. Or maybe you discover that this formality was always honored when Grandma was alive, and you no longer feel the need to enforce it.

When attempting to communicate your values to your children, you may find that explaining the beliefs that underlie your convictions, rather than issuing commandments, is more effective:

> What my mom did, and it worked for me, was this: Though we were Catholic, she never told me it was a sin to have premarital sex, but that it was for people who care for one another, to protect yourself, and to have more respect for yourself than to just go around having sex for sex's sake. And it worked. With one exception, all sex I had was within long-term relationships. And the one time I did go against her advice, I found out she was right!

Just remember, you have every right to your values, but your reward for raising critically thinking, intelligent children is that they have every right to theirs. As Harriet Lerner, author of *The Mother Dance*, reminds us: "As kids get older, parents need to be clear about their own values and beliefs and express confidence in their children's ability to make wise choices. Sex is one way kids separate from parents, so the more you clamp down like a sex cop, the more lawless your kids will become. Understand you can't legislate your child's sexuality and erotic energy. Don't expect your beliefs to become their beliefs, or your path to be their path. Not with sex or with anything else."

Now that you've brushed up on your own sexual literacy and you've reaffirmed certain values you'd like to convey, you're ready for your first day of class! If you remember that your kids have as much to teach you as you do them, you're ready for an ongoing, mutually beneficial dialogue about sex.

TIPS FOR TALKING TO KIDS ABOUT SEX

Your first job, one you should be prepared for after reading the preceding chapter, is to think about your child's sex education as a lifelong process and not one big nail-biting talk during puberty. Once you've mastered that philosophy, your task involves not only answering children's questions effectively but figuring out how to raise the subject for maximum effect.

The Opportunities

An inquisitive child may do all the work for you, setting the pace for his or her education with an endless stream of questions about sex. Whenever children come to you with sex questions, be certain to compliment them on their initiative, as this leaves the door open for further inquiries. Being receptive to children's questions about sex is good, but if you limit their education to waiting around for them to ask, you may miss the boat entirely:

> Be open and bring the subject up, don't wait for the kid to come to you. When I was sixteen and already having sex for nearly two years, my mom gave me a speech about doing jumping jacks if I felt I couldn't resist. She was so clueless.

Teachable moments

Your child will present you with any number of what educators and psychologists call "teachable moments," which provide ideal opportunities to impart information in a low-key manner. A toddler rubbing bath toys against her labia gives you the perfect introduction to a lesson on genital anatomy; a six-year-old watching animals mate at the zoo will be fascinated by an explanation of reproduction; or a teen's fondness for nighttime dramas can be the catalyst for a discussion of relationship dilemmas and responsibilities. By remaining attentive to your child's interests, you can use these metaconversations about sex to establish a comfort level with the subject matter and position yourself as an askable parent. Taking advantage of teachable moments requires that you be both vigilant and proactive.

> Respond to sexual things you see together in movies or TV—that can be the perfect time to talk about condoms or say "Hmm, that man is married, but he's having sex with some other woman. What do you think about that?" etc. Talk about sex as it really is—one of many aspects of adult life.

Many parents find that they're more successful approaching conversations about sex through the back door rather than making a grand entrance. This technique helps keep the tone casual, which contributes to a more natural dialogue between parent and child. Without the formality or seriousness of a sit-down conversation, the subject is treated as just another aspect of the child's life.

> Fit your sex talk into other conversational forums. Do not sit down to talk about sex—that's too uncomfortable for many folks. Make it a hit-and-run type of thing if that works for you—a little fact or tidbit here, change topic, another item later. And don't forget to keep that sense of humor!

The best and most important conversations happen when we're gathered to do something else. Cooking together, cleaning the house, playing a board game, walking. Direct questions never work.

Stay tuned

Chances are, if you had a secret camera rigged to your kid's jacket, the resulting footage would be every bit as riveting as a TV drama. By becoming intimately familiar with the characters in a favorite show, we come to care for them, cheer their struggles, and applaud their achievements. If we had this bird's-eye view into our kids' daily lives, we'd be more in tune with their daily dilemmas and, hopefully, more capable of relating to them. We're not suggesting invading your children's privacy with the latest technological gizmo, but do get to know them.

> Talk with them all the time about everything. Hanging around at bedtime, chatting, is a good habit to get into. Driving a child is a good time too. Encourage their questions but don't force them. Don't get freaked by things they talk about, sex or not. Let them see you as stable, objective, caring, and honest.

> Have a relationship with your child on every level. Eat dinner with your kids, play with your kids, read to your kids, participate in your kids' lives, know their friends, welcome them into your home. Don't stop doing this when they are teenagers even if you have to force them to slow down enough to spend time with you. Talking about sex with your kids won't be hard if you really know them and they really know you. They will value the relationship and value the advice even if they pretend not to.

Such involvement not only creates friendship and trust between you and your child, it also keeps you from being blindsided by the unexpected. You may have planned on talking to your teen about sex when she turns seventeen because that's when *you* first made out in a car, but if you know your daughter's peers are getting drunk and swapping oral sex at junior high parties, you'll probably decide to accelerate her education.

Make time

Parents often mask their embarrassment at being asked a sex question by brushing the child off, deflecting him or her to another parent, or forgetting to follow up with answers. But you have no better opportunity to talk to a kid about sex than when he or she approaches you with genuine curiosity; so hang up the phone, turn off the stove, or close your briefcase, and give your child your undivided attention.

How do you get a bunch of rowdy fourth graders to sit still for a lesson about sex? Ask Canadian sex educator Meg Hickling—she's been visiting schools for the past twenty-five years, dishing out her brand of "body science" with astonishing success. Meg stands before preschoolers, middle schoolers, and high schoolers, as well as parents, doctors, and teachers, but her message and manner are always the same: straightforward sex information delivered honestly, candidly, and with respect for individual curiosity and opinion. Parents and kids alike love her; their word-of-mouth referrals have landed her in classrooms all over Canada, and in the U.S. and Japan as well. She shares the secrets of her success:

It's All in the Approach
The first thing I say to fourth graders is, "This is not about how to have sex. This is about your body and how it works. I know you all think having sex is gross and you're never going to do it. Well, you never have to have sex in your life, but you're always going to have sexual health to think about. You're always going to have those parts. We're here to talk about body science."

A Little Humor Works Magic
I tell kids to think like scientists and that "scientists never say 'Ewwww,' they say 'Interesting.'" It works like a charm, the kids enjoy repeating it, and the teachers use that for the rest of the school year.

On Telling Preschoolers About Condoms
Kids find them on the playground and in the street and want to blow them up or use them as marble bags, so I explain what they're for, in a way that helps them to grow up feeling good about using condoms and expecting to use them. One of my favorite responses came when I was talking to tenth graders (I'd been talking to them since they were preschoolers). Eventually one of them said during my presentation about contraception: "What do you do

We have given our son a secret word as a red light to get our attention. If he needs to discuss something pronto, and I am on the phone/computer/or have company, he can just say that word and I will stop and discuss this issue. It really works!

If you can't make time at the right moment, make sure your child knows when you will be available, and make it soon. By prioritizing children's need for informa-

if you want to have a baby?" I was staggered, I'd truly not met a group before who'd grown up expecting to use condoms, and I said, "Have sex without a condom," and they went, "Oh gross, you put it in there bare-naked?!"

The Subject That Pushes Parents' Buttons Most: Masturbation

I call it the "M-word." Nobody wants to bring it up, but they all want to talk about it. They say, "We realize that it's normal and healthy, but we don't know what to say when he's sitting in front of the TV, uh, hanging on to it." I explain that masturbation in the strictest medical sense is anything we do that gives us pleasure and releases tension—twirling our hair, scratching our chin—anything we do when we're nervous or upset. That relaxes everybody. They ask, "Do you say to a three-year-old, 'That's masturbation, you can do it in the bedroom'?" and I say, "It's up to you, you can call it what you like, but the message needs to be that it's private."

The Joys of Sexuality

Children should grow up knowing that sexual activity is a healthy part of a healthy, committed relationship, so I'm always saying to parents, "For goodness' sake, celebrate the fact that you're still attracted to each other!" I joke with them and say, "The biggest secret in the whole world is that Saturday-morning cartoons were invented so parents can have sex." We don't celebrate healthy sexuality nearly enough in our society, we're so hung up on the horror we grew up with about our parents being sexual. If we had people talking to us when we were preschoolers, telling us, "This is what normal, healthy loving people enjoy," then we wouldn't have been grossed out when we found out that our parents were having sex.

Meg's book, *More Speaking of Sex*, is full of wonderful advice, frank talk, and more humorous anecdotes.

tion, you send the message that they have a right to know, and you make it easier for them to come to you in the future.

The Delivery

Get comfortable

Don't be afraid—they can smell your fear.

If your hands shake and your knees quake at the mere thought of talking to your child about sex, you might want to practice beforehand in front of a mirror or with your partner. When you want to broach the subject with your child, begin with baby steps — don't launch in about her or his sex life, but start raising the subject of sex in a casual way. Commenting on items in the news or discussing depictions of sex in the media can familiarize you with sex words and issues. The simple act of discussing sex on a more regular basis breeds familiarity and allows you to ease into a discussion of personal matters when it's appropriate.

> Start an open and ongoing conversation about sex and handle it the way you would anything else — try to stay one step ahead of your child's development and don't expect others to teach your child about sex. Give the right example (i.e., kiss and cuddle both with your children and your partner) and answer questions honestly and truthfully.

Be honest, be yourself

Candid sex conversations may never come easily to you, but leveling with your child about your feelings is better than avoiding the conversation out of discomfort. When you admit that you're embarrassed or a little nervous, you're honestly revealing your feelings, something your child will respect and hopefully model.

> You don't have to be good at it. You can say, "Okay, many people find this topic embarrassing. I am quite embarrassed myself here, but I thought we should have a little talk anyway." If the kid or the parent becomes too embarrassed, you can always agree to break off the talk and pick it up later.

As the following mom suggests, explain why you're uncomfortable, so as not to send the message that sex is naughty.

> Tell them right off the bat that you're uncomfortable because you don't know how to say what you want to say, not because you think that sex is bad.

Your nervousness may stem from a fear that you'll be asked questions you can't answer, thereby shattering your child's image of you as a walking encyclopedia. But you'll improve both your own and your child's sexual literacy if you entertain all questions, then seek out the answers to the ones you don't know. Your children deserve accurate sex information, so you shouldn't ever fake an explanation or refuse to answer a question.

Take a deep breath and just tell the truth. Even if you get embarrassed, red in the face, or stutter around. Give your children the respect of an honest, straightforward answer to their questions. Generally, keep yourself available to them by offering honest answers to all subjects, even if the answer is "I don't know."

We work hard not to be embarrassed by sexual issues around our kids, because children immediately pick up on parental discomfort. Sometimes I've had to take a deep breath, like the time my son, at age six, asked me what a "hooker" was at some big family gathering. He was watching a TV show, heard the word, found me, and asked. I told him, and he asked a few follow-up questions about prostitution, which I answered as straightforwardly as possible, all the while aware that a half-dozen relatives, some quite elderly, were listening in on this. Afterward, I got mostly positive feedback for my forthrightness.

As this mother notes, lying to your kids about sex will ultimately hurt you and them:

Be honest, because when your kids find the truth from other peers they are going to come back and ask you why you lied. And if you do lie, they will only be made fun of by the kids that do know.

Check the attitude

Most parents and kids agree that the best conversations about sex are those that are devoid of criticism and judgment. You can convey your opinions about sex and your child's behavior without humiliating, shaming, or scarring them.

Don't embarrass them. I remember from my own preadolescent experience that one personal shaming can have lasting effects.

Don't make kids feel ashamed. We say, "We don't touch someone else's penis, that's private" not "What the HELL are you doing!!??"

Many kids will either tune out or jump on the defensive when faced with a lecture. If your communication involves an exchange of ideas and feelings rather than a confrontation, you're more likely to retain their attention.

Open a dialogue. Don't plan a lecture, it will be ignored. Introduce the topic and let the conversation flow wherever it needs to. Listen. LISTEN.

Admit any discomfort and discuss it. Share your own feelings, but remember that it's appropriate to keep the details of your own sex life private. Communicate your values, but don't judge, or they will stop talking to you.

Similarly, try not to belittle a child's feelings. You may find grade school crushes amusing, but teasing your children only conveys the message that their feelings aren't legitimate. No, you don't need to emboss wedding invitations, but use the opportunity to validate their emotional discovery and provide some context. Given the amount of teasing that peers dish out, there's no reason for you to add to it.

Language

When it comes to a baby's sexual anatomy, we temporarily check our maturity at the door and regress to cutesy euphemisms for body parts whose real names make us uncomfortable. Do yourself and your kids a favor by brushing up on your genital anatomy and using accurate language from the get-go. If you use nicknames, you risk sending the message that genitals somehow aren't as "normal" as other body parts.

> Use proper terms. A penis is a penis, NOT a "dinglebanger." There is no shame in having these body parts and what they are really intended for. Vaginas are beautiful.

> I'm pretty liberated—or so I thought—but I had to force myself to go beyond saying "penis" and "vulva" or "labia" to say "clitoris." I thought that was pretty indicative of my own childhood years, when everyone knew what a penis was, but girls didn't know the names of their own parts.

Made-up names may sound adorable when kids are little, but they can be a hard habit to break, as this mom discovered:

> We thought it was cute that our daughter called penises "peanuts." And we really regret it. Now she won't call them anything but peanuts.

In addition to using proper sexual terminology, some parents find that developing a more detached, scientific approach helps them convey the message more effectively.

> Use third-person examples. ("Sometimes men and women . . .") I felt like I was describing an anthropological study. Still, it removes a certain amount of intimacy. Kids hate to think that you are doing the things you are describing.

Don't forget that your body is capable of communicating your reactions just as clearly as your words. You may be biting your tongue during a sex talk with your son, but if your face registers horror or shock during his disclosure, you're sending a pretty clear message.

> Don't get freaked by things they talk about, sex or not. Let them see you as stable, objective, caring, and honest.

> Kids are mostly all talk, but as parents you should LET THEM VENT. I've heard stories to curl your hair, but I acted calm till I was alone! They knew I'd lecture once, then accept them as people.

If you're worried about losing your composure during your sex conversations, try having them while you're doing something else—driving, sorting laundry, taking a walk—so you have a distraction at hand.

Agree on an approach

> When my son is old enough to ask, I think he is old enough for an honest answer. Sometimes, though, it is very tempting to say, "Ask Daddy!"

With sex, try to avoid the old "Go ask your mother/father" routine unless you have agreed in advance that only one of you will be providing the sex education. Otherwise, you're just creating confusion, advertising your discomfort, and setting up your coparent. Although many heterosexual households default to same-sex sex education—i.e., moms talk to girls, dads talk to boys—you might want to reconsider this convention. Your kids should get a range of perspectives, and if both parents can answer questions and broach the subject of sex comfortably, children won't identify one or the other as their sole confidant. Should you find yourself one day the only ear for an urgent issue, or even raising your child alone, this training will have proven valuable.

The Message

The content of your sex conversations depends largely on the age of your child, and we refer you to the previous chapter for a detailed discussion of your child's sexual development and the types of issues that may arise. What follows is some general advice about how to interpret your children's reactions to ascertain whether they're "getting the message."

Follow the leader

We parents fret about the right time and place to talk to our kids about sex. We worry about either overwhelming them with irrelevant sex facts or missing golden opportunities. Ultimately, your children will be the ones to set the pace of their sex education, and your ability to read their cues can make the difference in what and how they learn. You may be so committed to imparting all the technical information on schedule that you don't realize your child isn't processing any of it.

> If you tell your kids things before they are even curious, they tend to forget everything you told them!

> The other day my daughter asked me how a baby got into a uterus, and I started to explain to her about the penis, sperm, etc. She said to me, "Oh, not that again, Mama. I guess I really don't wanna know today after all." That was it for the sex-ed lesson that day.

That doesn't mean that giving them the information before they're ready is dangerous or futile; it's better to err on the side of too much rather than too little. Kids will simply process what they need and discard the rest. And ultimately, your efforts to talk about sex contribute to their comfort level with the subject.

> Make sure they know the basics, then see what needs addressing. What comes up a lot in our house is how guys talk about women—like how eleven- and twelve-year-old boys are all gonna talk this shit, but does he know the difference between that and reality. See what comes up in conversation, don't lecture, and pay careful attention to their discomfort level at talking about this stuff with you—stop talking before they stop listening.

You can usually take your child's questions at face value, but keep an eye on the reaction to make sure your response is on track. If your child looks puzzled, you're not answering the right questions. But don't restrict yourself to providing answers—you need to ask questions to make sure you're not making assumptions about what they know and what they want to know.

> Once, when walking down the street with my six-year-old niece, we heard the Salt 'n' Pepa song "Let's Talk About Sex." She said, "What are they talking about?" and I nervously expounded on sex. When I finished, she said, "Oh, I thought they were saying 'Let's Talk About *Six*,' because that's how old I am."

I remember a girlfriend's daughter once asking me where did her new kitten come from. I launched into a long explanation of eggs and sperm and birth only to have the girl say, "No no, I just want to know if the kitten came from the pound or the store!" Listen closely to what is being asked, and if you're not sure, get them to ask you again.

If your child looks scared, there may be more to the question, and you'll need to dig a little deeper. Oftentimes a question hides beneath a simple query. An eleven-year-old asking you about testicles may just want reassurance that the hair sprouting on his balls is normal.

Make it accessible

Your words have a better chance of penetrating if you can make them relevant to your child's life.

Don't overload them with biology and technical information. I try to compare it to something in my daughter's life, like how our neighbor is pregnant or how her father looks different from us.

Be a parent, not a friend

Friends may share your children's confidences, but they can't instill your values or promise your kids unconditional love. If you've taught your kids concepts like respect, honesty, responsibility, and justice throughout their lives, they've already absorbed a value system that enables them to make responsible decisions around sex. One way to ensure that your children understand your values regarding practical sex matters is to distinguish between facts and attitudes. Rather than simply telling your daughter "You're too young for sex," try explaining to her that "Just because it's physically possible to get pregnant once you have your period doesn't mean you're automatically mature enough for a sexual relationship. I believe you're not ready to deal with the possible consequences of sex, like pregnancy. What do you think?"

Responding to a challenge to your authority with "Why? Because I say so" might have worked occasionally on your toddler, but if you use it on a petulant teen, you're both in for trouble. Teens need to understand the logic behind your opinions, the values they're based on, and your expectations. You cannot make their decisions for them, but you can give them the skills to make well-informed decisions on their own.

Regardless of whether your children agree with you in word or in action, if they know that you love them, they will be more likely to learn from their mistakes and to make better choices in the future.

Reinforce that you will always love them, even if the decisions they make about sex don't necessarily agree with what you would want for them. And remember that they will make their own choices—you can't control their sex lives.

Don't try to be a friend; be a parent, but don't be a parent in a disapproving way. Let them know that you won't be disappointed no matter what happens. But be sure to follow through. And realize that you can't control them. They need to make their own way in life, and the best you can do is be there for them when they need to hold your hand through the tough times.

Follow Through

Respect privacy, keep confidences

If you want your children to confide in you, you need to prove yourself a worthy confidante. If your child asks you to keep a secret, keep it (unless you feel your child is in danger). One betrayal can cost you a lifetime of respect.

I kept a journal in my high school English class and was told by the teacher all our information was confidential. I liked having this teacher as confessor/counselor, but when I found out he blabbed to my physics teacher about my crush on a classmate, I never forgave him.

Similarly, no matter how tempted you are to read your teenager's journals or letters, don't do it. You may be going mad with curiosity about what he or she's been up to, but there's absolutely no excuse for such an invasion of privacy.

Try again

If your child spurns your attempt to talk about sex, try again at a later date. If he or she shows no interest in age-appropriate sex information, you might ask yourself whether you are subtly discouraging questions. Don't brush off a question if you're in a hurry, but tell your child when you'll be able to get back to it—and make sure you do. After a conversation, follow up with "Did I answer your question?" to make sure you got to the heart of the issue. If you don't know the answer to a question, research the answer and get back to your child, or look for the answer together (see the Resources section, page 340).

Accept the fact that your teen may brood or respond to your overtures with hostility. Consider the possibility that there may be another adult—a trusted aunt, uncle, or friend—in whom your child would rather confide:

If your child seems to be embarrassed to talk about sex, then do it at another time, or ask who else he or she would be comfortable talking to. But you should definitely be the first one to bring the subject up.

Use resources

You don't have to do it all alone! Regardless of your best efforts, your kids may be shy and embarrassed to talk with you, so it's great to have some backup. There are plenty of excellent written and visual sex materials for both parents and kids. Leave educational books and videos out, and bookmark Web pages for your kids. You may find that you're a resource not just for your kid, but for the entire block!

> I started with that funny book called *Where Did I Come From?* The book would disappear all the time. My kids would take it to friends' houses and finally I had to make a rule that the book stays at home.

> I liked using visual aids such as Miriam Stoppard's book *Questions Children Ask,* and even Betty Dodson's vulva drawings in her book *Sex For One,* as they help to structure the discussion and also help you not to forget important topics.

BE THE BRIDGE

Want one last doozy of a tip for improving your child's sex education? Go public. If you've made it this far in our discussion of kids' sex education, you know that they'll learn about sex from the cradle to the grave, but that you might not like all the lessons they're being taught. You can take a more active role in their sex education by getting involved in the different forums where sexuality is addressed — in schools, churches, hospitals, etc. Find out what is being taught, if anything, and offer to assist with or implement a program. As sex educator Meg Hickling says, "Kids may not remember who taught them math, but they'll always remember who taught them about sex." She and others, like the following mom, are engaging in grassroots efforts to expand children's formal sex education in every available arena.

> I am a religious education teacher (Catholic). This will be my eighth year of teaching eighth grade, and in the first semester we cover sexuality. My kids have all taken this class (to their great embarrassment). We discuss feelings and taking care of other people. We have had the kids role-play telling their parents they were pregnant (the kids role-playing the parents

What Parents Want Kids to Know About Sex

We asked, and here's what they said:

- Your body is beautiful, be proud
- You are the one who knows how to love your body the best
- Sex is not bad, dirty, or sinful
- Wait for sex, wait to have a kid
- Don't judge others
- Be careful and respectful of yourself and of partners
- Sex is not always about romance; the physical act can be fun and exciting
- Accountability
- Responsibility for your own and your partner's physical health
- Honesty
- Don't take sex too seriously
- Sex is sacred
- Sex is not always sacred
- Have boundaries and honor them
- Save yourself till marriage
- Nudity is beautiful
- Expressing affection is good
- Don't make the mistakes we did
- Beware of the sexual double standard for girls and boys
- Sex is about choices
- If you can't talk to a parent, read a book or talk to another adult

got really angry, and the ones playing the pregnant teens weren't too happy about telling their parents). Both in class and at home, we have tried to make the point that you should be smart, but if you are going to be stupid, at least be safe. This is a little harder in the church setting, but since the church also teaches you should follow your conscience, we have a little wiggle room.

What Parents Want Kids to Know About Sex

- Sex can be enhanced when the physical, emotional, and spiritual are in sync
- There are other ways to express love than sex
- Know the cause and effect of your actions
- Sexuality is fluid and always changing
- Sex is wonderful with a loving partner
- Sex is wonderful alone
- Don't be afraid to ask
- Don't be ashamed, and don't hide your sexuality
- Choose partners wisely
- Don't be promiscuous
- Respect women as thinking, strong people
- Say no if you don't feel ready
- Be with whomever makes you happy, regardless of gender
- Be monogamous
- Be nonmonogamous
- Be a generous and gentle lover
- Sex and love is more than intercourse
- Sex is consensual
- Don't be in a hurry
- Learn appropriateness
- Don't ever feel guilty about your sexual feelings

Until enough parents stand up for accurate, thorough sex information, children will continue to be disserved by a doomsday approach to sex that jeopardizes their health, safety, and happiness. Organizations like SIECUS offer sexuality-education programs geared to schools and churches, and the Web site SEX, ETC. (a site run by teens) offers guidelines for parents who want to bring more comprehensive sex education into the schools.

MAKE THE COMMITMENT

We asked our survey respondents what they wanted their children to know, learn, or feel about sex (see the sidebar for some of their responses). Why not take the time to answer this question for yourself? Once you have identified the information, attitudes, and values you want to bestow upon your children, you can take steps toward that goal. With a few practical tools, the willingness to take risks, and a commitment to your own sexuality, you're well equipped to raise sexually healthy children.

> The most important thing I want to communicate to my kids is that they are entitled to great sex too. That it's pleasurable, necessary, as elemental to life as breathing and eating. I want them to be their own people, especially when they become mothers (if they choose to be parents at all), and realize that a balance in all things is so important. In other words, they cannot live their lives FOR their children at the expense of themselves. Nor can they do that for a partner. I suppose, in essence, that's the virtue of "selfishness," because to truly be a good friend, lover, or parent you must first be happy with yourself and your life.

16

TEACHING BY EXAMPLE

YOU can talk to your kids about sex until you're blue in the face, but if your actions contradict your message, guess which they'll remember? When it comes to sex education, the cliché "Actions speak louder than words" rings decidedly true. Author Susie Bright sums up this sentiment nicely: "Be a good role model to kids. What you say is so secondary to what you do. If you want them to have a good sex life, you have a good sex life. If you want them to be comfortable talking about sex, are you? If you want them to have a good body image, have one yourself!"

This sounds great, but it ain't always easy. Maybe you feel fine about imparting age-appropriate sex information but get queasy when your kids express any curiosity about or awareness of your own sex life. Some parents panic at the thought of kids "catching them in the act"; some single parents avoid dating for fear their kids will realize they're having sex; and others evade or ignore children's questions when they get too personal. When your anxiety manifests itself to the point that you end up limiting physical affection with a partner, curbing sexual activity, or downplaying your sexuality, you've not only shortchanged your own sex life, you've also sent your kids the message that adult sexuality is nonexistent, which can have devastating effects.

Don't stop making sexuality a part of yourself because you've become a parent. Don't give your kids the unhealthy example of becoming a cold, asexual being. How are they supposed to see how a happy, healthy person relates in this world if Mom and Dad are examples of employees, civil servants, and parenthood, but devoid of human sexuality? How do kids learn what role sex plays in their lives when they start feeling sexual urges themselves? I never, EVER felt comfortable with my own sexuality until after becoming a mom, because my parents never touched or kissed (not once!) in front of me. They made sex dirty, ugly, and shameful. In my opinion, that is what happens when kids are left with the impression that sex is not part of life for adults, and they have feelings and desires that are at odds with that fact. They have no clue how to deal with it.

Most parents don't intentionally choose to self-censor their sexuality; they inadvertently succumb to embarrassment, discomfort, and genuine confusion. Even if you make every effort to model sex-positive behavior, you can still be taken off guard by an ill-timed question or intrusion from your child. But a little perspective and forethought will help you enjoy your sexuality, while also consciously—and realistically—addressing its impact on your children.

PROTECT YOUR PRIVACY

With kids' awareness of our sex lives, we're most troubled by a vague sense that we'll offend, shock, or harm our innocent ones with some inappropriate behavior. But if you've treated sexuality as a natural and integral part of their lives, they won't view yours as unnatural. If you've answered your child's sex questions honestly, thoroughly, and nonjudgmentally, they already know that you have sex.

If children request explicit details about your sex life, you don't have to provide them. You can maintain your privacy without skimping on your child's education. Your son may ask if you give Dad blow jobs, to which you can reply, "That's something private between me and your dad, but if you're asking what a blow job is, I can tell you."

Each of us has a different privacy threshold that dictates how much personal information we feel comfortable discussing with our children. As author Joani Blank points out: "It's important to legitimize people's sense of privacy—what they need and how much they need. I know moms who take baths with kids and show their genitals to their kids, but I never felt comfortable doing that. Some parents feel fine about that, but I didn't and I never felt guilty. If my daughter asked me, I'd say no, just as if she'd asked, 'Can I watch you and Dad have sex?' "

When a child does or says something you find intrusive, treating it as a privacy issue rather than a sex issue will avoid sending the message that sex itself is bad or shameful. And it can have humorous results, as Susie Bright discovered: "My daughter came in without knocking while I was making out with a lover. I told her that I was making love and wanted to be alone and that I would come check on her later. I was careful to make it nonchalant, and about privacy, rather than a sex issue. But she said, 'I want to watch.' And I told her that I wasn't a TV program for her entertainment!"

When children catch you by surprise, use the opportunity to reinforce the concept of privacy. Ask your child what sorts of things she feels private about and explain that you respect her privacy and are just asking that she respect yours. Eventually, your children will come to understand and view your sex life as something you enjoy, and they will give you the room to enjoy it.

> I'm sure my nine-year-old daughter knows that my boyfriend and I share a bed when we are together. She and I have talked about sex, so she knows that we are most likely "having sex." She understands that once she is in bed when my boyfriend is over, she should not go into my bedroom without knocking. She respects my privacy and I respect hers. My boyfriend and I take care not to be loud or vulgar when she is in her room.

> We don't flaunt our sexual selves in front of our kids, but they understand that a closed door means "leave us alone." They know we need that time to enjoy each other, and they are comfortable with it because we don't apologize for it, we don't explain it, and we don't make a big deal of it. If they hear us, or see us kissing, we don't react like we have been caught doing something ugly or wrong.

Privacy for some parents involves eliminating any signs of their sex life, but others find that a certain openness invites children's questions and creates a more natural opportunity for them to learn about sex. For example, a child's discovery of condoms or a diaphragm in a bedside drawer might inspire a conversation about contraception and sex for pleasure. We appreciate the way that this father honestly and intentionally answers his children's questions when it would have been much easier to respond without ever mentioning sex at all.

> Some of our sexual accoutrements (candles and a boom box in the bedroom) became fodder for sex education. "Why do you and Mommy have candles in your bedroom?" "Because we enjoy candlelight when we're making love." "Why do you and Mommy have a boom box in your bedroom? You never play it." "We play it when you're asleep, when we're making love. We like music then."

LIVE YOUR VALUES

Many of us think of values as a list of dos and don'ts that we rely upon to guide our children's development. But kids learn the most about your true values from your actions. Think about time spent at your job, with your partner, and your kids, and ask yourself whether you expend more energy on greed, jealousy, self-pity, and despair, or humility, generosity, respect, and kindness. Which of these attitudes do you think make you a better lover or help you develop a healthy sexual self-esteem?

You can stimulate your own sexual creativity by tapping in to the source of your passions. Figure out what brings you joy, do more of it, and you, your family, and your job will all benefit. Maybe it's dancing, listening to music, hiking, or baking exotic desserts, but if it brings you pleasure, you are in fact infusing your life with sexual energy. At the same time, take a closer look at how you've prioritized enacting your values. Make an effort to really put them into practice—not with token treats or hollow gestures—but in your daily behavior. Let a colleague run the meeting if that will convey respect, wow your partner with your thoughtfulness by doing more chores, explore generosity by volunteering. These things are what make us richer in mind, body, and spirit.

As parents, you can use your joy and generosity of spirit to imbue your children with passion. Not by lining up to buy Pokémon cards and Nintendo games, but by taking time out of your busy schedules in order to share moments of beauty and fantasy. Whether it's turning your kids on to the ballet, museums, country music, botanical gardens, architecture, cars, or cooking, when you expand children's horizons beyond animated cartoons, computer games, and plastic figurines, you unlock doors to their imagination and passion, thereby giving them the keys to creativity and eroticism.

Many parents find that their approach to sex education is an organic expression of their values. For example, these mothers believe their children are entitled to sexual fulfillment in the context of responsibility, safety, and respect, values that they impart both through words and actions.

> I have girls, so I'm greatly concerned that sex be good for them from the beginning. I can't believe it took me until I was thirty-three to find my G-spot (and what a spot it is!). I also can't believe that I settled for such bland sex for so long. I want them to be so well educated about sex, for it not to be taboo, and for them to expect and get good sex when the time is right. I want them to also understand how important it is to wait until they are mature and have a mature, loving partner so their early experiences will be good and memorable and safe.

I would like to give kids some of my own value system, which is that sexual expression is a wonderful gift, but not to be given without thought and emotion. Emotionally, I think it's important to have a level of maturity before becoming sexually active. I don't want them to regret their sexual actions (though I'm sure everyone has at least minor regrets), so I want them to give thought to things ahead of time. And the other big value is, of course, safety. My children will know about safe sex, they will know that they have non-judgmental access to birth control, and they will know where in our home they can just go grab a condom without anyone seeing it. I think the biggest barrier to safe sex for kids is that they are so often embarrassed to seek it, and so just go without. I don't want that for my children.

The fact that children will inevitably be exposed to sexually explicit materials such as adult magazines, soft-core advertising, erotic novels, and adult Web sites disturbs many parents. But rather than attempting the impossible feat of banning sexual imagery, these two fathers use the ubiquitous presence of sexual materials as an opportunity to educate their children about values:

I used to write for *Playboy*, so we had the magazine around the house. I never prevented my son from looking at it. But I made sure he understood that (1) Most women don't look like *Playboy* models. (2) Most women have mixed emotions about not looking like that. (3) Many women feel offended by girlie magazines as an invasion of privacy and a misrepresentation of who they are. (4) The *Playboy* version of sex is that sex is ONLY fun, which is simplistic. The best sex comes from a loving, trusting, intimate relationship.

I want my kids to learn that sex is much better than violence and should be more acceptable. I'd much rather them see a porno than a film showing violence as fun and appropriate. I also take them to nude beaches so they get used to real bodies (as opposed to those in *Playboy* and *Manpower*). This should help them be less judgmental of others.

We encourage you to take a closer look at how your own life reflects your values and to accept the challenge of adopting a style of sex education that allows you and your children to live and act in accordance with these values. We couldn't agree more with this mom's advice:

Don't lie, don't be a homophobe, and do not ever make it okay to be exploitative or disrespectful to others in a sexual (or nonsexual) setting.

Accept your children and teach them to accept themselves and others. Sex is a wonderful thing and our children deserve to learn that.

KEEP YOUR PERSPECTIVE

How does one remain oneself in front of one's children; that is, be sexual, act sexy, have art that deals with sexuality around, yet respect what is age-appropriate and right for children?

You may be completely committed to role-modeling positive sexual attitudes for your children. You may be confident in your right to sexual pleasure, and unselfconscious in your delight in sex toys and erotica. But you, like every other mother who reads this book, will inevitably encounter those moments of anxiety when your sex-positive philosophy collides with reality: Should I lock up the sex toys? Is it okay to leave that erotic photography book on the coffee table? And what should I do when the Scout troop comes over? Before you install the padlocks, draw the curtains, and bolt the door, take a step back and look at the big picture.

Child-proofing Your Pleasure Chest

We have greatly expanded our sexual oeuvre since parenthood. My partner sometimes worries about our daughter finding out about some of our non-traditional sex practices. So we keep our toys locked away. I feel that we need to establish a mutual respect with our daughter about private matters.

Like the mother quoted above, most parents choose to keep their sex accessories tucked well out of reach of their darling sons and daughters. Establishing a mutual respect for privacy is an admirable goal, but keep in mind that you won't have violated that goal if your kids spot a dildo on your bureau or catch sight of your vibrator cord sticking out from under the bed. Young children will accept your explanation that some toys are designed especially for grown-ups to enjoy while making love, and pubescent or adolescent children have probably known about your secret stash for some time.

Several years ago, the women-owned sex emporium Good Vibrations commemorated its fifteenth anniversary by soliciting customers' memories of their first vibrator experiences. A good 20 percent of these true-life tales revolved around the exciting discovery and enjoyment of a parent's vibrator. Doubtless the parents would have been horrified, but had they been more vigilant about hiding their toys, their kids would've missed out on a thrilling sexual discovery. Then again, this "don't ask, don't tell" approach can misfire:

Hide your vibrators really well! Last year, when my daughter was in first grade, I got a call from the principal telling me to come in because my six-year-old was brandishing my vibrator in class!

So if you truly want to protect your privacy, get a padlock for that treasure chest!

Hiding the Smut

Similarly, you may prefer keeping your sex books inaccessible to your children, but we'd encourage you to think twice before you put in a secret bookcase. Quarantining sex books is just one more way to reinforce the false notion that sex somehow belongs in a separate category from the rest of life's subject matter. As for erotic art and photography, your kids live in a world in which sexual imagery is used to sell clothing, CDs, and consumer appliances — don't they deserve to know that sexual imagery is sometimes an expression of creativity and eroticism that has no price tags attached?

This line of reasoning is much easier to embrace when you're hanging an erotic lithograph on the walls of your bedroom than when you're imagining your children accidentally cueing up your latest all-anal-action video rental. It's perfectly reasonable to hide your adult videos from your kids, but let them know that watching sexy videos is something adults enjoy (just as adults enjoy certain movies and TV shows that kids don't). Odds are good that your children are going to be exposed to porn, if not at your house, then at someone else's. Give them the message from an early age that adult videos aren't a secret decoder ring to the capital-T Truth about sex, but that they reflect adult sexuality about as well as cartoons reflect reality. As the father quoted below suggests, you can communicate your own values by letting your child know that porn is hardly a comprehensive depiction of eroticism.

> When my thirteen-year-old came home recently with a porno tape copied for him by the older brother of a friend, I didn't confiscate it or flip out. But I made sure he understood the shortcomings of porn's all-genital, nonsensual approach to sex.

HONOR YOUR PATH: NONTRADITIONAL SEXSTYLES

> How can I be open with my children and their questions without putting ideas into their head that lead to other parents calling to chew us out?

You may be worried that the details of your sexual tastes would raise a lot of eyebrows if word got out to the PTA. Moms in nontraditional relationships can be justifiably concerned about how "out" to be (and how to be out) in the public realm. We assume that if you're a lesbian or bisexual mom, you have a community and resources that allow you to be open about your sexuality at home. While our culture still has a long way to go toward accepting and extending full legal and economic support to gay and lesbian families, the fact is that queer families are a growing presence and political force. We were heartened by how many of our survey respondents have prioritized teaching their young children respect for diverse families. After all, the reality is that only a minority of American children are being raised in traditional families with a married mommy and daddy, so despite the weeping and wailing of political conservatives, our society is becoming more inclusive of diversity simply because it must. This said, do research your legal options and take steps to safeguard your parental rights; the National Center for Lesbian Rights (see the Resources section, page 340) offers state-by-state information on legal protection—including custody, adoption, and health and financial powers of attorney.

Other alternative forms of sexual expression can be even more marginalized. Parents exploring alternatives to monogamy face a huge societal bias against open relationships. Nonmonogamy, sometimes referred to as polyamory, is a mutual agreement to have sexual and emotional partners outside the primary relationship. Needless to say, it hasn't exactly caught on like wildfire in our culture, where we tend to have a much higher comfort level with the notion of affairs—all that nice, familiar secrecy, lies, and cheating!

Parents who incorporate aspects of power play into their eroticism also confront a wealth of stereotypes and negative attitudes. Power exchange is one of the most common themes in sexual fantasy, and we think it's likely that many of your fellow PTA members are exploring role-playing, bondage, discipline, dominance, submission, and S/M. However, despite the fact that images of fetish fashion and bondage accessories abound in popular culture—from advertisements to music videos to cult movies—any exploration of power play that's more than skin-deep is dismissed as "deviant" and "kinky."

So what impact does a nontraditional sexstyle have on your parenting? Not much. The privacy issues around your adult sexuality remain the same whether you're having three-minute intercourse in the missionary position in your own bedroom or heading out to an S/M play party. The ins and outs of your sexual activities are none of your kid's business; just communicate your entitlement to privacy as well as pleasure. As your kids become teenagers, you may want to share bare-bones information with them (such as that you're in a nonmonogamous relationship), but again, going into details is not necessarily appropriate.

You're also entitled (and we'd suggest obligated) to communicate realistic messages about alternative sexstyles to your children. Just as a lesbian mom will want to provide her children with the coping mechanisms of self-respect, independent thinking, and awareness that ignorance and intolerance of same-sex love are still painfully widespread, a mom who enjoys power play or is nonmonogamous will want to find ways to provide her children with positive messages to counteract the misapprehensions they're bound to pick up from the world around them. This doesn't mean confiding, "Your daddy and I enjoy dominant and submissive role-playing." It could just mean saying, "Lots of adults enjoy playing dress-up or fantasy games during sex, and there's nothing wrong with that."

Try to seek out and socialize with other nontraditional families, just so your children don't feel isolated. But there's no reason to create a greater charge around your neighbors' differences in sexual habits than you would around differences in TV viewing, dinner menus, or standards of cleanliness. You've probably discovered just how finely tuned kids' radar can be—they quickly develop the ability to discriminate between what are and aren't appropriate topics of conversation or behaviors in different contexts. For a child, there's not much difference between picking up that certain slang words are okay to say at your house but not at Grandma's, and picking up that Uncle Johnny can wear nothing under his chaps at the gay pride parade but shouldn't show up at the grade-school holiday pageant in the same outfit. Needless to say, as the parent, it's your job to make sure that Uncle Johnny is clear on these distinctions too.

TRUST YOUR JUDGMENT

You've probably noticed that we eschew pat answers in favor of philosophizing about the variety of questions that will arise as you walk the high wire of sex-positive parenthood in a sex-negative culture. Ultimately, our pat answers would be irrelevant, because you're the only one who can decide on the appropriate balance of discretion and disclosure for your household. Your philosophy is bound to evolve over the years; you may find that you take different tacks with different children depending on their personalities and your own development.

We do encourage you to trust your judgment and keep an eye on the big picture. After all, you may regret how you handle the occasional conversation, incident, or encounter related to sex—but isn't this true of other matters as well? There will always be plenty of opportunities to revisit the subject and try different approaches. If you're motivated by a sincere respect for sexuality and a sincere desire to communicate this respect to your children, you can't go wrong.

AUTHORS' NOTE

FINDING YOUR OWN ROLE MODELS

Your kids aren't the only ones who benefit from sex-positive role models, and you'll be well served by seeking out some of your own. Mothers deserve inspiration and validation for sexual self-expression. We need comrades to share our laughter and delight at the sexual pleasures we encounter; to share our frustration and rage at the sexual double binds we face; and to support us in each and every radical step we take. Partners and lovers can offer valuable support (and motivation!), but we urge you to cast your net wider. When you seek a sexual role model outside the domestic realm, you reinforce the fact that sexual discourse *belongs* in the public domain. We need to wrest control of this discourse back from the pandering politicians, fear-mongering members of the religious right, and titillating tabloid writers who preserve a lowest-common-denominator mode of sexual expression. Wherever you find women who trust their own judgment, reject labels, and act with integrity, the odds are good that you'll find women willing to speak out about their own authentic eroticism.

You may be particularly moved by women writers, artists, and teachers:

Joan Nestle, Dorothy Allison, Susie Bright, and other lesbians who wrote courageously about love and sex were inspirational to me and key in my sexual radicalism. I just have a lot of respect for women who are out there with their sexuality and their love of sex.

You may find inspiration among friends, family, and colleagues, or guidance from women in your church, community, or workplace.

Believe it or not, I've found our church and church friends to be a valuable sex resource. Watching other couples in committed, caring relationships has encouraged me over the years.

I have a close friend who is fifty-one, to my twenty-five, who is very accepting and expressive of her sexuality. I think having a role model of her acceptance and love for herself has done wonders for my view of my own sexuality.

Trust us, once you start looking, you'll find many amazing women testifying to the power and worth of our innate sexuality. And you'll become one yourself. Don't let a natural instinct to focus your creative energies on your children prevent you from giving your erotic life its due. Your children are going to grow up and move on; if you sow the seeds of self-awareness, uncensored fantasies, sensual playfulness, and sexual independence now, you'll enjoy a harvest of pleasure that's beyond compare. We wrote this book for mothers—it's going to be up to you to write your very own *Grandmother's Guide to Sex*.

NOTES

CHAPTER 1: SEXUAL SELF-IMAGE

1. Shahrukh Husain, *The Goddess* (Boston: Little, Brown and Co., 1997), p. 11.
2. Sarah Dening, *The Mythology of Sex* (New York: Macmillan, 1996), p. 48.
3. For a summary of this history, see Elaine Pagel's groundbreaking book, *The Gnostic Gospels* (New York: Random House, 1979).
4. Dening, p. 13.
5. Winifred Milius Lubell, *The Metamorphosis of Baubo: Myths of Woman's Sexual Energy* (Nashville: Vanderbilt University Press, 1994), p. 139.
6. See John D'Emilio and Estelle B. Freedman, *Intimate Matters: A History of Sexuality in America,* Second Edition (Chicago: University of Chicago Press, 1997).
7. Erna Olafson Hellerstein, Leslie Parker Hume, Karen Offen, eds., *Victorian Women* (Stanford: Stanford University Press, 1981), p. 181.
8. Barbara Ehrenreich and Deirdre English, *For Her Own Good* (New York: Doubleday, 1978), p. 244.
9. Susie Bright, *Full Exposure* (San Francisco: HarperSanFrancisco, 1999), p. 20.
10. Michie Mee, "Sexy Mamas," SexTV, February 2000.

CHAPTER 2: SEXUAL SELF-ESTEEM

1. Laura Fraser, "Body Love, Body Hate," *Glamour*, October 1998, p. 281.

2. Ibid, pp. 282–3.

3. Quoted in an interview with Moira Brenna, "The Opposite of Sex," *Ms.*, August/September 1999, p. 64.

4. Marty Klein, Ph.D., and Riki Robbins, Ph.D., *Let Me Count the Ways: Discovering Great Sex Without Intercourse* (New York: Jeremy P. Tarcher/Putnam, 1998), p. 147.

5. Joan Jacobs Brumberg, *The Body Project: An Intimate History of American Girls* (New York: Random House, 1997), p. 212.

6. *The Works of Aristotle the Philosopher, in Four Parts*, 1831, quoted in John D'Emilio and Estelle B. Freedman, *Intimate Matters: A History of Sexuality in America*, Second Edition (Chicago: University of Chicago Press, 1997), p. 46.

CHAPTER 3: SELF-LOVE

1. S. A. Tissot, quoted in Walter Kendrick, *The Secret Museum: Pornography in Modern Culture* (New York: Viking, 1987), p. 89.

2. According to the nineteenth-century American health reformer John Kellogg, who promoted clean living, self-restraint, and a bland diet (like the cereals he invented).

3. Deidre English and Barbara Ehrenreich, *For Her Own Good* (New York: Doubleday/Anchor, 1978), p. 123.

4. Memorable words from *All My Children*'s Tad Martin while advising an acquaintance to get over his troubled childhood.

CHAPTER 4: THE EBB AND FLOW OF DESIRE

1. Barbara Smuts quoted in Natalie Angier, *Woman: An Intimate Geography* (New York: Houghton Mifflin, 1999), p. 335.

2. Associated Press, "Study finds dysfunction in sex lives is widespread," *The New York Times*, February 9, 1999.

3. Teresa Riordan, "Patents: Viagra's success has brought to light a second big market for sexual dysfunction therapies: women," *The New York Times*, April 26, 1999.

4. Natalie Angier, "Science is finding out what women really want," *The New York Times*, August 13, 1995. Ellen Laan also makes an explicit connection between her results and the fact that women sometimes lubricate vaginally during rape. Obviously, this automatic physiological response doesn't indicate that women are turned on by being raped.

5. Angier, pp. 200–1.

6. Jack Morin, Ph.D., *The Erotic Mind* (New York: HarperCollins, 1995), p. 6.

CHAPTER 6: SEX AND CONCEPTION

1. "As part of welfare reform in 1996, Congress passed, and President Clinton signed into law, a federal program that allocates cash—a total of $50 million per fiscal year—to states that teach abstinence-only-until-marriage as the expected standard for school-age children." Carolyn Mackler, *Ms.*, August/September 1999, p. 69.

2. One journalist researching sex-selection technology in America found a two-to-one preference for girls. Lisa Belkin, "Getting the Girl," *The New York Times Sunday Magazine*, July 25, 1999.

3. If sex selection was merely a matter of timing, women using frozen sperm—who have to inseminate within twenty-four hours of ovulation—would logically produce a much higher percentage of boys than girls. In fact, the sex ratio among children born through donor insemination is not that disparate. For example, at The Sperm Bank of California, the ratio of all deliveries since 1982 is approximately 47 percent female and 53 percent male.

4. Peggy Orenstein, "Are You My Father?," *The New York Times Sunday Magazine*, June 18, 1995.

5. A term popularized by Jane Mattes, who literally wrote the book on the subject and went on to form a national network of "Single Mothers by Choice" support groups.

6. According to the American Society for Reproductive Medicine (www.asrm.org).

7. As a result of her research measuring stress levels among 133 infertile heterosexual couples, Maryl Walling-Millard coined the term "infertility stress syndrome," which she concluded is comparable to post-traumatic stress disorder. She also found that female partners had higher stress levels than male partners, regardless of which partner was infertile. Maryl Walling-Millard, "Infertility Stress Syndrome: A Study of Preadoptive and Adoptive Parents" (Ph.D. dissertation, The Professional School of Psychology, San Francisco, 1993).

CHAPTER 7: SEX DURING PREGNANCY

1. Ariel Gore, *The Hip Mama Survival Guide* (New York: Hyperion, 1998), p. 139.

2. Stephen Schwartz, "Electric Fields Linked to Leukemia," *San Francisco Chronicle*, October 1, 1998. Although a report by the National Institute of Environmental Health Sciences found "limited evidence" for a link between residential exposure to EMF and increased risk for childhood leukemia, it "concluded overwhelmingly that there is inadequate evidence" that residential EMF exposure has adverse effects on pregnancy.

3. Gore, p. 27.

4. Susie Bright, *Susie Bright's Sexual Reality* (San Francisco: Cleis Press, 1992), pp. 100–1.

5. See Jack Morin, *The Erotic Mind* (New York: HarperCollins, 1995).

6. Paula Bomer, "Knocked Up, Getting Off," from a piece that originally appeared in Word, 1998 (www.word.com/desire/bomer).

7. Sheila Kitzinger, *Ourselves as Mothers: The Universal Experience of Motherhood* (Reading: Addison-Wesley, 1994), p. 128.

8. Bright, p. 102.

9. Sheila Kitzinger, *Woman's Experience of Sex* (London: Dorling Kindersley, 1983), p. 209.

10. Niles Newton, "Interrelationships Between Sexual Responsiveness, Birth, and Breast-feeding," quoted in Elisabeth Bing and Libby Colman, *Making Love During Pregnancy* (New York: Bantam Books, 1977), p. 121.

CHAPTER 8: THE FOURTH TRIMESTER

1. While oxytocin is most frequently discussed in relation to female physiology—such as the uterine contractions of labor or the "letdown" of milk—it affects male physiology as well. Both men and women experience increased oxytocin levels after orgasm. Evidence suggests that oxytocin and prolactin levels go up for fathers postpartum (presumably they increase for nonbiological mothers also).

2. Estimates as to how many girls experience child sexual abuse range from one in three to one in eight. According to a 1992 report from the National Center for Victims of Crime, one out of every three women will be sexually assaulted in her lifetime.

CHAPTER 9: HOW TO GET THE INFORMATION YOU NEED

1. One meta-analysis of twelve different international studies determined that the participation of doulas—experienced laywomen who provide physical, emotional, and informational support both before, during, and after birth—resulted in reduced length of labor, fewer surgical deliveries, decreases in induced labor, a less painful experience for the mother, increased breast-feeding, and better mood and self-esteem postpartum. K. D. Scott, et al., "The Obstetrical and Postpartum Benefits of Continuous Support During Childbirth," *Journal of Women's Health and Gender-Based Medicine*, December 1999.

2. C. MacArthur, M. Lewis, and E. G. Knox, *Health After Childbirth* (London: University of Birmingham and HMSO, 1991), referenced in Sheila Kitzinger, *The Year After Childbirth* (New York: Charles Scribner's Sons, 1994), p. 23.

3. Per the 1990 U.S. Census.

4. J. O'Farrell, "Childbirth and the Disabled Woman," *New Generation*, March 1993, referenced in Sheila Kitzinger, *The Year After Childbirth*, p. 10.

5. Natalie Angier, *Woman: An Intimate Geography* (Boston: Houghton Mifflin, 1999), p. 76.

6. Geoffrey Cowley, "Gender Limbo," *Newsweek*, May 19, 1997. While this article puts the frequency at one in every two thousand births, author Phyllis Burke quotes a researcher who estimates the frequency to be over three times as high (1.7 for every thousand births), Phyllis Burke, *Gender Shock: Exploding the Myth of Male and Female* (New York: Anchor Books, 1996), p. 221.

7. David Steinberg and Helen Behar, "A Talk about Differences, Sex, and Power," an interview with therapist and educator David Hingsburger, *Spectator* magazine, January 30, 1998. David Steinberg's *Spectator* columns are posted by the Society for Human Sexuality (www.sexuality.org/davids.html).

8. The Canadian therapist David Hingsburger has written and produced several relevant resources, including a book entitled *Just Say Know*, on reducing sexual abuse, and videos on topics including masturbation, condom use, and safe sex (his male masturbation video has the wonderful title *Hand Made Love*). All are available through Diverse City Press; see the Resources section (page 341) for details.

CHAPTER 10: SURVIVING SCARCITY

1. John Gottman and Nan Silver, *Seven Principles for Making Marriages Work* (New York: Three Rivers Press, 1999).

CHAPTER 11: DESIRE REVISITED

1. Jack Morin, Ph.D., *The Erotic Mind* (New York: HarperCollins, 1995), p. 268.

2. Lenore Tiefer, *Sex Is Not a Natural Act and Other Essays* (Boulder: Westview Press, 1995), pp. 11–12.

3. Sheila Kitzinger, *Ourselves as Mothers: The Universal Experience of Motherhood* (Reading: Addison-Wesley, 1994), p. 7.

4. See Sarah Blaffer Hrdy, *Mother Nature: A History of Mother, Infants, and Natural Selection* (New York: Random House, 1999) for a well-balanced discussion of how mothers are not the only individuals capable of meeting their infant's needs.

5. Carolyn Pape Cowan and Philip A. Cowan, *When Partners Become Parents: The Big Life Change for Couples* (Lawrence Erlbaum Associates, 1999).

6. Harriet Lerner, *The Mother Dance* (New York: HarperCollins, 1999), p. 37.

7. A summary of recent studies on the subject of parental division of labor can be found in Raymond Chan, Risa Brooks, Barbara Raboy, and Charlotte Patterson, "Division of Labor Among Lesbian and Heterosexual Parents: Associations with Children's Adjustment," *Journal of Family Psychology*, Vol. 12, No. 3, 1998, pp. 402–419. The researchers found that while "both lesbian and heterosexual couples reported relatively equal divisions of paid employment and of household and decision-making tasks, lesbian biological and nonbiological mothers shared child-care tasks more equally than did heterosexual parents."

8. Ibid, p. 403.

9. Dr. Patricia Love and Jo Robinson, *Hot Monogamy* (New York: Dutton, 1994), p. 70.

10. In discussing loss of desire in long-term relationships, he comments, "I haven't seen a couple—nor have any of the colleagues I've informally surveyed—who were able to rebuild a sexual connection after they had stopped thinking of each other in an erotic way for five or more years." *The Erotic Mind*, p. 283.

11. See Alan R. Hirsch, *Scentsational Sex: The Secret to Using Aroma for Arousal* (Los Angeles: Element Books, 1998).

12. Blumstein and Schwartz, *American Couples: Money, Work, Sex*, 1983, summarized in *The Erotic Mind*, p. 277.

CHAPTER 12: THE SILVER LINING

1. Natalie Angier, "In the history of gynecology, a surprising chapter," *The New York Times*, February 23, 1999, discussing Rachel Maines, *The Technology of Orgasm: "Hysteria," the Vibrator and Women's Sexual Satisfaction* (Baltimore: Johns Hopkins Press, 1999).

2. Per a 1997 press release from the Lawrence Research Group, reporting results of the National Sexual Health Survey of almost eight thousand Americans, ages eighteen to ninety. The general survey was funded by National Institute of Mental Health, and the sex-toy questions were funded by the Lawrence Research Group, publisher of the Xandria Collection catalog.

3. Sheila Kitzinger, *Ourselves as Mothers: The Universal Experience of Motherhood* (Reading: Addison-Wesley, 1994), p. 11.

CHAPTER 13: SEX AND THE SINGLE MOM

1. Lauri Umansky, "Breast-feeding in the 1990s: The Karen Carter Case and the Politics of Maternal Sexuality," in *Bad Mothers: the Politics of Blame in Twentieth-Century America*, Molly Ladd-Taylor and Lauri Umansky, eds. (New York: New York University Press, 1998), p. 299.

CHAPTER 14: KIDS ARE SEXUAL, TOO

1. In her book *Flight of the Stork: What Children Think (and When) About Sex and Family Building*, psychologist Anne Bernstein points out that children are often misled by the very books written to enlighten them about reproduction, largely because these books mix information about flowers, animals, and people in such a random way that children under five become as confused as the four-year-old who told the author that "to get a baby, go to the store and buy a duck." (Indianapolis: Perspectives Press, 1994), pp. 23–32.

2. Heather Corinna, "Everything I Really Needed to Know (about masturbation) I Learned in Kindergarten," Scarlet Letters, spring 2000 (www.scarletletters.com).

3. A Mayo Clinic study of one thousand two- to twelve-year-olds concluded that most sexual behaviors in young children—masturbation, flashing underwear in public, "playing doctor"—are perfectly normal and should not be interpreted as indicative of abuse. "Sexual Behavior in Children: What's Normal?" April 24, 1998 (www.mayohealth.org).

4. Ariel Gore, *The Hip Mama Survival Guide* (New York: Hyperion Press, 1998), p. 110.

5. Nearly two thirds of teenagers think teaching "Just say no" is an ineffective deterrent to teenage sexual activity. Roper Starch Worldwide, *Teens Talk About Sex: Adolescent*

Sexuality in the Nineties (New York: Sexuality Information and Education Council of the United States, 1994), p. 18.

6. Meg Hickling, *Speaking of Sex* (Northstone Publishing, 1996), p. 89.

7. "Pap tests urged for all sexually active teen girls," *San Francisco Chronicle,* March 2, 1999.

8. B. A. Cromer, "Family Planning Services in Adolescent Pregnancy Prevention: The Views of Key Informants in Four Countries," *Family Planning Perspectives,* Nov./Dec. 1999.

9. The National Campaign to Prevent Teen Pregnancy fact sheet (www.teenpregnancy .org).

10. Ron Stoghill II, "Where'd You Learn That?," *Time,* June 15, 1998.

11. In another study, 50 percent of teens said they trust their parents for reliable and complete information on birth control (versus 12 percent who trust a friend). Statistics from the National Campaign to Prevent Teen Pregnancy fact sheet (www.teenpregnancy.org).

12. The National School Boards Foundation (www.nsbf.org) surveyed 1,735 households and found that parents and children alike view the Internet as a positive force in children's lives, despite recent negative headlines about on-line violence, pornography, predators, and commercialism. It also found that three out of four kids will be on the Internet by the time they're teens, and that most kids go on-line at home.

13. L. J. Magid, "Child Safety on the Information Highway" (Arlington, VA: National Center for Missing and Exploited Children, 1994). You can download a copy of the tips from www.safekids.com and www.safeteens.com.

14. Michael Levine, "Summary of Findings Concerning Weight and Shape Concerns in Late Childhood and Adolescence" (paper presented at the thirteenth national NEDO conference, Columbus, OH, October 3, 1994), as reported on About Face (www.about-face.org).

15. Debra Haffner, *From Diapers to Dating* (New York: Newmarket Press, 1999), p. 204.

16. A survey of 2,100 eleven- to seventeen-year-old girls revealed that girls want schools to move beyond abstinence-based training and basic biology lessons to help them better understand the complex social and emotional nature of relationships. The American Association of University Women's Foundation report: "Voices of a Generation: Teenage Girls on Sex, School and Self," February 2000 (www.aauw.org).

17. Michael Resnick, et al., "Protecting Adolescents from Harm," *Journal of the American Medical Association,* 1997, as referenced on SIECUS (www.siecus.org).

18. According to the fact sheet from the National Campaign to Prevent Teen Pregnancy, all six studies of abstinence-only programs failed to show any effect on delaying the onset of intercourse. Referencing D. Kirby, *No Easy Answers: Research Findings on Programs to Reduce Teenage Pregnancy* (Washington, D.C.: National Campaign to Prevent Teen Pregnancy, 1997), p. 25.

19. "Study calls high school condom giveaway a success," *San Francisco Chronicle,* April 14, 1998.

RESOURCES

Recommended Reading

FAMILY BUILDING

Adopting After Infertility, by Patricia Irwin Johnston (Perspectives Press, 1992). Outlines the process of deciding to adopt and the ongoing issues of adoptive families.

Bigger Than the Sky: Disabled Women on Parenting, edited by Michele Wates and Rowen Jade (The Women's Press/Trafalgar Square, 1999). Disabled women speak out about their fight for the right to be mothers.

The Complete Single Mother, by Andrea Engber and Leah Klungness (Adams Publishing, 1995). The founder of the National Organization of Single Mothers dishes up practical advice on time and money management, talking about a missing parent, child support, adoption, legal concerns, dating, and finding support.

Considering Parenthood: A Workbook for Lesbians, by Cheri Pies (Spinsters Ink, 1985). An interactive guide to decision-making about whether and how to become a parent.

The Fertility Sourcebook, by M. Sara Rosenthal (Lowell House, 1998). Covers male and female infertility, available medical interventions, and interpersonal issues.

Helping the Stork: The Choices and Challenges of Donor Insemination, by Carol Frost Vercollone, Heidi Moss, and Robert Moss (Macmillan, 1997). A practical guide to the issues and challenges of DI.

The Hip Mama Survival Guide, by Ariel Gore (Hyperion, 1998). A fast-paced, funny, and nontraditional guide to pregnancy, childbirth, and parenting.

The Lesbian and Gay Parenting Handbook: Creating and Raising Our Families, by April Martin (HarperCollins, 1993). Written by a psychotherapist (and mom), this affirming and comprehensive guide is filled with resources and first-person stories.

The Lesbian Parenting Book: A Guide to Creating Families and Raising Children, by D. Merilee Clunis and G. Dorsey Green (Seal Press, 1995). Two lesbian therapists (and parents) cover the how-tos of everything from conception and adoption to "coming out" to children and families and addressing homophobia in age-appropriate ways.

The Long-Awaited Stork: A Guide to Parenting After Infertility, by Ellen S. Glazer (Jossey-Bass, 1998). Includes practical advice on discussing assisted reproduction and adoption with children, and reassurance for parents who may continue to struggle with loss in the aftermath of infertility.

The Mother Trip, by Ariel Gore (Seal Press, 2000). A collection of short personal essays from the inimitable founder of *Hip Mama* magazine.

Single Mothers by Choice, by Jane Mattes (Random House, 1994). The founder of this national support group discusses the options, pitfalls, and rewards of choosing single motherhood.

Taking Charge of Your Fertility: The Definitive Guide to Natural Birth Control and Pregnancy Achievement, by Toni Weschler (HarperCollins, 1995). An accessible and detailed guide to understanding your body's fertility signs.

Two of Us Make a World: The Single Mother's Guide to Pregnancy, Childbirth, and the First Year, by Prudence and Sherill Tippins (Henry Holt, 1996). Practical advice for single mothers-to-be, with a focus on financial and legal planning.

The Ultimate Guide to Pregnancy for Lesbians: Tips and Techniques from Conception Through Childbirth, by Rachel Pepper (Cleis Press, 1999). An informative guide that focuses on the author's experience with donor insemination and pregnancy.

Waiting in the Wings: Portrait of Queer Motherhood, by Cherrie Moraga (Firebrand, 1997). Chicana writer and activist Cherrie Moraga blends diary entries from her pregnancy and her son's first years with essays on motherhood, partnership, and families.

PREGNANCY AND POSTPARTUM

Laughter and Tears: The Emotional Life of New Mothers, by Elisabeth Bing and Libby Colman, Ph.D. (Henry Holt, 1997). From the first hours after giving birth through the end of the first year, this book covers the highs and lows of the transition to motherhood.

Making Love During Pregnancy, by Elisabeth Bing and Libby Colman (Bantam, 1977). Out of print, but if you can find this seventies-era treasure, you'll relish the quotes from heterosexual couples describing their sex lives during pregnancy.

Sheila Kitzinger has written numerous books related to pregnancy, breast-feeding, and childbirth, all of which provide valuable tips on asserting your rights as a health-care consumer. These are two of the most popular and readily available:

The Complete Book of Pregnancy and Childbirth (Knopf, 1996). An authoritative guide to both medical and cultural trends.

The Year After Childbirth: Enjoying Your Body, Your Relationships, and Yourself in Your Baby's First Year (Charles Scribner's Sons, 1994). A sympathetic guide to weathering the physical, emotional, and situational changes postpartum.

SEX EDUCATION FOR KIDS

Bellybuttons Are Navels, by Mark Schoen (Prometheus Books, 1990). Two children taking a bath learn the correct names for all their body parts.

Did the Sun Shine Before You Were Born, by Sol and Judith Gordon (Prometheus Books, 1992). Drawings of multicultural families illustrate the discussion of conception, pregnancy, and birth.

Heather Has Two Mommies, by Leslea Newman (Alyson Publication, 1989). Picture book about a daughter with lesbian moms.

How Babies and Families Are Made: There Is More Than One Way!, by Patricia Schaffer (Tabor Sarah Books, 1988). Combines basic information on reproduction with a straightforward explanation of the different ways in which families are created, including adoption, donor insemination, and IVF.

How You Were Born, by Joanna Cole (Mulberry Books, 1994). A classic guide to conception, pregnancy, and birth, updated with stunning color photos.

It's Perfectly Amazing: A Book About Eggs, Sperm, Birth, Babies, and Families, by Robie H. Harris, illustrated by Michael Emberley (Candlewick Press, 1999). An upbeat, comprehensive sex-ed book with splendid cartoon illustrations.

A Kid's First Book About Sex, by Joani Blank (Down There Press, 1983). A lively presentation of sex information for young children—one of the few books that discusses sexuality as distinct from reproduction. Illustrated.

Mommy, Did I Grow in Your Tummy?: Where Some Babies Come From, by Elaine R. Gordon (E. M. Greenburg Press, 1992). Explains infertility and the many ways of becoming a family, including IVF, donor sperm, donor egg, and surrogacy.

My Dad Has HIV, by Earl Alexander, Sheila Rudin, and Pam Sejkora (Fairview Press, 1996). Seven-year-old Lindsey tells about her dad's life and illness in a serious yet hopeful way.

One Dad, Two Dads, Brown Dad, Blue Dads, by Johnny Valentine and Melody Sarecky (Alyson Publications, 1994). A Dr. Seuss–like introduction to gay parenting and racial diversity.

The Playbook for Kids About Sex, by Joani Blank (Down There Press, 1982). An interactive workbook that encourages sexual awareness in children (text is the same as in *A Kid's First Book About Sex*).

What's the Big Secret?: Talking About Sex with Girls and Boys, by Laurie Krasny Brown and Marc Brown (Little, Brown and Company, 1997). Designed to be read aloud with children. Covers the basics of sexuality and reproduction.

Asking About Sex and Growing Up, by Joanna Cole (William Morrow, 1988). Q&A format with good questions and thoughtful answers.

Captain Bio: HIV Attacks (Tim Peters and Company, 1988). A comic book that presents the facts about HIV.

The Care and Keeping of You: The Body Book for Girls, by American Girl Library (Pleasant Company Publications, 1998). Easy-to digest information and wonderful color illustrations designed to prepare girls for the changes of puberty. No sex ed here, but lots of advice on body image, self-esteem, and navigating physical changes, including menstruation.

Caution: Do Not Open Until Puberty!: An Introduction to Sexuality for Young Adults with Disabilities, by Rick Enright (Devinjer House, 1995). Guidance for physically disabled adolescents who want to understand their sexuality and discuss it with their families.

It's Perfectly Normal: Changing Bodies, Growing Up, Sex and Sexual Health, by Robie H. Harris, illustrated by Michael Emberley (Candlewick Press, 1994). Sex-education book with a particular focus on the changes of puberty, by the writing and cartooning team behind *It's Perfectly Amazing!*

Period; Periodo, by JoAnn Gardner-Loulan, Bonnie Lopez, and Marcia Quackenbush (Volcano Press, 1991). Classic guide to menstruation, available in English or Spanish.

The Period Book: Everything You Don't Want to Ask but Need to Know, by Karen and Jennifer Gravelle (Walker Publishing Company, 1996). Information for girls on the physical, emotional, and social changes that accompany puberty, cowritten by a teenager.

What's Going on Down There?: Answers to Questions Boys Find Hard to Ask, by Karen Gravelle (Walker Publishing Company, 1998). Straightforward information for boys on the changes of puberty.

What's Happening to My Body? Book for Boys; What's Happening to My Body? Book for Girls, by Lynda Maderas (Newmarket Press, 1987). Written for preteens, these informative guides to the changes brought on by puberty are reassuring without being condescending.

SEX EDUCATION FOR TEENS

Changing Bodies, Changing Lives, edited by Ruth Bell (Times Books/Three Rivers Press, 1999). Following the model of *Our Bodies, Ourselves,* this comprehensive guide to puberty and adolescence is filled with quotes from teenagers.

Deal with It: A Whole New Approach to Your Body, Brain, and Life as a gURL, by Esther Drill, Heather McDonald, and Rebecca Odes (Pocket Books, 1999). From the creators of the gURL.com Web site, a comprehensive guide to physiology, relationships, and sex, written by and for young women.

Easy for You to Say: Q&As for Teens Living with Chronic Illness or Disability, by Miriam Kaufman, M.D. (Key Porter Books, 1995). Q&A format with straightforward advice on a range of sexual and medical issues.

Free Your Mind: The Book for Gay, Lesbian and Bisexual Youth and Their Allies, by Ellen Bass and Kate Kaufman (HarperCollins, 1996). Addresses common issues, including sexual health, and empowers gay youth to accept and celebrate their sexual orientation.

The Go Ask Alice Book of Answers: A Guide to Good Physical, Sexual, and Emotional Health, by Columbia University's Health Education Program (Owl Books, 1999). Q&A from the popular sex-information Web site.

How Sex Works, by Elizabeth Fenwick and Richard Walker (Dorling Kindserly, 1996). A comprehensive, respectful guide for teens, illustrated with color photographs.

"I'm Pregnant, Now What Do I Do?," by Robert W. Buckingham and Mary P. Derby (Prometheus Books, 1997). Offers firsthand accounts and a comprehensive discussion of a pregnant teen's options: adoption, abortion, and becoming a parent.

Just Say Yes; Di Que Sí, by Coalition for Positive Sexuality (Coalition for Positive Sexuality, 1997). Pamphlet (in English and Spanish) covering safer sex, pregnancy, abortion, and sexual responsibility, with effective use of streetwise language.

Out with It: Gay and Straight Teens Write About Homosexuality by Youth Communication (Paula Fell Cartoons, 1996). Essays by teens of all sexualities.

Two Teenagers in Twenty: Writings by Gay and Lesbian Youth, edited by Ann Heron (Alyson, 1994). A collection of essays (only some relate to sex) by gay and lesbian teens.

TALKING TO CHILDREN ABOUT SEX AND FAMILY BUILDING

All About Sex: A Family Resource on Sex and Sexuality, edited by Ronald Filiberti Moglia, Ed.D. and Jon Knowles (Planned Parenthood Federation of America, 1997). Family sourcebook on sexuality and family planning.

Does AIDS Hurt?: Educating Young Children About AIDS, by Marcia Quackenbush, M.S., M.F.C.C., and Sylvia Villarreal, M.D. (ETR Associates, 1992). A guide to discussing AIDS in age-appropriate ways for teachers, parents, and health-care providers.

Flight of the Stork: What Children Think (and When) About Sex and Family Building, by Anne Bernstein, Ph.D. (Perspectives Press, 1994). Explains how children organize information on sex and reproduction at different developmental stages.

From Diapers to Dating: A Parent's Guide to Raising Sexually Healthy Children, by Debra Haffner (Newmarket Press, 2000). Written by the president of SIECUS.

Making Sense of Adoption: A Parent's Guide, by Lois Ruskai Melina (Harper & Row, 1989). A classic guide to navigating adoption that includes material on how to discuss "where I came from" with children adopted or conceived through assisted reproduction.

Sex Is Not a Four-Letter Word!: Talking with Your Children Made Easier, by Patricia Martens Miller (Crossroad Publishing Company, 1994). Places sexuality education and acceptance of all sexual orientations within a religious (Judeo-Christian), ethical framework.

Sexuality: Your Sons and Daughters with Intellectual Disabilities, by Karin Melberg Schwier and David Hingsburger (Paul H. Brookes Publishing Co., 2000). A guide to interacting with children of any developmental ability in ways that encourage self-esteem, appropriate behavior, identification of abuse, and the development of relationships.

More Speaking of Sex, by Meg Hickling, R.N. (Northstone Publishing, 1999). Thorough, engaging, and often humorous sex advice for parents of kids of all ages.

The Underground Guide to Teenage Sexuality: An Essential Handbook for Today's Teens and Parents, by Michael J. Basso (Fairview Press, 1997). Answers teens' questions about health and sexuality.

Understanding Your Child's Sexual Behavior: What's Natural and Healthy, by Toni Cavanagh Johnson, Ph.D. (New Harbinger Publications, 1999). Explains children's stages of sexual development and expression and helps parents distinguish between natural sexual behaviors and problem behaviors or signs of abuse.

SEX INFORMATION AND ENHANCEMENT

Women's Sexuality

Becoming Orgasmic, by Julia Heiman and Joseph LoPiccolo (Simon & Schuster/Fireside, 1986). A structured series of exercises designed for women who have never had orgasms.

The Black Women's Health Book: Speaking for Ourselves, edited by Evelyn C. White (Seal Press, 1994). Over fifty African-American women address a variety of issues affecting their health, with some discussion of sexual health.

Cunt Coloring Book, by Tee Corinne (Naiad Press, 1989). Line drawings of women's genitals — for you to color in.

Femalia, edited by Joani Blank (Down There Press, 1993). Over thirty full-color photographs of women's genitals.

For Yourself: The Fulfillment of Female Sexuality, by Lonnie Garfield Barbach (Penguin Group/Signet, 1975). The classic guide to achieving orgasm and enhancing sexual responsiveness.

The Good Vibrations Guide: The G-spot, by Cathy Winks (Down There Press, 1999). Information on the G-spot, female ejaculation, and tips and techniques for pleasurable exploration.

The G-Spot and Other Recent Discoveries About Human Sexuality, by Alice Kahn Ladas, Beverly Whipple, and John D. Perry (Bantam Doubleday Dell, 1982). The book that launched a thousand curious fingers.

New Ourselves, Growing Older, by Paula Brown Doress and Diana Laskin Siegal (Simon & Schuster/Touchstone, 1996). Specific to the concerns of women over forty.

New View of a Woman's Body, by the Federation of Feminist Women's Health Centers (Feminist Health Press, 1991). This self-help classic includes color photographs of women's genitals.

Our Bodies, Ourselves for the New Century: A Book by and for Women, by the Boston Women's Health Collective (Simon & Schuster/Touchstone, 1998). Covers all aspects of general and sexual health.

Sex for One: The Joy of Self-loving, by Betty Dodson (Crown Publishers/Harmony Press, 1996). A thorough — and thoroughly infectious — guide to the joys of masturbation, illustrated with Dodson's erotic line drawings.

The Survivor's Guide to Sex: How to Have an Empowered Sex Life After Child Sexual Abuse, by Staci Haines (Cleis Press, 1999). How to rebuild a fulfilling sex life, identify dissociation, handle triggers, and cultivate sexual pleasure.

The Ultimate Guide to Anal Sex for Women, by Tristan Taormino (Cleis Press, 1997). Covers all aspects of anal eroticism.

When the Earth Moves: Women and Orgasm, by Mikaya Heart (Celestial Arts, 1998). Tips on enjoying and enhancing the experience of orgasm, with quotes from hundreds of women.

Men's Sexuality

The New Male Sexuality: The Truth About Men, Sex and Pleasure, by Bernie Zilbergeld (Bantam Books, 1992). Practical advice on common sexual concerns.

Sex: A Man's Guide, by Stefan Bechtel and Laurence Roy Stains (Rodale Press, 1996). Well-researched information on a range of topics.

Sexual Solutions: A Guide for Men and the Women Who Love Them, by Michael Castleman (Simon & Schuster/Touchstone, 1983). Well-written information and advice geared to men in heterosexual relationships.

Manuals and More

Anal Pleasure and Health, by Jack Morin (Down There Press, 1998). The foremost guide to enjoying anal stimulation.

Big, Big Love: A Sourcebook on Sex for People of Size and Those Who Love Them, by Hanne Blank (Greenery Press, 2000). A wonderful affirmation of fat people's sexuality and an excellent resource for anyone who has body-image issues related to size.

The Erotic Mind: Unlocking the Inner Sources of Sexual Passion and Fulfillment, by Jack Morin, Ph.D. (HarperCollins, 1995). A fascinating exploration of the nature of arousal that guides readers to uncover what really turns them on and why.

Exhibitionism for the Shy, by Carol Queen (Down There Press, 1995). Tips for dressing up, showing off, talking sexy, and communicating your desires with a partner.

Good Vibrations: The New Complete Guide to Vibrators, by Joani Blank with Ann Whidden (Down There Press, 2000). Learn how to select, enjoy, and introduce your partner to a vibrator.

Guide to Getting It On!: A New and Mostly Wonderful Book About Sex, by Paul Joannides (Goofy Foot Press, 1998). Covers a variety of sexual interests and activities with enthusiasm and humor.

Health Care Without Shame, by Charles Moser, Ph.D., M.D. (Greenery Press, 1999). Geared primarily toward those with alternative sexual lifestyles, this book offers invaluable advice on talking to health-care providers about sexuality.

Hot Monogamy: Essential Steps to More Passionate, Intimate Lovemaking, by Dr. Patricia Love and Jo Robinson (Penguin/Plume, 1994). Exercises for monogamous couples who want to improve sexual intimacy and technique.

I'm Not in the Mood: What Every Woman Should Know About Improving Her Libido, by Judith Reichman, M.D. (William Morrow, 1998). Highlights the effect of hormones — specifically testosterone — on libido, and discusses physiological as well as emotional factors in offering solutions to waning desire.

Intimate Resources for Persons with Disabilities, by Susan Wheeler and Linda Crabtree (Sureen Publishing, 1999). An extensive collection of informational, educational, and consumer resources.

Let Me Count the Ways: Discovering Great Sex Without Intercourse, by Marty Klein, Ph.D. and Riki Robbins, Ph.D. (Jeremy P. Tarcher/Putnam, 1998). Exposes the "cult of intercourse" for the oppressive, sex-negative monolith that it is and offers tips for exploring your own unique sexuality.

The New Good Vibrations Guide to Sex, by Anne Semans and Cathy Winks (Cleis Press, 1997). The best, most comprehensive sex manual ever written — trust us!

101 Grrreat Quickies (1997); *101 Nights of Grrreat Romance* (1996); *101 Nights of Grrreat Sex* (1995), by Laura Corn (Park Avenue Press). Unseal each page of these creative heterosexual couples' books to discover suggestions for exploring sensuality and building intimacy.

Sex Over Fifty, by Joel D. Block, Ph.D., and Susan Crain Bakos (Prentice Hall Press, 1999). A thorough guide including tips, techniques, and health information.

Talk Sexy to the One You Love, by Barbara Keesling, Ph.D. (HarperCollins, 1996). Learn to create and enjoy an erotic vocabulary.

The Whole Lesbian Sex Book, by Felice Newman (Cleis Press, 1999). A comprehensive sex manual for women who love women.

The Woman's Guide to Sex on the Web, by Anne Semans and Cathy Winks (HarperSanFrancisco, 1999). Annotated guide to over two hundred of the best sex information and entertainment Web sites created by and for women.

CULTURAL STUDIES/SEXUAL POLITICS

The Body Project: An Intimate History of American Girls, by Joan Jacobs Brumberg (Random House, 1997). Details how and why American girls have less self-esteem and more dissatisfaction with their bodies now than one hundred years ago.

For Her Own Good: 150 Years of the Experts' Advice to Women, by Deidre English and Barbara Ehrenreich (Anchor Books/Doubleday, 1978). Written with wit and verve, this classic of women's history reveals the toll medical "expertise" has taken on women's bodies and minds.

Gender Shock: Exploding the Myths of Male and Female, by Phyllis Burke (Anchor Books/Doubleday, 1996). A provocative and highly readable attack on our rigid gender system.

Intimate Matters: A History of Sexuality in America, second edition, by John D'Emilio and Estelle B. Freedman (University of Chicago Press, 1997). A compelling read about the evolution of American sexual attitudes over the past four centuries.

Mother Nature: A History of Mothers, Infants, and Natural Selection, by Sarah Blaffer Hrdy (Random House, 1999). A renowned feminist anthropologist and primatologist examines how millennia of evolutionary forces have shaped maternal behaviors and strategies.

Sex Is Not a Natural Act, by Lenore Tiefer (Westview, 1995). A collection of short, smart essays that skillfully expose the assumptions underlying our cultural construction of sexuality.

All of Susie Bright's essay collections will make you laugh, provoke you, pique your curiosity, and — best of all — inspire you to think about sexuality in a whole new way.

Full Exposure: Opening Up to Your Sexual Creativity and Erotic Expression (Harper-SanFrancisco, 1999).

Susie Bright's Sexual State of the Union (Simon & Schuster, 1997).

Susie Bright's Sexwise (Cleis Press, 1995).

Susie Bright's Sexual Reality: A Virtual Sex World Reader (Cleis Press, 1992).

Susie Sexpert's Lesbian Sex World (Cleis Press, 1990).

Woman: An Intimate Geography, by Natalie Angier (Houghton Mifflin, 1999). A fascinating, wide-ranging excursion through the biology of the female body.

Sexuality Resources

SEX INFORMATION AND ENHANCEMENT ON-LINE

Clean Sheets
http://www.cleansheets.com
A quality sex zine, equal parts erotica and commentary.

Erotica Readers Association
http://www.erotica-readers.com
An excellent forum for women and men interested in writing, reading, or talking about erotica; includes links to selected erotica sites.

Healthy Sexuality
http://www.healthgate.com/healthy/sexuality
Timely articles on an impressive array of subjects related to sex and relationships.

Heartless's Holey Haven
http://www.grownmencry.com/hhh/HHH.html

An irreverent look at women's sexuality, featuring frank, funny essays filled with tips and techniques.

Jane's Net Sex Guide
http://www.janesguide.com
Jane is the Ralph Nader of on-line adult commerce: She reviews hundreds of adult sites, provides consumer tips, and exposes fraudulent practices. And she's a mom.

Johan's Guide to Aphrodisiacs
http://www.santesson.com/aphrodis/aphrhome.html
This entertaining encyclopedic site dishes up tips, recipes, and the history behind aphrodisiacs' reputed powers.

Scarlet Letters: The Journal of Femmerotica
http://www.scarletletters.com
High-quality, high-spirited erotica, articles, and advice from a women-run site.

Society for Human Sexuality
http://www.sexuality.org
The largest on-line archive of sexuality materials, sponsored by the University of Washington, is a gold mine of useful information.

PROFESSIONAL RESOURCES

American Association of Sex Educators, Counselors, and Therapists (AASECT)
P.O. Box 238
Mount Vernon, IA 52314
Phone: 319/895-8407
http://www.aasect.org
Can provide list of AASECT-certified therapists and counselors; publishes *Journal of Sex Education and Therapy.*

Sexuality Information and Education Council of the United States (SIECUS)
130 West 42nd Street, #350
New York, NY 10036
Phone: 212/819-9770
http://www.siecus.org
This organization is a national treasure; its annotated bibliographies on dozens of subjects—including general sexuality, adolescent sexuality, sex and disability, religious perspectives, teaching materials, sexual orientation, sex and pop culture, and child sexual abuse—are posted on the SIECUS Web site or available by mail. Particularly useful to parents who need help talking to kids about sex, or who want to bring comprehensive sexuality education programs into the schools.

The Society for the Scientific Study of Sex (SSSS)
P.O. Box 238
Mount Vernon, IA 52314
Phone: 319/895-8407
http://www.ssc.wisc.edu/ssss
Publishes *Journal of Sex Research.*

American Social Health Association
P.O. Box 13827
Research Triangle Park, NC 27709
Phone: 919/361-8400
Fax: 919/361-8425
http://www.ashastd.org
A private, nonprofit organization, ASHA provides up-to-date information on STDs via its telephone hotlines and Web site. The well-maintained site has an exceptional links page.

The Body: An AIDS and HIV Information Resource
http://www.thebody.com
Posts articles and information about safer sex, including a forum where questions from HIV-positive moms are answered by medical experts in the fields of pediatric AIDS and HIV treatment.

Circumcision Information and Resource Pages
http://www.cirp.org
Includes medical and historical articles, as well as information for parents and educators.

Dimensions Magazine
P.O. Box 640
Folsom, CA 95763-0640
Phone: 916/984-9947
http://www.dimensionsmagazine.com
This print magazine and Web site explores sexuality and relationships for BBW (big, beautiful women) and their admirers.

Gender Issues
http://songweaver.com/gender
A directory site with extensive links to transgender resources and information.

HIV InSite: Gateway to AIDS Knowledge
http://hivinsite.ucsf.edu
The University of California San Francisco's comprehensive resource site includes a section on pregnancy, childbirth, and HIV.

Intersex Society of North America
P.O. Box 3070
Ann Arbor, MI 48106-3070
http://www.isna.org
National organization with the goal of ending shame, secrecy, and unwanted genital surgeries for people born with atypical sex anatomy.

Largesse, the Network for Size Esteem
P.O. Box 9404
New Haven, CT 06534
Phone/Fax: 203/787-1624
http://www.eskimo.com/~largesse
This activist resource site lists fat-positive publications for adults and kids.

RAINN (Rape Abuse and Incest National Network)
252 10th Street N.E.
Washington, D.C. 20002
Phone: 800/656-HOPE
http://www.rainn.org
Sponsors the only national hotline for survivors of sexual assault; free confidential counseling around the clock; Web site with statistics and resources.

Safer Sex Page
http://www.safersex.org
This friendly, comprehensive site takes a multimedia approach to sex education and dispenses information on risk management, birth control, and every kind of safer-sex supply.

Sexual Assault Information Page
http://www.cs.utk.edu/~bartley/saInfoPage.html
Directory of information and referrals to Web sites concerning child sexual abuse, incest, rape, sexual assault, and sexual harassment.

SexualHealth.com
http://www.sexualhealth.com
An excellent site offering a wide range of sexuality resources for people with physical disabilities, illness, or other health-related problems.

Parenting Resources

FAMILY BUILDING

American College of Nurse Midwives
818 Connecticut Avenue N.W., Suite 900
Washington, D.C. 20006
Phone: 202/728-9860
Fax: 202/728-9897
http://www.midwife.org
The Web site for this national organization has extensive links related to pregnancy, medical issues, women's health, and parenting.

American Society for Reproductive Medicine
1209 Montgomery Highway
Birmingham, AL 35216-2809
Phone: 205/978-5000
Fax: 205/978-5005
http://www.asrm.org
Publishes fact sheets, booklets, and guidelines related to infertility, reproductive medicine, and biology.

Depression After Delivery
P.O. Box 1282
Morrisville, PA 19067
Phone: 800/944-4PPD or 215/295-3994
Resource for women with postpartum depression.

Fertility Plus
http://www.fertilityplus.org
A nonprofit, peer-based Web site that offers information on trying to conceive. Great articles and resources.

Mana: Midwives Alliance of North America
Phone: 888/923-MANA
http://www.mana.org
Professional organization for all midwives; offers referrals by phone.

National Center for Education in Maternal and Child Health
2000 15th Street North, #701
Arlington, VA 22201
Phone: 703/524-7802
http://www.ncemch.org
Publishes research and public policy recommendations.

National Center for Lesbian Rights
870 Market Street, #570
San Francisco, CA 94102
Phone: 800/528-NCLR or 415/392-6257
http://www.nclrights.org
NCLR advances the rights and safety of lesbians and their families through litigation, public policy advocacy, free legal advice and counseling, and public education.

Parents with Disabilities Online!
http://www.disabledparents.net
A one-stop resource for parents with physical disabilities, this site has excellent annotated links and is the home of the Parent Empowerment listserve.

RESOLVE: The National Infertility Association
1310 Broadway
Somerville, MA 02144
Phone: 617/623-0744
http://www.resolve.org
A nonprofit providing support and information to people who are experiencing infertility.

Single Mothers By Choice
P.O. Box 1642, Gracie Square Station
New York, NY 10028
Phone: 212/988-0993
http://www.parentsplace.com/family/singleparent
National organization with regional chapters.

These two sperm banks welcome single women and lesbians and offer donors who are willing to have their identities released to adult offspring:

Pacific Reproductive Services
444 Deharo Street, #222
San Francisco, CA 94107
Phone: 415/487-2288
http://www.hellobaby.com

The Sperm Bank of California
2115 Milvia Street, #201
Berkeley, CA 94704
Phone: 510/841-1858
http://www.thespermbankofca.org

PARENTING, SEX, AND SEXUALITY

Advocates for Youth
1025 Vermont Avenue NW, #200
Washington, D.C. 20005
Phone: 202/347-5700
Fax: 202/347-2263
http://www.advocatesforyouth.org
Creates programs (including peer counseling) and promotes policies to help young people make informed and responsible decisions about sexual health.

Children of Lesbians and Gays Everywhere (COLAGE)
3543 18th Street, #17
San Francisco, CA 94110
Phone: 415/861-KIDS
http://www.colage.org
Support and advocacy organization by and for children of lesbian, gay, bisexual, and transgender parents.

Committee on Sexuality
Advocating for People with Developmental Disabilities
21450 Bear Creek Road
Los Gatos, CA 95030
http://www.w3ddesign.com/committee
Committee of professionals, parents, and disabled that focuses attention on the sexual needs and rights of developmentally disabled people.

Family Pride Coalition
http://www.glpci.org
A site for gay, lesbian, bisexual, and transgender parents, with links to local groups, event listings, and resources. Articles serve as excellent guides for all parents on discussing diversity, values, and sexuality.

The Gay, Lesbian, and Straight Education Network
http://www.glsen.org
National organization dedicated to ending discrimination against lesbian, gay, and transgendered youth in the schools.

Mother's Voices
165 W. 46th Street, #701
New York, NY 10036
Phone: 888/MVO-ICES or 212/730-2777
Fax: 212/730-4378
http://www.mvoices.org
A national nonprofit mobilizing mothers as educators and advocates for HIV prevention, research, and treatment. Resources and statistics about teen sexual activity and disease transmission posted on the Web site underscore the importance of talking to kids about sex.

National Information Center for Children and Youth with Disabilities (NICHCY)
P.O. Box 1492
Washington, D.C. 20013-1492
Phone/TTY: 800/695-0285
Fax: 202/884-8441
http://www.nichcy.org
A national information and referral center; publishes pamphlet on sexuality education for children with disabilities.

Parents, Families, and Friends of Lesbians and Gays (PFLAG)
1101 14th Street N.W., #1030
Washington, D.C. 20005
Phone: 202/638-4200
Fax: 202/638-0243
http://www.pflag.org
National organization of families with gay children.

Planned Parenthood Federation of America (PPFA)
810 7th Avenue
New York, NY 10019
Phone: 800/829-PPFA or 800/230-PLAN (to contact your local Planned Parenthood)
Fax: 212/245-1845
http://www.plannedparenthood.org
Birth control and family planning are just the tip of the iceberg; Planned Parenthood offers excellent sex-education articles, resource materials, and advice for parents and teachers about how to raise sexually healthy kids, much of which is available on their voluminous Web site.

Talking with Your Kids About Tough Issues
http://www.talkingwithkids.org
Designed to help parents initiate dialogue on issues such as sex, drugs, violence, and HIV.

RESEARCH

Alan Guttmacher Institute
120 Wall Street
New York, NY 10005
Phone: 212/248-1111
http://www.agi-usa.org
Dedicated to protecting reproductive choice around the world, this organization's public policy reports on family planning, STDs, and sexual behavior are available on-line.

Association for Research on Mothering
Room 726, Atkinson College
York University
4700 Keele Street
Toronto, Ontario M3J 1P3
Phone: 416/736-2100 X 60366
Fax: 905/775-1386
www.yorku.ca/crm/index.html
This organization of feminist researchers publishes *The Journal of the Association for Research on Mothering.*

The Henry J. Kaiser Family Foundation
http://www.kff.org
Extensive research into all avenues of family life (what do kids learn from sex in the media, do abstinence-only programs work, etc.) makes this a great resource for factoids and stats.

Sex Education Coalition
http://www.sexedcoalition.org
Organization of educators, health-care professionals, trainers, and legislators dedicated to providing information concerning sexuality education.

ON-LINE COMMUNITIES

CyberMom Pillow Talk
http://www.TheCyberMom.com
A popular Web site with discussion boards about dozens of topics related to sexuality.

Hip Mama
http://hipmama.com
The on-line version of this progressive zine features provocative essays and interviews related to parenting and teen motherhood, and is home to thriving discussion boards.

Parenthood
http://www.parenthoodweb.com
A good general information site.

ParentsPlace
http://www.parentsplace.com
Offers countless discussion boards on a multitude of topics, including donor insemination and single parenting.

ParentTime
http://www.parenttime.com
Discussion boards, articles, and advice.

SusieBright.com
http://www.susiebright.com/forum
Susie's site features excerpts from her sex-positive articles and essays, along with discussion boards on a wide range of topics, including sex and parenting.

Web Sites for Kids and Teens

About-Face
http://www.about-face.org
An in-your-face look at culture's overemphasis on physical appearance. The site hopes to engender positive body-esteem in girls and women of all ages, sizes, races, and backgrounds.

Coalition for Positive Sexuality
http://www.positive.org
The Coalition—a group of high school students and adults—gives teens vital sex information and affirmation for their ability to make intelligent decisions about sexuality and reproductive control. Great graphics and streetwise language make the site and its discussion boards a popular destination among teens.

Dr. Paula's Site
http://www.drpaula.com
Pediatrician Dr. Paula's site offers a section in which teens can learn about sexuality, orgasm, masturbation, sexual pressure, talking with parents, contraception, and physiology.

Elight
http://www.elight.org
A site by and for gay teens, featuring prose, poetry, and a supportive community.

Go Ask Alice!
http://www.alice.columbia.edu
Maintained by Columbia University, this site was launched to provide accurate and frank information to a student population and now boasts one of the most extensive archives of sex Q&As available on-line.

iwannaknow.org
http://www.iwannaknow.org
Information for teens on puberty, sexuality, sexual health, and STD prevention, sponsored by the American Social Health Association (ASHA).

It's Your Sex Life
http://www.itsyoursexlife.com
A youth guide to sexual health—primarily contraception, STDs, and talking to partners about safer sex.

Kotex and Tampax's Being Girl
http://www.kotex.com
http://www.beinggirl.com
Great resources for girls going through puberty, these sites offer help charting menstrual cycles, advice about cramps, answers to common questions about puberty, help with self-esteem, and active discussion boards.

Loveline
http://www.drdrew.com
Popular MTV expert dishes out advice on a variety of youth issues, including sexual health, relationships, and sexual orientation.

Scarleteen: Sex Education That's for Real
http://wwwscarleteen.com
Accurate sex advice for young women and men delivered in a friendly, nonjudgmental manner. A labor of love courtesy of adult Webmistress Heather Corinna (see her on-line magazine, *Scarlet Letters*).

SEX, ETC.
http://www.sxetc.com
This fantastic site has articles written by teens on a variety of sex subjects, including sexuality education, circumcision, first sex, defending virginity, peer pressure, and dating. Great links, archives of all past issues, and helpful information for parents and educators as well.

Teen Advice On-line
http://www.teenadviceonline.org
Covers a range of issues relevant to teens, including sex, sexuality, and dating. Material provided by peer counselors—teens from all over the world who volunteer to participate by writing articles and answering questions.

Teenwire
http://www.teenwire.com
Planned Parenthood's site for teens features information on sexual health, along with articles written by teens.

Shopping Guide

SEX TOYS, BOOKS, AND VIDEOS

Blowfish
Mail order only
P.O. Box 411290
San Francisco, CA 94141
Phone: 800/325-2569
Fax: 415/252-4349
http://www.blowfish.com

Come As You Are
Mail order only
701 Queen Street West
Toronto, Ontario M6J 1E6 Canada
Phone: 416/504-7934
Fax: 416/504-7490
http://www.comeasyouare.com

Condom Sense
Mail order only; primarily safer-sex supplies
WWWarehouse, Inc.
2015 Polk Street
San Francisco, CA 94109
Phone: 888/702-6636
http://www.condoms.net

Eve's Garden
Retail store and mail order
119 W. 57th Street, #420
New York, NY 10019-2383
Phone: 800/848-3837
http://www.evesgarden.com

Focus International, Inc.
Mail order only; sexual self-help videos
1160 E. Jericho Turnpike
Huntington, NY 11743
Phone: 800/843-0305

Good Vibrations mail order
938 Howard Street #101
San Francisco, CA 94103
Phone: 800/289-8423
http://www.goodvibes.com

Good Vibrations retail stores
1210 Valencia Street
San Francisco, CA 94110
Phone: 415/974-8980

2504 San Pablo Avenue
Berkeley, CA 94702
Phone: 510/841-8987

Grand Opening!
Retail store and mail order
318 Harvard Street #32
Brookline, MA 02146
Phone: 617/731-2626
http://www.grandopening.com

Libida
Women's Web site and mail order
http://www.libida.com

Toys in Babeland
Retail stores and mail order
711 E. Pike Street
Seattle, WA 98112
Phone: 800/658-9119
http://www.babeland.com

94 Rivington Street
New York, NY 10002
Phone: 212/375-1701

The Xandria Collection
Mail order only
165 Valley Drive
Brisbane, CA 94005
Phone: 800/242-2823
http://www.xandria.com

A Woman's Touch
Retail store and mail order
600 Williamson Street
Madison, WI 53703
Phone: 608/250-1928
http://www.a-womans-touch.com

SPECIALTY

Corolle dolls (French anatomically
correct baby dolls)
http://www.corolledolls.com
Corolle's Web site lists retail outlets
throughout the U.S.

Diverse City Press
33 des Floralies
Eastman, Quebec JOE 1P0
Canada
Phone: 450/297-3080
http://www.diverse-city.com
Publishes educational materials, including
sex resources, for people with
developmental disabilities and their
caregivers.

Nolo Press
950 Parker Street
Berkeley, CA 94710
Phone: 800/992-6656
http://www.nolo.com
Publishes legal self-help books, including
guides for lesbian and gay couples,
unmarried couples, and couples building
child-custody agreements.

Tapestry Books
P.O. Box 359
Ringoes, NJ 08551
Phone: 800/765-2367
http://www.tapestrybooks.com
One-of-a-kind catalog of books on
adoption, infertility, and assisted
reproduction—for adults and children.

INDEX

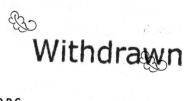

ABOUT THE AUTHORS

ANNE SEMANS and CATHY WINKS, authors of the bestselling *The New Good Vibrations Guide to Sex* and *The Woman's Guide to Sex on the Web*, and contributors to the *Hip Mama* Web site, have spent more than ten years writing and speaking about sex and working at the Good Vibrations sex-toy store. Both authors live in San Francisco.